Shaping Up for a Healthy Pregnancy

Barbara B. Holstein, MS

Life Enhancement Publications
Champaign, Illinois

Library of Congress Cataloging-in-Publication Data

Holstein, Barbara B., 1952–
    Shaping up for a healthy pregnancy.

    Bibliography: p.
    Includes index.
    1. Prenatal care. 2. Exercise for women.
3. Pregnancy. 4. Postnatal care. I. Title.
RG525.H55   1988   618.2'4   87-37857
ISBN 0-87322-926-6

Developmental Editor: Lisa Busjahn
Production Director: Ernie Noa
Projects Manager: Lezli Harris
Copy Editor: Claire Mount
Assistant Editor: Julie Anderson
Typesetters: Brad Colson, Sonnie Bowman
Cover Design: Hunter Graphics
Text Design: Keith Blomberg
Text Layout: Denise Peters
Printed By: Versa Press

ISBN: 0-87322-926-6

Printed in the United States of America

10 9 8 7 6 5 4 3 2 1

Life Enhancement Publications
A Division of Human Kinetics Publishers, Inc.
Box 5076, Champaign, IL 61820
1-800-342-5457
1-800-334-3665 (in Illinois)

Dedication

Dedicated to the loves of my life.

Contents

Preface

Shaping Up for a Healthy Pregnancy is a book about teaching exercise for pregnant women. It focuses on the physiologic changes of pregnancy and how those changes can affect a woman's capacity for and enjoyment of exercise.

Over the years, I have come to believe that education is a healing process for pregnant women. As teachers, our task is to help women integrate all that they learn and feel during the prenatal months. We must learn to work carefully and thoughtfully both to unify the physical and emotional experience of pregnancy and to heal the separation of body, mind, and spirit.

Our cultural memory of pregnancy and childbirth is a mixed bag of confusing messages. In recent decades, women who have borne children in America have been deprived of food and water, drugged into unconsciousness, strapped onto beds, and required to remain in the hospital for many days after childbirth. This history of intervention sadly reflects a widespread misunderstanding of the essence of female biology and human birth.

In the 1960s, in the face of institutional mismanagement of female health care and increased obstetrical interventions during childbirth, women began to emerge as outspoken leaders and participants in their own revolution of attitudes and expectations about health care. The original *Our Bodies Ourselves* (1971), which came to us from the Boston Women's Health Book Collective, is now a monument to female consciousness-raising about female health and our definitions of womanhood.

As a result of feminism and the women's health movement (of which the childbirth education movement should be considered an important part), women have begun to move out from under negative medical control and claim their rights to the control of their own bodies.

In the current decade, women's health concerns have at last been recognized by health and fitness professionals. The field of health education for women now covers a broad spectrum of issues including illness prevention, health enhancement, self-care, and positive reproductive options. Research on female exercise physiology has emerged as a new and important field. With it has come a new interest in maternal exercise physiology. Much of what is pertinent in this field is summarized for you in this text.

Childbirth education, with which women prepare to be active participants in birth, was a novelty in this country 30 years ago. Now it is a priority among childbearing women. National organizations of childbirth educators have thousands of members. In many states hospitals have been mandated to provide childbirth education. The importance of preparation and information about birth, the quintessential female experience, is undeniable.

This is an exciting time. Educating pregnant women about their bodies and encouraging them to experience themselves as strong, beautiful, and healthy people who are capable of working hard, exercising daily, and giving birth with confidence is truly a joyous task. This manuscript has grown from my experience teaching prenatal and postpartum exercise classes and childbirth education. Originally, I intended to introduce women to carefully-planned movement experience that would encourage a full range of safe motion and creative exploration of the body's changing capacity for exertion. I felt that through learning techniques for maintaining and improving muscle tone and flexibility, women would experience an enhanced sense of self during a time of rapid weight gain and unprecedented physical and emotional changes.

Almost right away, I sensed that the women in my classes wanted more than just exercises. They wanted information. They wanted to know about their bodies. They wanted to know if their aches and pains were legitimate. They wanted to know how to prepare for birth. They wanted to talk about being pregnant. In each class, I witnessed the emergence of a forum where ideas were shared, questions were asked, and respect and friendship blossomed. This book reflects the holistic blend of information and caring that prenatal teaching requires.

I have divided the book into four parts. Part I prepares the instructor by describing the philosophic basis for the holistic approach to prenatal care. The integration of wisdom from both scientific and natural healing techniques is emphasized. We look at female anatomy and physiology in simple, concrete, and usable terms. The guidelines for prenatal exercise published by the American College of Obstetricians and Gynecologists (ACOG) are thoroughly examined and explained in terms that make the material accessible and useful.

Part II examines the basic methods for monitoring individuals and their responses to exercise. Changes in the mother's body as well as fetal growth are used to help define and describe the adaptations in maternal activities that occur throughout pregnancy. A number of specific endeavors will be evaluated, and necessary modifications for safe participation will be discussed.

Part III contains materials on the design and teaching of specialized prenatal exercise classes. It includes discussions of self-image, exercises to promote positive birthing experiences, and emergency procedures. This section also presents techniques for teaching relaxation and creative visualization, as well as the practice of mantras and massage. Chapter 13 is about women with special needs, and in it I make an effort to raise our collective consciousness about the challenges faced by these women.

Part IV addresses the new mother and her exercise requirements. The material is organized around my own classroom style. It continues the theme of the ecologically balanced, educational, and experiential reality of healthy childbearing. You will find a glossary at the back of the book.

Welcome to the field of maternal fitness education. I sincerely hope that your experience working with pregnant women is as rich and rewarding as mine.

Acknowledgments

I begin by saying thank you to all of those people who have advised me and put up with all of my antics: To my husband, David, and to my children, Benjamin and Daniel, who have probably watched too much television as I have tried to finish this manuscript; to my parents, the professors Blumberg, whose lives and dedication to scholarship have been a life-long inspiration.

To my friends and editors: Dr. Joel Potash, a physician and trusted advisor who was always available to answer a question and to lend an editorial hand; Dorothy Peckham, a remarkable writer and childbirth educator; and Dani Riposo, a gifted and generous teacher. To my editor and friend Lisa Busjahn whose caring and swift editorial pen have made this whole experience a helpful, healing one.

Thank you to Dr. Bernie Oliver, for recommending that I send my manuscript to this publishing house; to Sue Wilmoth for recognizing the importance of sharing pregnancy and exercise information and acquiring this book for publication; to Sally Mericle for being so gifted an artist; to Laurie Deyo for being such a lovely pregnant model; to Helen Domer, whose daily counsel has been priceless; to Dr. Joan Roberts, Dr. Norbert Reicher, Leslie Shipps, Denise and Rick Davies, Seska Dune, Chris Kennedy, Judy Granatstein, Sally White, Paula Heiman, Judy Gettino, Denise Trionfero, and John and Kim Townsend, for their friendship and support.

Part I

Education
as Healing

Becoming One

No dance teacher can teach
the student to dance.
Rather, the student must
loosen her body and let go
of ego.
She must become the Dance.
No one can teach a woman
what it is like to be pregnant
or give birth.
Rather,
The woman, her body and her child
blend together
to be born.
She and they become One.

Barbara Holstein

Chapter 1

The Healing Educator

Throughout this book we will look at ways in which movement can be a healing experience and how you, as a teacher of prenatal exercise, can work to be a healer for pregnant women.

All of us committed to women and women's health are healers. The cures we offer are information, support, and caring. If you consider your influence and the information you have to share with expectant mothers as healing, you afford yourself a wonderful opportunity for professional and personal growth.

Prenatal education is the key to healthier mothers and healthier babies. Prenatal exercise is an essential element in the matrix of health education, for with it come changes in behavior and physiology that can directly enhance a woman's experience of pregnancy.

The Ecosystem Approach to Care

Health and fitness education are part of a network of support services for pregnant women that make up a health care *ecosystem*. An ecosystem is a web of interwoven relationships between the environment and the human beings who inhabit it (Capra, 1982). In a healthy ecosystem, persons can experience health and well-being on multiple levels: social, emotional, physical, intellectual, and spiritual. An ecosystems approach to prenatal education is an integrated, holistic approach to childbearing. The pregnant woman is understood as a whole person, central to a living network of family and employment and educational systems. Her education will occur at many levels, and each interaction

between teacher and learner should promote optimum awareness and recognition of the potential for wellness.

When it comes to how we feel about our bodies, each of us has ways of thinking that reflect our opinions and our experiences. When it comes to health and healing, most of us think about doctors and medicines, because in our experience they have been the major components of health care. This approach to health care is called the *traditional model*. It defines the medical specialist as the vital element in the healing process; the only activity required of us is going to the doctor to get medicine or treatment. As a prenatal health educator, I have found myself faced with a new imperative: the creation of a new process, a new way of knowing and believing about pregnancy, health, and healing. To do this creating, I have examined the difference between managing health and choosing health. By comparing the traditional and ecosystem models, I have come to understand their differences in both philosophy and practice.

The traditional model has also been referred to as the mechanistic model, the biomedical model, or the linear model. It is ecologically unsound because it isolates roles and, consequently, isolates individuals from one another, from themselves, and from access to self-help. The traditional model emphasizes narrow definitions of health and illness. Natural female functions—menstruation, childbearing, and menopause—have long been given negative connotations. In childbearing, there is a pattern of intervention rather than an acceptance of the body's natural processes. In the traditional model, medical personnel provide treatment, drugs, and therapies that remove pain and speed birth. Medications artificially tranquilize the patient, who is not encouraged to seek tranquility from within.

In contrast, the ecosystem model is participatory. It assumes that health is a goal toward which women and men can choose to move. Healers working within this holistic model do not support passive acceptance of traditional medical protocol and procedures. Rather, they encourage the redistribution of power and decision making, for example, about childbearing, away from the single medical care giver and among all of those who care for the expectant woman. This promotes collaboration among care givers and leads to personal and individualized planning. Members of a healthy ecosystem know that healers and healing are a blend of body and soul, wisdom and choice.

When we think about a holistic approach to healing we see that the traditional model of health care is very control-oriented. Services in most medical facilities are carefully overseen and regulated, with fairly rigid perspectives on behavior and order. This has had an important impact on how women have come to think about birth. For many women, the issue of control during pregnancy and childbirth has become extremely important. The Lamaze method of childbirth, based on Pavlovian learning theories, emphasizes that a women can control the pain of childbirth by training herself to respond to labor with a specific set of behaviors. The application of learning theory to birth is illustrative of the manner in which birth has been stripped of its natural intimacy.

Focuses on the Individual

In contrast, in the ecosystems model of health, and in the model of exercise and health education that underpins this text, control is not the goal. Understanding and responding with skills that promote healing and self-awareness is the purpose of the ecosystems approach to maternal education.

Health educators—exercise teachers, childbirth educators, and prenatal specialists—working within the ecosystems framework will find that they are able to focus on the individuality of each woman with whom they work. Instead of relying on standard procedures, they will continually evaluate lectures, demonstrations, exercise routines, and meditations to determine whether they meet the needs of participants. As they move away from emphasizing pregnancy and childbirth as crises, they will discover activities that promote nurturing and support (see Table 1.1). Eventually, the institutionalization of childbearing will be replaced by a

Table 1.1   Contrasting Systems of Healing

Traditional model	Ecosystems model
The physician acts with unquestioned authority. The relationship with the pregnant woman is tightly structured and clinical.	The healer is self or those who offer comfort or information. The relationships among healer, individual, and family are characterized by harmony, warmth, and affection.
Definition of female function requires moving health care from the home to the hospital.	Definition of female functioning supports essential intimacy of health and home, encourages individual decisions about values, works toward creative solutions for personal problems.
Defines weakness as a disease and tries to cure it.	Observes weakness, examines support systems, and encourages self-healing.
Considers pain negative.	Considers pain a message about disharmony.
Creates cycle of fear of failure and mistrust of the body.	Promotes being in touch with the body and the capacity to meet the challenges of the body.

continuum of intimate and creative solutions to the drama and challenge of giving birth.

By viewing prenatal health care and maternal health education in this holistic way, we can understand and describe the shift in our values away from fear and powerlessness and toward successful problem solving and self-awareness. The cycle of fear, mistrust, and pain, which have for so long dominated our images of birth, will be replaced by an appreciation of a transformation of knowledge and being.

The essence of the ecosystems approach is warmth, harmony, and self-esteem. It promotes the redistribution of power and reevalutes definitions of health and female functioning. The ecosystems model does not deny sickness, nor does it deny pain. It defines both as messages of the body. The system encourages self-awareness, shared responsibility, and self-esteem. The question is, How can you as an instructor, group leader, educator, and healer help women to use this system to their benefit?

By definition, a teacher who embraces and accepts the ecosystems model of health educator is a healer. The ancient Latin meaning of the word *healer* is teacher; as a healer/teacher, you act as a catalyst, helping women to integrate elements of the health ecosystem, empowering individuals to initiate important personal health and behavior-related change.

Encourages Active Participation

This model also promotes active, healthy participation in physical fitness, games, and sports for all people, including pregnant women. Movement education and the range of activities it implies is a powerful tool for promoting self-knowledge. You will find that when you encourage women to learn about themselves through movement, you support their intuitive efforts to move toward wholeness and independence. By helping them to strengthen their bodies and learn about the options for childbearing that contribute most to self-image and self-esteem, you act as a healer.

Part of the role of the teacher in the ecosystems model is to encourage women to seek positive, strong female images with which to identify. It is important to work with women to help them see that we have all been hampered by narrowly defined sex roles and historically biased views about women. These traditionally defined roles and attitudes have prevented many women from developing patterns of personal strength and dignity regarding their bodies and their health. Jean Shenoda Bolen, author of *Goddesses in Every Woman* (1984), writes about understanding female psychology through examining the goddess archetypes of Greek and Roman mythology. The text is particularly helpful for women to wish to identify and explore the noble, powerful elements of our female heritage, while facing less desirable characteristics with a willingness to overcome and mature beyond them.

The challenge we face is to accept ourselves as healers. This requires that we take responsibility for ourselves and for others and that we become educated about our beautiful, strong, female bodies. This means we must accept ourselves as healthy women who wish to redefine health and fitness education.

The transformation of belief away from the traditional model of healing and toward the ecosystems model requires a commitment to the integrity of the individual and to education. I believe that the success of this model will be its reflection in the joyous freedom, competence, and success of those who learn from it.

Integrating Exercise With Preparation for Childbirth

The realms of healing intersect at the juncture of medicine, spirit, and education. The integration of body and mind, wisdom and cure is the genuine goal of prenatal education. It is appropriate for childbirth educators, nurse practitioners, and midwives to incorporate fitness education into preparation for childbirth, and it is important for fitness teachers to become part of the prenatal education program. This model of maternal health education should incorporate a female-oriented approach to teaching about the body, mind, and birth, with emphases on

- Body awareness: Body awareness is more than anatomy. It includes teaching about the functional ability of the body systems to manage pregnancy, labor, and delivery. It promotes self-esteem and enhances respect and admiration for female physiology.
- Body fitness: During pregnancy, fitness means more than building muscles. It includes exercises that promote strength and flexibility for birth, nutrition, and fitness as an integral part of one's lifestyle throughout the life span. These activities promote body confidence.
- Stress reduction and health education: Relaxation is important for labor and delivery, for coping with workday stress, for reducing high blood pressure and quitting smoking, for reducing alcohol and drug consumption, and for improving eating habits.

Education for childbirth must teach about the dignity of the body. This is a lesson that must be integrated into daily life with carryover into improved self-concept and lifestyle management. The new emphasis on fitness-related discussions and activities can be pivotal to a woman's experience of health and wellness during pregnancy and may be critical to her ability to function within the range of quality and dignity during the birth experience.

Current Priorities and Approaches

Current models of childbirth preparation place the pregnant woman in the center of a network of support services and personnel that include a medical care giver, other medical support persons, friends, family, employment, and education. For 20 years, childbirth educators have worked to build this interactive model of childbirth preparation as a natural, conceptual framework whose outcome can be measured through positive client, agency, and medical feedback. Results of much research indicate that childbirth education has had a positive effect on women's experiences of birth in American hospitals through successfully influencing the behavior of staff and patients and effecting important changes in institutional policy. Yet, much work remains, for we do not know whether childbirth education has permanently influenced and improved the level of body wisdom and wellness of the women who enroll in its classes.

I believe it is important that childbirth educators assume responsibility for empowering women *beyond* birth. Preparation for labor and delivery can no longer be a unidirectional process that ends at birth. Rather, it must be seen and practiced as an educational continuum that nurtures body pride, body confidence, and body power.

Childbirth education cannot be simply an initiation into obstetrical practices. The importance of instruction about medications and surgical procedures must not so overwhelm instructors that there is no time to get down on the floor and place their hands on a mother's belly and talk to her about how it feels when the baby moves.

Providers of services and educational opportunities for pregnant women can no longer afford to ignore the importance of disability prevention, wellness, or fitness education. We all need to recognize that beyond the birth experience, education on health, fitness, and wellness must be appreciated and promoted for its reciprocal effects on all aspects of family life.

The adaptation of childbirth preparation programs to these perspectives may require flexibility and change in many educators' professional practices. But childbirth and fitness educators able to transcend the traditional medical-educational models may discover new options and exciting new professional identities in the field of women's health. This new ecosystems option enhances the range and potential of the unique services and settings available to women preparing for birth.

Research has shown that behavior is one of the key elements in preventing disease and disability. Choices about exercise; diet; personal hygiene; the use of alcohol, tobacco, or drugs; and adaptations to stress all directly affect individual and family health. The health of both a woman and her family may depend on the behaviors and choices that she makes. Encouraging behavioral change toward a healthier lifestyle should be a central goal of childbirth education.

Summary

During pregnancy, women are hungry for information about their health. They have a seemingly vast potential for self-awareness and self-understanding and a capacity for self-exploration that may not be present during the nonpregnant state. If we continue to think in terms of the ecosystem model, the efforts of the healing educator must be toward promoting insight, understanding, creativity, and problem solving. The educator is in a position to promote acceptance and appreciation of the pregnant female and her body. And the healing educator is able to show support and understanding for the intimacy that brings both women and men to her classroom.

Teaching and sharing movement experiences and creating a trusting, comfortable group can be joyous. The greatest pleasures of prenatal teaching can be felt when you help women to explore new ways of planning for birth and coping with fear. When you work to heal fear and anxiety about childbirth, you offer women the opportunity to experience pregnancy and birth as positive. Though pregnancy remains a journey into the unknown, a strong, healthy body and trusting, cooperative relationships with others are the foundations for an ebullient and powerful encounter with self.

Learning Body Skills

Movement skills are essentially body skills. Pregnancy and childbirth are both experiences of the body. As women come to feel pride rather than dread or shame, they can view both the changes in their bodies and the birth itself as positive and healthy. Women need to learn to move and to enjoy their bodies. You can encourage them to train their bodies and their minds to perform new and challenging tasks. Fear of failure plagues many pregnant women. By challenging them to experience themselves and to learn new skills you work to heal that fear.

Women do their best when they are trusted and when they have confidence in themselves and their own abilities (see *Joy*; Schutz, 1967). As you encourage women to talk about how they feel and what they think, they will learn that they have both freedom and responsibility to make decisions. They will learn to listen to themselves and to see other women as allies. This is why it is so important that pregnant women have the opportunity to learn about female physiology, fitness, and birth. Knowledge is power. By offering it to the women in your classes, you free them to use the tools that an ecosystem education provides.

As an educator and healer you deal specifically with the interplay of body and mind and with the transformation of concern and fear into informed perspectives. As women, we have the responsibility to accept the realities of our knowing and healing potential. Even our caring, and our willingness to act on our caring, distinguishes us as partners, working to heal the fear, to put aside the myths, and to discover the truths about our bodies. In the next chapter we will explore how to integrate prenatal physiology into understanding and teaching exercise. This balance of information and intuition leads us to wholeness.

Chapter 2

Major Body Systems Changes During Pregnancy and Implications for Exercise

The ecosystem model of prenatal health education values the understanding of maternal physiology, and promotes the integration of this knowledge into the teaching process. This chapter provides an introduction to the physiologic changes of the major body systems during pregnancy and the implications for exercise as a result of these changes. We will consider the interactive and balanced functioning of these systems as part of our effort to understand and promote a healthy and holistic approach to prenatal fitness. Patricia Estok (1985) wrote of the relationship between body changes and exercise during pregnancy as follows: ''Exercise is health promoting. . . . Helping women understand how body mass, hemo-dynamic, respiratory, and musculoskeletal changes and other factors alter capacity for exercise can be a part of prenatal education programs'' (p. 6).

I have always believed that educating women about their bodies should be a top priority. In my work with pregnant women, childbirth educators, and exercise specialists, I have discovered that many women know a great deal about how their bodies work. I attribute this to the enormous impact of the women's health and fitness movements, and it pleases me greatly. In this chapter,

I will share with you how to enhance the link between body fitness and body wisdom with regard to the changes of pregnancy. Those who are interested in additional reading about prenatal exercise physiology should refer to Artal and Wiswell (1986).

Integrating the Medical and Holistic Models

There are many ways to explain the interdependence of the human body's systems. The traditional mechanic's view is that the body is a processing plant, or an engine, equipped to process fuel and perform its necessary work (Artal & Wiswell, 1986). According to this line of thinking, each of the body's systems is a separate entity, and the body functions like a well-oiled machine.

The holistic view defines the body as an organism composed of synergistic systems. These complex systems work together to give the body its shape, form, and energy. When teaching pregnant women about synergy, I point out that the babies they are carrying within them are complete human beings, with functioning organs and systems of their own.

The maternal and fetal systems are intimately tied to one another; in fact, mother and baby share a remarkably balanced, interactive existence. The dependence of the fetus on the mother and the capability of the maternal system to support the fetus is the perfect example of a synergistic, human ecosystem.

In the traditional, mechanical model, the body is an object consisting of separate, distinct, and identifiable masses and materials. The holistic perspective defines the body as an experience: The body is lived, it is experienced, and that experience is subjective and personal. For pregnant women, this definition of the body is profoundly meaningful.

It is important to integrate both the traditional and the holistic views of the body as we examine some of the physiological changes of the female body during pregnancy. Each part of the human organism is intimately dependent upon the other parts, and the balanced functioning of the various body systems is the result of this complex interdependence. Though we will look at the systems separately, keep in mind their interdependence and the delicate balance that exists among them. These interdependent parts include the respiratory, cardiovascular, gastrointestinal, metabolic, musculoskeletal, and endocrine systems, all of which are dealt with in the following sections.

Respiratory Function

From the first cry of the neonate to the last breath of life, the oxygen a human breathes is life-sustaining nourishment. Breath is the elemental life force. I frequently talk with pregnant women about their breath and how each full, deep respiration nourishes their bodies and their babies. The concept of oxygen as food that filters through to the baby makes sense to most women. At rest, all of the cells in the body require oxygen. During exercise, those cells require an increased amount of oxygen. The mechanical process for providing the cells with that needed oxygen is called *respiration*, or breathing.

The respiratory system is composed of the lungs, the passageways that lead to them, and the structures of the chest. The nasal passages and throat allow for air flow, whereas the 12 pairs of ribs, the sternum (breast bone), and the intercostal muscles provide the shape of the thoracic cavity and provide protection for the elastic lung tissue.

Pulmonary means having to do with the lungs. As the uterus grows and places pressure on the diaphragm, pulmonary functioning is altered. The diaphragm is a dome-shaped sheath of muscle that separates the thoracic (chest) and abdominal cavities. During normal respiration the diaphragm is drawn down during inhalation, allowing the lungs to expand, and it rises during exhalation. As a result of the pressure from the enlarged uterus, the diaphragm cannot be drawn down as far during inspiration, leading many women to feel that they cannot inhale deeply enough. Interestingly enough, the female torso compensates for this crowding by allowing the rib cage to flare out, providing adequate room for the lungs. However, as pregnancy progresses and until lightening, which is the settling of the baby's head down into the pelvis during the last days or weeks of pregnancy, a woman breathes less deeply.

For some, the pressure on the diaphragm creates a tendency to hyperventilate. Hyperventilation occurs when a person breathes too rapidly or exhales without deep enough inhalation. The body eliminates carbon dioxide too quickly, causing a tingly feeling, light headedness, dizziness, or nausea. Because deep inhalation may be uncomfortable for women in advanced stages of pregnancy and during labor, they should be reminded to breathe slowly and evenly, inhaling as deeply as possible and lengthening the exhalation.

Knuttgen and Emerson (1974) identified four major pulmonary changes during pregnancy:

1. A decrease in functional residual capacity (the amount of air left in the lungs after respiration).
2. Increased inspiratory capacity (the amount of air breathed in).
3. Increased vital capacity (the maximal amount of air that can be expelled following a maximal inspiration).
4. No increase in total lung capacity (the volume of air in the lungs) (p. 552).

The amount of air breathed in during pregnancy actually increases, and there is a 30%-40% increase in the tidal volume (the amount of air inhaled in a single breath). As pregnancy progresses from Week 16 to Week 40, actual oxygen consumption increases by 15%-20%. Lung capacity remains constant, but the pregnant woman has a smaller oxygen reserve. The cause for this reduced reserve has not been determined, but it may contribute to the breathlessness pregnant women experience when participating in vigorous exercise.

We all know how it feels to be breathless. It happens when the muscles have used all the available oxygen, and a period of slowed activity is necessary to allow the breathing rate to return to normal. This slower level of activity increases the amount of oxygen available to the muscles and repays the *oxygen debt*, which can be incurred as a result of strenuous exercise.

Research by Collings, Curet, and Mullin (1983) indicated that on the basis of submaximal exercise, mothers who exercise during pregnancy can achieve an improved aerobic capacity (the amount of work or exercise that can be done) and improved functional aerobic levels (the amount of work that can be done at submaximal levels). Nonexercising pregnant women usually experience a decline in functional aerobic capacity. Edwards, Metcalfe, Dunham, and Paul (1981) showed that pregnant women who exercise demonstrate a faster adjustment to aerobic stress than pregnant women who don't exercise.

Implications for Exercise

If you were to observe a nonpregnant individual during strenuous exercise, you would see a natural tendency to lift the rib cage, thereby increasing chest volume. Because of the size of the uterus, a pregnant woman may not be able to lift the rib cage far enough to improve ventilation capacity. The heaviness that many women feel as the uterus pushes up against the diaphragm may be relieved to some extent by performing movements that lift the arms out to the sides and up over the head (Figures 2.1 and 2.2).

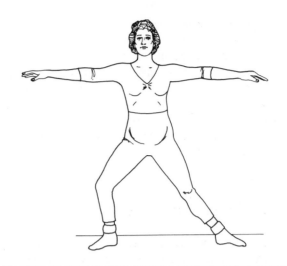

Figure 2.2. When both arms are raised, as in the sideways lunge, the pregnant women is able to breathe more deeply.

Because hyperventilation and breathlessness are common in late pregnancy, even among women who exercise regularly, fitness instructors should not expect women to exercise to the point where they are gasping from overexertion. Unfortunately, though the need for oxygen increases steadily throughout gestation, a woman's ability to increase her oxygen uptake during strenuous exercise may not keep pace with her needs. It is reasonable to suggest that pregnant women avoid high levels of aerobic activity, which may lead to *dyspnea*, or labored breathing. Although mild hyperventilation is considered normal, strenuous exercise-induced hyperventilation should be avoided.

The implications of respiratory changes also involve certain precautions. For example, some women exhibit a tendency to hold their breath during strenuous activities. Doing this increases pressure in the thoracic cavity and compresses the large veins that return blood to the heart and subsequently provide oxygen to the brain. The result of the reduced oxygen supply can be dizziness or fainting. Holding one's breath during strenuous activity is referred to as Valsalva's maneuver, and pregnant women should avoid the breath-holding response to stress or exercise.

Pregnant women may experience stitches because of respiratory changes. A stitch is a cramp that occasionally accompanies exercise. It occurs as a result of minor immobility of the diaphragm or a lack of oxygen to the intercostal muscles. Lifting one's knees, blowing out crisply, and massaging beneath the rib cage can relieve a stitch. Cramps as a result of stretched uterine ligaments will be discussed in the next chapter.

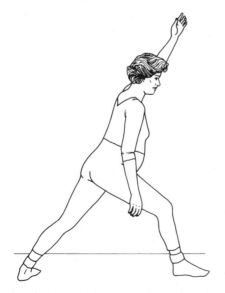

Figure 2.1. The forward lunge strengthens the body while promoting balance and alignment. With the arm raised it promotes improved respiration.

Related to pulmonary function, nasal stuffiness, runny noses, and occasional nosebleeds are common during pregnancy. They occur because of estrogen-induced edema and vascular congestion of the nasal mucosa. Though long walks in all seasons are encouraged, the pregnant woman may find that the changes in humidity from outside to inside will aggravate any stuffiness or nosebleeds she experiences.

Cardiovascular System

The cardiovascular system is responsible for pumping blood throughout the body. Pregnant women are fascinated when they are told about the changes in the cardiovascular system during pregnancy, and the old line, "Your heart beats for two," suddenly takes on new significance. The heart is a muscle and its walls thicken, most notably the left ventrical wall, as it works harder to handle the increased blood volume of pregnancy. The heart lengthens in both longitudinal and transverse directions, and as the uterus exerts pressure on the diaphragm, the heart becomes displaced upward and to the left.

The cardiovascular system—the heart and all the veins and arteries—is under considerable stress during pregnancy. During the prenatal months blood volume increases by an average of 30%-45%, and the heart has to work much harder to pump the blood through the veins and arteries. The largest vessels in the body are arteries, which transport the blood directly from the heart to the smaller vessels. The hormones of pregnancy cause the tone of all the body's vessels and arteries to soften considerably, allowing the veins themselves to stretch to accommodate the increased blood volume. Sluggish circulation, varicose veins, and sometimes a degree of edema (swelling) may occur as a result of these changes.

Blood volume is the amount of blood circulating in the body. Blood volume increases steadily in the first trimester and more rapidly in the second trimester. The rate of increase slows during the last weeks of pregnancy. Pulse may show no change or a normal increase approaching 20% or 10-15 beats per minute (bpm). Blood flow to the mother's internal organs increases as their work load increases. Circulation to the uterus and kidneys increases whereas cerebral flow, for example, is unchanged. Research has shown that there is less margin of cardiac reserve for performance of muscular work as pregnancy progresses. That means

that the heart is less able to adapt to increasing demands by increasing output or raising blood pressure. Sustaining high levels of activity or participating in activities that require sudden bursts of movement may prove difficult and tiring during pregnancy.

Exercise instructors should keep this in mind when considering the duration and intensity of a workout. It is important to encourage the expectant woman to be aware of what her body is telling her in terms of exertion. A pounding heart or irregular heart beats may be critical signs that indicate that the woman should reduce her pace. After pregnancy it may take up to six weeks for cardiac output and blood volume to return to normal.

Anemia in Pregnancy

Anemia may exist before pregnancy or be due specifically to the pregnancy. Iron-deficient anemia, which is frequently accompanied by a folic acid deficiency, is a condition that causes a woman to tire easily due to the decreased oxygen-carrying capacity of her blood. Folic acid is a member of the B complex vitamins. An anemic woman may not tolerate exercise well, especially when extra demands are placed on her oxygen consumption requirements.

Veins and Capillaries

Sixty thousand miles of veins and arteries form a two-way system within the body that carries nutrients and waste products to and from the organ and muscle systems. The tiny endings of the veins and arteries are capillaries, and in these tiny thin-walled capillaries the body exchanges oxygen for carbon dioxide. It is at these exchange points that the body is nourished. In a normal pregnancy, venous capacity increases and circulation is generally improved.

Impaired Circulation: High Blood Pressure

Blood pressure is a measurement of the force that the flow of blood through the body exerts on the blood vessels. High blood pressure during pregnancy is a potentially lethal disease that may be a chronic condition or may develop for the first time during pregnancy, frequently during the second half of pregnancy. In a normal pregnancy, as blood volume increases, vasodilation, which is the softening and increased dilation of the blood vessels, occurs most likely in response to the hormone progesterone. Blood pressure drops or remains the same. In hypertension, a woman develops vasoconstriction and her blood vessels constrict or narrow, causing her blood pressure to climb.

The onset of high blood pressure during pregnancy is referred to as pregnancy induced hypertension (PIH). The disease can progress rapidly, increasing a woman's risk of heart attack, stroke, or kidney failure. During pregnancy, high blood pressure can impair the circulation to the fetus through the placenta, causing serious problems for the fetus. There are usually no early symptoms of high blood pressure, though sudden swelling or fluid retention, severe headaches, or blurred vision may indicate serious problems (referred to in the medical literature as *preeclampsia, eclampsia,* or *toxemia of pregnancy*). Women should have their blood pressure checked regularly throughout gestation.

Impaired Circulation: Low Blood Pressure in Pregnancy

Low blood pressure is referred to as *hypotension*. Orthostatic hypotension in pregnancy is a drop in blood pressure related to posture. It may occur as a result of the pooling of blood in the lower extremities after long periods of sitting or standing or when the pregnant woman reclines. In the reclined or supine position, the pressure of the heavy uterus on the vena cava decreases the rate of blood flow to the heart and the brain. The vena cava is a major vein that consists of two systems that return blood from the body to the heart. The inferior vena cava is located on the right side of the back wall of the abdomen. It returns blood to the heart from the lower torso and lower extremities. The superior vena cava returns blood from the brain and upper extremities to the heart. Dizziness, pallor, and nausea may be symptoms of orthostatic hypotension. During pregnancy the chances of these symptoms occurring may also be related to increased pressure on the femoral veins.

Varicose Veins

Varicose veins are the result of softening of the venous tissue and malfunctioning of the tiny valves inside the veins that help pump the blood back to the heart. Varicosities can occur in the legs, vulva, or rectum, where they are called hemorrhoids. During pregnancy, prolonged periods of standing or sitting encourage the blood to pool in the legs, making the work of returning the blood to the heart more difficult. Varicose veins can be very painful. Exercise can help stimulate circulation by increasing muscular pressure on the veins. Many women wear support hose to create pressure on the veins in the legs.

Implications for Exercise

The pregnant woman's cardiovascular system undergoes significant adjustments during gestation, and the risks and benefits of cardiovascular exercise are of great concern. Research has found that during exercise there is a significant rise in maternal blood pressure and pulse, both of which may remain elevated for up to 15 min following an activity. The ACOG exercise guidelines for pregnant women (1985), which we will discuss shortly, clearly indicate that intelligent limits be set on the length and intensity of exercise sessions. The group leader must limit the length of all workouts, and each participant must take her pulse after a strenuous routine. Any woman who feels dizzy or experiences a pounding feeling in her chest or palpitations (irregular heart beats) must stop exercising. It is advisable for her to walk for several minutes before sitting down to rest. She should definitely keep her head above the level of her heart, that is, she should not bend over or put her head down until her pulse has returned to normal. Stress on the cardiovascular system during pregnancy warrants that a woman not strive to maintain any preset level of cardiovascular fitness, but rather, exercise only to her comfortable capacity. Pulse rate will be discussed further in chapters 4 and 5.

As you have seen, there are a number of significant changes in the cardiovascular system during pregnancy. Through organizations like ACOG, medical science is beginning to address these changes in ways that are more compatible with a woman's total life-style. As advocates of women's health education, we share a commitment to heal through education. Awareness of this information can help us to teach and broaden our own definitions of health.

Gastrointestinal Changes

The gastrointestinal system includes the stomach and the intestines, and, like the other major systems in the body, it adjusts to the increased work of gestation. Whereas cardiovascular activity increases during pregnancy, the main change in the gastrointestinal system is that activity actually slows down.

Many of the discomforts of pregnancy can be attributed to the changes in the gastrointestinal system. Symptoms of nausea, morning sickness, or vomiting may be related to increased hormone production. Any woman who is affected by vomiting must guard against dehydration, or excessive fluid loss. Under extreme circumstances, when dehydration is a result of environmental factors, it can lead to decreased blood volume and premature labor. As pregnancy progresses, gastrointestinal symptoms such as heartburn and indigestion may be attributed to the displacement of the stomach and intestines. Heartburn occurs as a result of the relaxation of the esophageal sphincter (the muscle that partially or completely opens and closes the esophagus) and the reflux action of acidic secretions from the stomach into the lower esophagus or as a result of the enlarging uterus' putting pressure on the stomach or duodenum. Intestinal motility may be delayed, sometimes causing bloating, flatulence, and constipation. This is because of the smooth muscle softening effects of progesterone, which is produced by the placenta, the organ through which the fetus is nourished. It may also be related to diet.

The gallbladder, which is a small sac attached to the liver, tends to empty more slowly during pregnancy, occasionally leading to some discomfort or to the formation of gallstones.

Implications for Exercise

Exercise may help to stimulate the pregnant woman's appetite, and she should be encouraged to eat a nutritious snack an hour before and an hour after exercise. Exercise can reduce the gastrointestinal distress of pregnancy by stimulating the sluggish intestines and creating a refreshing feeling of vitality. Training in contraction and release of the perineal muscles, those muscles which comprise the perineum, the central tendon between the vagina and the anus, and practicing the pelvic tilt exercise may also stimulate the bowel (for an anatomical view of the perineum see Figure 3.3 in chapter 3). Women who find they are straining to have a bowel movement should be advised to put their feet up (perhaps on a small footstool) and change positions while seated on the commode.

Dietary sensitivities may be responsible for some gastrointestinal problems. Some women develop digestive difficulties related to carbohydrate absorption, frequently referred to as lactose intolerance. Milk products may cause cramping and diarrhea for those women. For others, dried fruit, beans, bananas, cabbage, and brussels sprouts may be the culprits. Careful dietary and nutritional counseling should become an integral component of prenatal care.

Metabolic Changes

Metabolism refers to the physical and chemical processes by which energy is produced and life is sustained. Within the body, metabolism is the process by which nutrients are made available to the cells. Metabolic functions release the energy from complex nutrients and transform it into usable chemical structures like amino acids, which are needed to build and repair the cells. Most metabolic functions accelerate during pregnancy to meet the growing needs of mother and fetus.

The energy cost of pregnancy is estimated to be 300 cal a day (Artal & Romen, 1986, p. 61). A pregnant woman is often advised to increase her caloric intake by about 300 calories each day. This additional food energy covers the added cost of the developing fetus, the buildup of maternal tissues, and the increased activity of the maternal metabolism. Research has shown that caloric need changes during pregnancy. The middle months are the most demanding whereas the final weeks are least demanding in terms of caloric need. Yet, throughout pregnancy, excellent nutrition as well as nutritional supplements is recommended.

Nutrition Suggestions

Each woman should receive nutritional guidelines and support from her care giver. As an exercise instructor, you should be able to suggest strategies for improving the quality of a woman's diet. Some suggestions might include avoiding soft drinks and caffeinated beverages and eating enough roughage, including uncooked fruits and raw vegetables. You might suggest that women begin to read the labels on the canned and packaged foods they buy, if they do not do so already. This way they can choose to avoid those with unnecessary or excessive chemicals or preservatives. Women should avoid eating when they are anxious, eating to soothe cravings, and eating to make others eat. Some women crave nonfood items because of dietery insufficiencies, superstition, or even tradition. It is dangerous for anyone to eat bleach, laundry starch, clay, or dirt. Yet pregnant women have been known to crave such items. Food should be viewed as a gift to the self, essential to the healthy functioning of the body and to the growth of the baby. Women who are encouraged to consume a well-balanced diet feel a sense of comfort and self-control about their appetites and their ability to nourish themselves and their babies.

A well-balanced diet includes eating a variety of foods to ensure an adequate supply of all nutrients. During pregnancy women need an enriched supply of all nutrients, especially calcium, iron, folic acid, protein, and vitamin C. Remind pregnant women that eating well is the best way to ensure a healthier life, for themselves and for their babies. Table 2.1 will help you provide suggestions when women ask you how to improve their diets.

Table 2.1 Food Sources for Necessary Nutrients

Nutrient	Recommended daily allowance
Calcium	1,200-1,400 milligrams (mg)
Salmon (canned), 1 cup	408 mg
Yogurt, 1 cup	400 mg
Milk (low fat), 1 cup	297 mg
Cheese (cheddar), 1 oz	204 mg
Collard greens, 1 cup	304 mg
Tofu, 4 oz	146 mg
Broccoli, 1 cup	132 mg
Cheeseburger on a bun, 4 oz	115 mg
Pecans, 1 cup	79 mg
Enriched spaghetti with tomato sauce, 1 cup	47.5 mg
Iron	30-60 milligrams (mg)
Lean meat, 7 oz	5.8 mg
Baked beans in molasses, 1 cup	5.4 mg
Spinach (cooked), 1 cup	4.0 mg
Turkey, 7 oz	2.8 mg
Peas (cooked), 1 cup	2.6 mg
Pecans, 1 cup	2.5 mg
Sunflower seeds, 1 oz	2.0 mg
Peanut butter, 3 tbs	1.8 mg
Whole wheat bread, 2 slices	1.8 mg
Protein	75-100 grams (g)
Poultry (roasted), 7 oz	60 g
Cottage cheese (low fat), 1 cup	32 g
Cheeseburger on a bun, average serving	15.5 g
Tofu, 4 oz	10 g
Cheese (cheddar), 1 oz	7 g
Egg (cooked), 1	6 g

Nutrient	Recommended daily allowance
Whole wheat bread, 2 slices	4 g
Pecans, 1 cup	10 g
Sunflower seeds, 1 oz	7 g
Folic acid	800 micrograms (mcg)
Asparagus (cooked), 1 cup	218 mcg
Fortified cereal, 2 oz	250 mcg
Romain lettuce, 1 cup	98 mcg
Egg (cooked), 1	24 mcg
Orange juice, 1 cup	52 mcg
Whole wheat bread, 2 slices	28 mcg
Sweet potato (baked), 1	26 mcg
Pecans, 1 cup	26 mcg
Vitamin C	80 milligrams (mg)
Broccoli (cooked), 1 cup	134 mg
Fruit juice, 1 cup	90 mg
Strawberries, 1 cup	86 mg
Cantaloupe, 1 cup	68 mg
Grapefruit, 1/2	39 mg
Tomato, 1	34 mg
Potato (baked), 1	20 mg
Pecans, 1 cup	2 mg

Artal and Romen (1986) point out that there are two ways to meet the increased caloric needs of pregnancy. A woman can either add that much food to her diet or decrease her activity level and use less caloric energy. I definitely advise women with healthy, normal pregnancies to increase their caloric intake and to enjoy physical activity. Pregnancy is not the time to stop moving!

Weight gain, related to increased caloric consumption and the increased weight of the fetus, breasts, and uterus, should be steady throughout pregnancy with expected gain in the range of 24 to 34 lb. Pregnant women should be aware that proper nutrition and reasonable, steady weight gain are directly related to fetal well-being.

Appetite Changes

Many women report significant changes in appetite during pregnancy, noting that after any initial queasiness in the first trimester, they feel hungrier during the middle months of pregnancy and are able to eat more than they normally do. This may be due to the increased presence of progesterone, which is known to increase heat production and therefore caloric expenditure.

Because pregnant women often feel very hungry, they may be tempted to eat sweets, like candy bars, before exercise classes. This raises the level of glucose in the bloodstream very quickly and appears to provide quick energy. Unfortunately, blood sugar levels drop just as quickly once the glucose is utilized. During exercise, when the body is using and demanding more energy, women who have not eaten or who have eaten foods that are high in sugar content may experience this sudden drop in blood glucose level; the resulting symptoms include nervousness; shakiness; hunger; and cool, clammy skin, leading in serious cases to disorientation, fainting, convulsions, or coma.

Nutritional support for pregnant women ranks at the top of most care givers' lists of subjects that need more attention. As an exercise instructor, you should be aware of the importance of a well-balanced diet and remind women to eat a small high-fiber, high-carbohydrate snack before exercising (e.g., an apple, dried apricots, a banana, or a whole wheat muffin) and to avoid a high-sugar snack such as a candy bar.

Heat Production and Metabolic Function

The metabolic activity of the cells in the body is constantly producing heat. During exercise, when more oxygen is consumed, more heat is produced. The problems of increased heat production are of particular concern to the pregnant woman who exercises. The normal core temperature of the body is about 100.4 °F or 38 °C. Prolonged exercise (i.e., 30-60 min) can raise the body's internal core temperature a full degree centigrade. Although still in its early stages, preliminary research has suggested that hyperthermia of the fetus, that is, exposure of the fetus to excessively high temperature in pregnancy, may be responsible for some neural tube defects, which are congenital defects of the spine or brain.

Pregnant women react quickly to the heat produced during exercise. They tend to perspire freely and should not be encouraged to keep going if they are uncomfortably warm. Overheating and dehydration have immediate effects on the fetus as reflected in an increased fetal temperature. Research has shown that when the fetus experiences an increased temperature its recovery time (the period it takes for its temperature to return to normal) is much longer than maternal recovery rate. Perspiration is the body's method of self-cooling. Remember, the fetus cannot perspire! Also, remind women to consume small amounts of fluids before, during, and after exercise. Constantly replacing fluids lost by perspiration and evaporation helps keep the body cool, prevents dehydration, and slows the rate at which the core temperature rises.

As you can see, sharing with expectant mothers this information about metabolic changes during pregnancy can be critical to their well-being. Knowledge of these functional and metabolic changes makes them aware of the rapid changes that may occur as they exercise or perform other activities. The level of awareness you, as an exercise instructor and/or health educator, display of this knowledge will be reflected in the expectant mother's own level of awareness.

Please remember to show sensitivity with regard to a mother's feelings during exercise or other activities; this will speak volumes about the importance of paying attention to one's own body signals. Part of your role is to encourage a mother to be aware of her body's physiological changes during activities and, if necessary, to support her decision to discontinue activities. The best teacher will encourage each woman to take control of her own experience and to trust herself, her decisions, her intuition, and her body.

Waste Production and Kidney, Ureter, and Bladder Changes

The kidneys, ureters, and bladder undergo major changes in structure and function during pregnancy (Olds, London, & Ladewig, 1984). Just as the other major organs adjust to the additional workload, the kidneys also work harder to filter blood and maintain a balance of salt, water, and other elements of the body.

The bladder is affected by both the hormones of pregnancy and the presence of the fetus. High levels of progesterone may affect the muscle tone of the bladder, reducing its contractile action as well as sphincter control. Very early and then again late in pregnancy, pressure from the uterus on the bladder may significantly reduce retention capacity, causing many bothersome trips to the bathroom. Women should not reduce fluid consumption to control this functional change. It is normal unless signs of a bladder infection—pain, a burning sensation, or bleeding—accompany urination. The urethra, the narrow tube through which urine is drained from the bladder, may alter in shape due to uterine pressure, and tone may be reduced. This may also create an increased potential for urinary tract infection.

Although the kidneys increase slightly in size and renal (kidney) function is altered considerably, these changes appear to have no major effects on exercise. Studies attempting to show that posture affects kidney function have been inconclusive (Olds, London, & Ladewig, 1984). However, late in pregnancy kidney function, which is measured by urine flow and sodium excretion, can be reduced if a mother remains in a supine position (Pritchard & MacDonald, 1980). This is another reason to advise women to rest in the lateral recumbent position. (For location of kidneys, see Figure 2.3.)

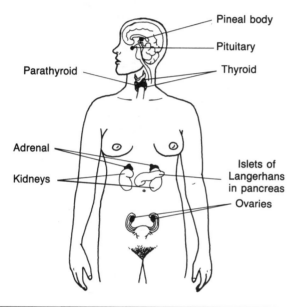

Figure 2.3. The endocrine system shown with location of the kidneys.

In the third trimester, many women experience reduced mobility in the wrists, fingers, and ankles due to increased intravascular fluid retention. Resting in the left lateral position and gentle exercise may help to relieve stiffness or minor swelling. Sudden or severe edema may be a symptom of hypertension or may be related to kidney disease.

Although physical exercise does not directly affect urinary tract health, persistent urinary tract infections or stress incontinence (the leaking of urine during routine activities, exercise, coughing, or sneezing) can influence any woman's choices about and enjoyment of exercise.

Women should be taught how to exercise the muscles that contribute to urinary tract health. The kegel exercise, which is described in more detail in chapter 10, teaches women to contract and release the pubococcygeal muscle, which supports the urethra and the neck of the bladder, to insure continued maintenance of bladder control. The pubococcygeal muscle acts like a sling to support the organs of the lower pelvis, particularly the vesicle outlet of the urethra, the neck of the bladder, the vagina, and the anal sphincter. Women should develop a clear knowledge of how to empty the bladder completely by contracting and releasing the pubococcygeus after urinating. The exercise and teaching program used to increase awareness and tone of this muscle group is an essential component of your class.

Adequate fluid intake also contributes to good urinary tract health. You should ask each woman to have a small drink of water before exercise, to take a bathroom break during class, and to have another drink of water after exercise. Proper hydration should produce profuse, light-colored urine. Dark, scant urine indicates inadequate fluid consumption. A pregnant woman should drink up to a quart of fluid each day to keep up with expanding blood volume. This does not mean that she needs to drink milk. Water and juice are fine.

The musculoskeletal system undergoes the most visible changes during pregnancy. The strength and balance of the musculoskeletal system can be tied directly to exercise. I will discuss this connection in the following pages.

The Musculoskeletal System

The musculoskeletal system is composed of bones, ligaments, muscles, tendons, and cartilage. It is the body's support system, giving it shape and defining its structure and the form and vitality of movements. Throughout pregnancy, this system responds to the body's changing alignment, center of gravity, and hormonal balance. Careful use of the body, excellent nutrition, attention to body mechanics, and strengthening of the body tissues create the energy, power, vitality, and liveliness of the synergistic musculoskeletal system.

Most people think of the skeletal system as a fairly rigid, static system of interlocking bones. The big surprise about the skeletal system is that it is very much alive and lively. Bones change shape and size continuously throughout the life cycle. They respond to nutritional changes, pregnancy, and exercise. Bones are strengthened through exercise.

The bones come together at joints, which can be nonmovable, like those in the skull; slightly movable, such as the vertebrae of the spine; and freely moving, as in the joints of the fingers, hips, and knees. Freely moving joints are encased in a synovial membrane. When a joint moves the membrane secretes a fluid that lubricates and protects it.

Bands of fibrous tissue called ligaments connect the bones together at the joints. They attach to the bones on each side of a joint, give the joint its strength, and limit its motion. All ligaments, although quite resilient, can be strained, and once injured take some time to heal. Tendons are tough, fibrous tissues that attach muscles to the bones. Muscles are attached to bones at the origin, the point closest to the midline of the body, and the insertion, the point furthest from the midline. A muscle contracts or lengthens between its origin and insertion. We will discuss the joints and muscles that are most affected by pregnancy in chapter 3.

Muscular aches and spasms occur in people of all ages and are typical of pregnancy. Increased weight, the presence of relaxin, an important hormone produced during pregnancy, and the nutritional demands of pregnancy may influence muscular pain. Muscle cramps in the calves and feet are common during pregnancy. Diminished or impaired absorption of calcium may contribute

to the occurrence of leg cramps. The involuntary tightening of the muscles can be very painful. Anyone who experiences leg cramps should extend the leg, flex the foot, and knead the cramping muscle. Exercises that flex the foot and stretch the backs of the legs may be helpful (Figures 2.4 and 2.5). Avoid pointing the toe during these exercises.

Backache, abdominal achiness, and sore hips are common during pregnancy and reflect the strain undergone by the supportive and connective tissues of the muscular system. During pregnancy the stretching of the broad ligament, the uterosacral ligament, and the round ligaments that support the lower abdomen and the growing uterus can cause backache and abdominal cramps that can be particularly uncomfortable. Shifting the weight of the uterus by moving slowly may help to ease the abdominal cramping. Sleeping with the belly well supported by pillows may reduce the spasms that occur at night. These aches and pains should not be confused with uterine contractions, which we will discuss in the next chapter. However, contractions of the uterus can be mild, achey, and dull or quite strong and painful. Uterine cramping during exercise should never be ignored.

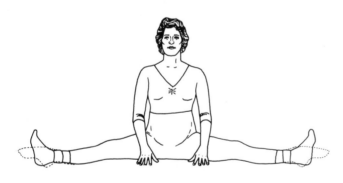

Figure 2.4. Flexing the foot helps to avoid or alleviate muscle cramps.

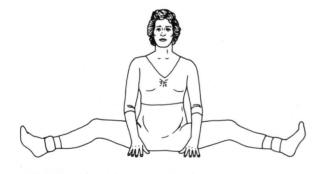

Figure 2.5. Exercises that alternate extension with flexion improve awareness of position and range of movement.

Musculoskeletal Changes and Adaptations in Pregnancy

The spinal column has three natural curves. The cervical, thoracic, and lumbar curves are places where the spine flexes to help absorb the shock of impact and gravitational pull. As pregnancy progresses, there is an accentuation of the lumbar curve in the lower back accompanied by a forward tilt of the pelvis. This is called lordosis. In an effort to maintain an upright position, women tend to lock, or hyperextend, their knees, which results in an awkward backward lean. This maladaptive postural shift is responsible for much lower back pain. Another postural variation occurs when the thoracic curve is accentuated and the shoulders are allowed to round forward: This is called kyphosis. Some women experience neck and shoulder aches, and upper backache, all of which occur as the anterior flexion of the neck increases. Scoliosis is a lateral, or sideways, curve in the spinal column. Scoliosis can be a congenital problem or it can develop as a result of years of poor postural habits.

Carpal Tunnel Syndrome

Women who suffer from carpal tunnel syndrome describe it as numbness in the forearms, hands, and fingers that occurs at night or a pins-and-needles sensation that occurs throughout the day. About one third of all pregnant women have symptoms of carpal tunnel syndrome in either one or both hands. Most cases are fairly benign, though women with severe discomfort may require a care giver's attention. The cause of carpal tunnel syndrome appears to be pressure on the median nerve as it passes through the carpal tunnel in the wrist. Other nerves may be affected. The pressure is probably a result of fluid retention.

Another cause of these symptoms may be posture. The anterior orientation of the expanding uterus displaces a woman's center of gravity, aggravating the lordosis in the lower spine and contributing to the anterior flexion of the upper spine. Unfortunately, in some women the pressure of this incorrect alignment leads to weakness and numbness of the arms, hands, and wrists.

Any woman experiencing severe back pain, pain in her arms, or pain or loss of sensation in her legs during pregnancy should consult her care giver.

Implications for Exercise

There are several implications for exercise during pregnancy as a result of our understanding of the musculoskeletal system. First, more than 15 min of standing aerobic exercises may be too demanding late in pregnancy. Standing exercise sessions should be interspersed with exercises that allow the mother to assume more comfortable positions (e.g., sitting, side lying, or kneeling on hands and knees). This will protect the body's supportive tissue as well as reduce the potential for fatigue.

Walking, a favorite exercise, is advisable when attention is paid to correct, erect posture. The sternum should be lifted slightly, and those with a tendency to allow the pelvis to tilt forward, which increases the curve in the lower back, should be aware of tucking in the buttocks and pulling up on the abdominal muscles. Shoulders and iliac crests should be level.

To protect the ligaments of the knees, lengthy, deep, unsupported flexion, during which the pelvis goes below the level of the knees (e.g., deep squatting exercises done for long periods of time) should be avoided. Squatting exercises to prepare for birth should be supported as much as possible and should not be held for more than 20 seconds. When seated with soles of the feet together, pregnant women should avoid pushing down and out on the inside of the knees in an attempt to increase flexibility of the hip. This prevents unintentional

injury of the softened cartilage and supportive tissues of the symphysis pubis and hip joints. The hurdlers stretch, which requires one leg to be bent backwards at the knee, may promote injury to the softened cartilage of the symphysis pubis and the ligaments of the knee.

Explanations of the musculoskeletal changes of pregnancy should be shared with women to increase their ability to feel involved in and comfortable with their pregnancies. It will also help them to be more aware of how they move and stand so they can avoid unneccesary strain or injury. I will look more closely at the muscles and bones of the body in the next chapter.

Endocrine Changes

The female endocrine system is composed of nine glands that produce the hormones that regulate grown, the metabolic functioning of the cells, reproduction, and the maintenance of a pregnancy. The pineal, thyroid, parathyroid, hypothalamus, pituitary, adrenals, pancreas, and ovaries play a major role in controlling and adjusting the many sensitive female physiologic functions related to reproduction. During pregnancy, the developing placenta also produces hormones that support the fetus, and it is considered a vital endocrine organ. Hormones are the chemical messengers of the body, and a woman's hormonal system undergoes substantial adaptation during pregnancy.

Functions of the Endocrine Glands

It has been found that in addition to increases in the metabolic rate, most of the endocrine glands enlarge during pregnancy. The thyroid and the hypothalamus contribute to the regulation of temperature. Because pregnant women have an elevated basal temperature they will perspire quite readily to maintain a relatively stable core temperature. The parathyroid, which produces and adjusts levels of calcium in the bloodstream, also enlarges. And the pituitary, which produces the follicle stimulating hormones (which in turn stimulate ovulation), also controls the mechanism for the release of oxytocin. Oxytocin is the hormone that stimulates uterine contractions and, after childbirth, the ejection of milk from the breasts. (There is some debate over the role of the hypothalamus and the production of oxytocin.) Another pituitary secretion is prolactin, the hormone that initially stimulates lactation. The adrenal glands control both blood sugar levels and the balance of salt and fluids in the body. The also control the biofeedback mechanisms that regulate the body's reaction to stress. The pancreas adjusts to support and maintain the pregnancy through the increased production of insulin. Problems related to the production of insulin are discussed later.

The ovaries, of course, are the organs that produce the egg whose fertilization and growth is maintained by the entire endocrine system. The site of the release of the egg is called the corpus luteum. After ovulation the corpus luteum cells behave much like a temporary endocrine gland, producing progesterone and estrogen until, if a pregnancy takes place, the placenta can take over its function while the corpus luteum continues to produce estrogen, progesterone, and relaxin (Artal & Wiswell, 1986, p. 69). The ovaries enlarge and elongate during pregnancy.

Changes in the Breasts

The changes in the size and function of the breasts during pregnancy occur as a result of the hormones estrogen and progesterone. These changes are initiated to permit the production of milk. There is a proliferation of milk-producing cells and an increased blood supply to the breasts.

Breast sensitivity increases in the early weeks of pregnancy, and many women feel a tingling, tightening sensation along with some tenderness. Some women find this painful but the discomfort is usually minor. Usually during the second trimester of pregnancy the breasts begin to produce a substance called colostrum, which nourishes the infant during the initial 24-72 hr after birth. The hormone prolactin goes into production after delivery and is responsible for the production of milk for the nursing infant. Because of the increased size and weight of the breasts, women should wear comfortable bras that provide excellent support during exercise.

Hormones Produced by Exercise

Exercise promotes the production of several hormones that affect alertness as well as mood. These hormones include the catecholamines, adrenaline and noradreniline, and the endorphins. The catecholamines stimulate alertness, and the endorphins produced during exercise appear to reduce the subjective experience of pain. In fact, endorphins may be credited with the increased tolerance for pain during childbirth because their natural opiate-like structures permit chemical bonding with the opiate receptors, producing a natural analgesia. Research has shown that these chemicals can be produced through the imagination, that is, through pleasurable stimulation, visualization, and anticipation of pleasure (Achterberg, 1985). This suggestion poses key instructional issues for the childbirth educator for, if exercise stimulates the presence of these hormones and if women can become acquainted with the chemically induced pleasure produced by exercise, the experience of delight and pride in bodily achievement can become the central focus in preparation for labor and delivery. If women feel proud of their bodies and view them as sources of positive experiences, then they can come to view birth as a powerful opportunity in which to experience self. In addition, if we can promote the use of positive visualization and imaging during birth, which I will discuss further in chapters 11 and 12, women may be able to enhance the production of endorphins during labor, reducing the perception of pain and promoting the euphoria that frequently follows delivery.

Diabetes: An Endocrine Disorder

Gestational diabetes mellitus is an endocrine disorder of carbohydrate metabolism and is related to a decreased ability to produce adequate insulin when needed. Insulin is produced in the islets of Langerhans and may be affected by increased levels of estrogen and progesterone in the maternal system. Insulin is the catalyst for glucose metabolism and helps to control the level of glucose in the bloodstream by enabling the muscles to absorb and use it for energy. Women with too much insulin at one time suffer from hypoglycemia, or low blood sugar. Those who are not producing adequate insulin may suffer from hyperglycemia, or high levels of blood sugar.

Diabetes mellitus occurs in 1 out of 300 pregnancies. It is a complex disease with many symptoms. Chronic thirst, excessive urination, weight loss, excessive hunger, and a history of large babies may be clues to its diagnosis. Implications for exercise depend directly on the severity of the maternal condition. Control of diabetes varies also. Those women whose diabetes requires insulin injections have a form of diabetes that may be difficult to manage during pregnancy. Others may have a milder form of diabetes that can be controlled through diet and exercise. Gestational or pregnancy-induced diabetes makes its first appearance during pregnancy. The woman with gestational diabetes may be asymptomatic—that is, she may not have any serious signs, symptoms, or problems of which she is aware. However, careful monitoring of blood-glucose levels in the pregnant woman with gestational diabetes, as determined by her care giver, is essential because control of the disease, even in its milder forms, can be critical to the survival of the fetus. After pregnancy, many women with gestational diabetes show no signs of diabetes.

The early symptoms of hypoglycemia and hyperglycemia may seem to overlap, even though they are in fact opposite problems. The teacher should be alert to a woman complaining of unusual shakiness, nervousness, or weakness that may accompany hunger, thirst, leg cramps, and confusion. These are symptoms of hyperglycemia. Other symptoms to watch for include complaints of blurred vision, headache, disorientation, unusual perspiration, and rapid respiration, which may indicate hypoglycemia. In an extreme case, a woman with diabetes may have a convulsion or go into a coma.

In the event that exercise is not supported by adequate caloric intake, the pregnant woman, even when not affected by diabetes mellitus, may develop symptoms like those above. If a woman begins to exhibit the symptoms of hypoglycemia described above and if she indicates that she has not eaten, you should be prepared to offer her 1/2 cup of fruit juice, 1 tsp of honey, two cubes of sugar dissolved in water, or three to five Lifesavers. Ask her to contact her care giver immediately.

A woman who indicates that she has diabetes may require specialized care and should include you in conferences with her care givers during which her exercise plan can be discussed and an emergency care plan arranged.

Exercise does seem to increase the effective uptake of insulin. However, mothers with diabetes must pay close attention to how they feel and what they eat. They should learn to read their own symptoms. A pregnant woman with diabetes must discuss all exercise routines with her care givers. Her exercise routine should not vary from day to day but should remain relatively constant. She should never exercise alone. As an exercise specialist, you should provide a full description of your program or the woman's regular exercise regimen so there can be a careful assessment of exercise stress. Fatigue may become a factor for the mother with diabetes, and the balance between rest and physical activity is crucial. Changes in her exercise routine or excessive exercise without adequate caloric intake may create a situation that is life-threatening for mother and fetus. It is probably advisable for anyone with diabetes, whether or not they require insulin, to monitor their own blood sugar before, during, and after exercise with a finger stick glucose monitoring device. Uteroplacental insufficiencies, as identified by a care giver, may be indicators of problems that require the cessation of exercise.

The Placenta

The role of the placenta is so important that it is considered by some to be the major endocrine organ of pregnancy. It produces hormones to sustain and support the pregnancy, and fetal survival depends on a healthy, functioning placenta.

Though mother and fetus do not share blood, most nutrients, medications, or toxins in the maternal bloodstream pass through the placenta and the umbilical cord and will be found in the fetal circulatory system.

Hormonal Activity and Exercise

It is known that exercise affects hormone productions and that different hormones affect exercise. Three hormones that may affect a woman's capacity to exercise are relaxin, progesterone, and estrogen. Relaxin inhibits uterine activity and seems to be the causative factor in the softening of the connective tissues in the skeletal system. Progesterone appears to have a wide range of effects. In large quantities it creates a feeling of fatigue and may be responsible for the increased need for sleep that so many pregnant women experience. It also affects the uterine environment, enriching and thickening it to support the fertilized egg, and the development of the lobules of the breasts. Its presence may cause a rise in maternal basal temperature as well as a rise in respiratory rate. Estrogen, produced by the ovaries, placenta, and corpus luteum, also promotes the successful maintenance of the pregnancy. It may contribute to the morning sickness some women experience. Estrogen stimulates the growth of the uterus and the enlarging and readying of the breasts for lactation.

Implications for Exercise

Women with endocrine system abnormalities may have difficulties conceiving and/or maintaining a pregnancy and may be advised not to exercise. There have been some studies to determine whether fetal response to exercise can be affected by placental health and circulatory efficiency but these have not evaluated endocrine functions of the placenta during exercise.

Pregnant women who develop diabetes may be advised that some studies have reported that the beneficial effects of exercise for the individual with diabetes include maximized oxygen uptake, decreased blood pressure, and the potential for improved glucose control. However, documentation of long-term effects of exercise during a diabetic pregnancy is not complete.

Is It Safe to Exercise During Pregnancy?

When a healthy pregnant woman exercises regularly and monitors her own heart rate and her body's responses to exercise stress, the chances are good that it is safe to exercise during pregnancy. Perhaps the most confusing aspect of the research on pregnancy and exercise is that it is highly technical and somewhat inaccessible to the average reader. In this section I will try to summarize some of the most important research findings.

Most of the research on pregnancy and exercise has addressed one of five questions:

1. How does exercise affect the fetus in utero?
2. How does prenatal exercise affect the fetus at birth?
3. What are the effects of exercise on the mother?
4. Are there practical applications of these research findings?
5. Does prenatal exercise have any effect on the length of labor?

The epidemiological and laboratory studies of pregnant women have attempted to determine at what level maternal activity interferes with fetal development. Review of the research shows that infant *Apgar scores* and birth weights have been conscientiously recorded in hundreds of births to mothers who exercise. An Apgar score, which is given twice in the minutes just after delivery, is a method for providing a quick evaluation of an infant's condition at birth. The infant is given a score from 0 to 10 that rates its muscle tone, heart rate, respiratory effort, reflex irritability, and color. Infants who score below 8 may require special care. Infants born to mothers who exercise have not shown any significant incidences of lowered Apgar scores.

The last 10 years have seen the advent of highly accurate fetal monitoring systems, and observation of the human fetus during maternal exercise also has been successful. The problems with invasive testing of human subjects persist, however, and efforts to determine the exact effects of blood flow shunting away from the uterus are still inconclusive. Sheep, goats, guinea pigs, and rabbits have all been tested but the results have been contradictory depending on the species and intensity of exercise. Evidence of fetal hypothermia has been demonstrated in animal studies. Evidence of neural tube defects, preterm deliveries, and small-for-gestational-weight offspring has been revealed in animals exercised until exhaustion.

No studies are available on injuries due to exercise during pregnancy. The normal softening of the body's musculature may be responsible for joint pain experienced and described anecdotally by female athletes. Avoiding sudden changes in direction, level, and speed as well as prolonged weight-bearing flexion may help to eliminate some injuries. We might speculate that injury to the symphysis pubis, which can occur in runners, may be potentially more serious in the pregnant runner.

Exercise strengthens the body's muscles and bones. It has been found that aerobic training before conception and a prenatal maintenance program improves a woman's functional cardiopulmonary levels. Women with improved physiologic health tend to feel better, report fewer discomforts, and may suffer reduced incidences of hypoglycemia. Studies as to the length of labor and trained women's ability to tolerate labor better than untrained women are inconclusive. Fetuses born to women who exercise are usually full term with normal birth weights.

Research at a Glance

Following is a brief summary of current research to answer some important questions about exercise during pregnancy.

What Are the Effects of Exercise on Fetal Well-Being in Utero?

Healthy pregnant women underwent mild exercise programs to evaluate the effects of maternal work. Fetal breathing movement, scanned by sonograms, often increased in response to carbon dioxide and glucose in the maternal bloodstream. Fetal heart rates usually increased slightly in response to maternal exercise. The data suggest that there are no cardiovascular signs of fetal distress immediately after moderate maternal exercise (Marsal, Gennser, & Lofgren, 1979; Pijpers, Wladimiroff, & McGhie, 1984; Platt, Artal, Semel, Sipos, & Kammula, 1983).

Does Exercise Effect Fetal Well-Being at Birth?

Research has shown that fetal heart rate climbs slightly during maternal exercise and may take up to 22 min to return to normal, but affected fetuses have not exhibited distress at birth. In the three studies of exercisers, joggers, and nonexercisers, no correlations were found between moderate exercise and fetal well-being at birth, birth weight, or Apgar scores. One study of 336 women who participated in regular vigorous exercise showed a slight increase in incidences of low birth weight but did not indicate low Apgar scores (Collings, Curet, & Mullin, 1983; Dale, Mullinax, & Bryan, 1982; Hauth, Gilstrap, & Widmer, 1982; Jarrett & Spellacy, 1983; Lotgering, Gilbert, & Longo, 1984).

How Do Pregnant Women Respond to Aerobic Exercise?

Research has shown an increase in aerobic capacity in exercising pregnant women and a decrease in aerobic capacity in nonexercising women. Four major observations about pulmonary function include decreased functional residual capacity, increased ventilation, increased vital capacity, and unchanged total lung capacity. In addition, pregnant women have an accelerated respiratory response during moderate exercise. Women who exercise show a faster adjustment to exercise stress, although adjustments may not occur efficiently under vigorous exercise stress. Finally, oxygen consumption and oxygen debt are greater later in pregnancy.

Far less margin of reserve was observed in terms of cardiac output; when under stress the heart could not increase output to meet increased demand (Edwards, Metcalfe, Dunham, & Paul, 1981; Knuttgen & Emerson, 1974; Pernoll, Metcalfe, Schlenker, Welch, & Matsumoto, 1975).

Can Exercise Testing Be Applied to Routine Obstetrical Care?

Experimental research to determine whether uteroplacental insufficiency or fetal stress can be measured from responses to maternal exercise has been inconclusive. Exercise does not seem to be a factor in preterm delivery; women who have participated in sports and fitness activities may have a decreased risk of preterm delivery. Factors shown to be related to preterm delivery include bleeding during pregnancy, low maternal weight gain, alcohol and substance abuse, and history of miscarriage or infertility (Berkowitz, Kelsey, Holford, & Berkowitz, 1983; Pomerance, Gluck, & Lynch, 1974).

What Is the Relationship Between Exercise and the Length of Labor?

Research has shown that training improves cardiac output and decreases resting heart rate but has no effect on the length of labor. Aerobic training may improve stamina and reduce the tendency toward hypoglycemia, which may enhance the individual's ability to withstand labor; however, fitness training does not appear to affect the length of labor (Morton, Paul, & Metcalfe, 1985; Snyder & Carruth, 1983).

Summary

Traditional advice to women regarding the impropriety of exercise during pregnancy appears to have little or no factual basis. While moderation is always good advice, at this time the evidence for drastic reduction of maternal physical activity during a normal healthy pregnancy does not exist. The healthy and well-integrated body adapts miraculously and mysteriously to pregnancy and exercise. There is a great deal more to be learned from the study of prenatal exercise physiology. I highly recommend that those of you who are exercise instructors take the time to explore this fascinating field in more detail.

In the next chapter we will take a look at female anatomy and the actions of the muscles most directly affected by pregnancy. Learning about the muscles of the body and the structures of reproductive anatomy is especially important to instructors who work with pregnant women.

Chapter 3

Female Anatomy

In this chapter we will look closely at the musculo-skeletal system, the structure and related organs of the torso and pelvis, and the muscles that directly affect a woman's ability to carry her pregnancy and successfully deliver her baby. I will discuss the muscles whose strength and flexibility enable a woman to maximize her active participation in and control of childbirth.

The information presented in this chapter should help you to understand and teach about the structures of female anatomy and their relevance to choices about exercise. The overview of the muscles of the torso, shoulder girdle, pelvic girdle, and hip joint is provided to enhance your understanding of and ability to determine the range, options, and choices of exercises you may suggest to pregnant women. If you are interested in a more detailed review, refer to Luttgens and Wells (1982).

Most women enjoy learning about their bodies, and during pregnancy they want to be in tune with, pay attention to, and listen to their bodies for cues about their health. Those of you who teach women about childbearing and exercise should be able to respond with sensitivity to the pregnant woman's need to know about her body and should be comfortable using and explaining the vocabulary of female anatomy. To facilitate your understanding of the terms used in this chapter please refer to the glossary at the back of the book.

The Pelvis: Baby's First Cradle

The female pelvis is shaped to carry and protect a fetus in utero and, in most cases, to allow the fetus to pass down and through the birth canal to be born. It is a stable, bony structure that absorbs much of the impact of movement. Its shape is bowl-like, with high, flaring sides. The passage through which the baby must travel during birth is surrounded by the pelvic bones and is referred to as a canal. The entrance to the canal is called the pelvic inlet and the exit is referred to as the pelvic outlet.

The proper name of the pelvis is the os innominata. It is actually composed of three bones that are fused together and form the bowl shape of the pelvis: the ischium, the pubis, and the ilium. The major pelvic bones are shown in Figure 3.1.

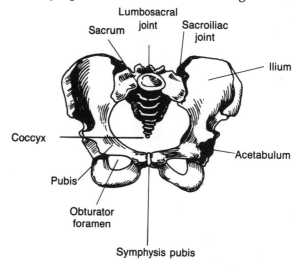

Figure 3.1. The major pelvic bones.

The front of the pelvis is formed by the joining of the two pubic bones at the symphysis pubis. This arch-shaped juncture is united by two main ligaments and a fibrocartilage disk. Normally there is little or no movement at this joint. During pregnancy there is some softening of the cartilage, and the pubic bones may separate from 1 to 12 mm to allow enlargement of the pelvic cavity. Excessive separation may lead to pain and difficulty in walking.

The front of the pelvis has two large openings formed by bony bars called rami. Blood vessels, nerves, and muscles pass through these openings, referred to as the obturator foramem. The back of the pelvic girdle is formed by the coccyx, a tiny bony structure, and the sacrum, the triangular wedge-shaped bone of the lower back. The coccyx is attached to the sacrum at the sacrococcygeal joint. The fifth lumbar vetebra of the spine meets the pelvis at the lumbosacral joint. The sacrum is joined to the hip bones at the sacroiliac joint, a very stable, sliding joint. The entire pelvis is supported by the long thigh bones, the femurs, at the hip joints.

The hip joint, which is formed by the articulation of the head of the femur in the acetabulum, is one of the strongest joints in the body. Despite its weight-bearing responsibilities it is also one of the most flexible. At the point where the head of the femur meets the acetabulum of the pelvis, three ligaments of heavy fibrocartilage wrap around and support the joint. Figure 3.2 shows the anterior view of the ligamentous support of the hip.

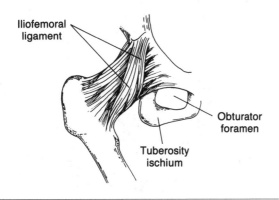

Figure 3.2. The right hip joint with iliofemoral ligament. The ligaments of the hip joint make it very strong and flexible.

The strength and flexibility of the iliofemoral and pubofemoral ligaments on the anterior and the ischiofemoral ligament on the posterior make the hip very difficult to dislocate.

Stretching to Increase Flexibility

Throughout pregnancy the hormones progesterone and relaxin contribute to the increased flexibility and softening of the ligamentous support of the sacroiliac, symphysis pubis, and hip joint. Special care should be taken to avoid damaging these ligaments during exercise. As mentioned earlier, to promote exercise safety you should avoid choosing those activities that require repetitious or prolonged unsupported flexion and forceful outward and downward pressure on the flexed femur when seated. You should avoid leading rapid, ballistic stretches, which include bobbing or bouncing motions and which depend on the momentum and weight of the body to stretch the muscles. During pregnancy women should perform stretching gently and slowly to prevent injury. This method, called static stretching, gently and gradually stretches the tissues. No stretches should be taken to the maximum point of resistance. Pregnant women should not feel pain when practicing stretching exercises. It is also sensible to discourage women from anticipating a rapid return to vigorous stretching exercise immediately after childbirth to avoid postpartum injury.

Mobility of the Pelvis

Strong ligaments weave in and out of the pelvis, giving it support and allowing it to move. Although its mobility is limited, it moves as a unit, rotating up and down or to the left and right. Proper training during pregnancy can directly affect its mobility during delivery by enabling a woman to exercise direct control over the tension and flexibility of the abdominal and pelvic muscles.

The sacrum, which forms the back wall of the pelvis, has fairly limited mobility. It does, however, move slightly forward and backward. When the torso is flexed forward, the sacrum goes forward with the spinal column and the coccyx extends slightly backward. In this position the outlet of the pelvic canal can be positioned to be open and at its widest angle for childbirth. Exercises that mimic the C curve of birth (chapter 10) enhance a woman's understanding of and ability to achieve this maximally opened position.

Almost every muscle that you use for the flexion or extension of the torso and thigh is attached at some point to the pelvis. Those that cause the abduction, or opening, of the thighs and flexion of the trunk are the most important in terms of exercise and childbirth. We will discuss those muscles in greater detail shortly. The muscles that contribute to adduction, the movement of the thigh in toward the midline of the body, should be strengthened and gently stretched to promote flexibility for childbirth.

The Pelvic Floor Muscles

The pelvic floor muscles encircle the pelvic outlet and extend from the sacrum and coccyx to the ischium and the symphysis pubis (see Figure 3.3). A pair of muscles referred to as the levator ani, forms the sling that supports all the organs of the lower abdomen, including the uterus, vagina, rectum, urethra, and bladder. These muscles are in two layers; the outer layer is referred to as the perineal layer, the inner as the pelvic diaphragm.

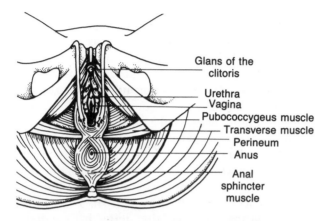

Glans of the clitoris
Urethra
Vagina
Pubococcygeus muscle
Transverse muscle
Perineum
Anus
Anal sphincter muscle

Figure 3.3. The pelvic floor muscles support and encircle the urethra, vagina, and anus. These muscles are in two layers. The outer layer is referred to as the perineal layer, the inner as the pelvic diaphragm.

The levator ani includes the pubococcygeal and iliococcygeal muscles. The pubococcygeus is the most dynamic of the pelvic floor muscles. It acts as a sling for the vagina and supports the rectum. The iliococcygeus serves as a support layer. Proper exercises to strengthen and relax the perineum are an essential component in any prenatal routine.

The perineum is a diamond-shaped space below the pelvic floor that is divided into two triangles: the urogenital triangle and the anal triangle. The deep transverse muscles of the perineum come together at the midline of the urogenital triangle, encircling the urinary meatus (opening of the urethra) and the opening of the vagina, and forming the vaginal and urethral sphincters (Olds, London, & Ladewig, 1984, p. 67). The central point of the perineum is called the perineal body. It lies between the posterior angle of the vagina and the anus.

During delivery, the perineum and its muscles stretch to allow the fetal head to descend and emerge. Tears, bruises, or small lacerations of the perineum can occur during childbirth. A rapid birth or uncontrolled pushing can contribute to the incidence and severity of tears. A slow, controlled delivery and complete relaxation of the perineal muscles can help to prevent tearing during birth.

The following exercises and precautions help to reduce the possibility of a tear of the perineal body during birth:

- Pelvic floor exercises, referred to as kegel exercises (chapter 10).
- The physiologic pushing technique (chapter 11).
- The feather-blowing technique (chapter 10).
- Perineal massage before and during labor (chapter 12).
- Childbirth in a lateral sims (side-lying) or upright position rather than the lithotomy (back-lying with feet up in stirrups) position.
- Warm towels against the perineum during labor and manual support for the perineal tissue as the baby's head crowns.

Many medical practitioners perform episiotomies to prevent perineal tears. An episiotomy is an incision made at the mouth of the vagina either laterally, to the side, or medially, downwards toward the anus. It is occasionally made on an angle or in the shape of a J. The incision is usually about 1-1/2 in. long, and it goes through the skin as well as the muscle of the perineum. It is usually performed as the baby's head distends the perineum. At this time the skin is stretched very tightly and the episiotomy can be done without an injection of local anesthesia.

Women who work closely with their care givers, pursue perineal support and massage during labor, feel the baby's head with their own hands as the baby is born, and are able to relax and respond with gentle breathing techniques during birth rarely need episiotomies. Women who are able to relax and release their vaginal muscles fully, who are not encouraged to lie on their backs with their legs up in stirrups, and who are not rushed do not need episiotomies.

Routine performance of episiotomy is unnecessary. There is no evidence to prove that it is better than the slight tears that may occur during a normal birth. Cases of extreme concern may warrant an emergency widening of the vaginal outlet, but routine interference may be harmful and disruptive in the average birth.

The Uterus

The female reproductive tract is protected by the strong bones of the pelvis. The uterus, which is a pear-shaped muscle, nestles within the lower abdominal cavity, surrounded in front by the bladder and behind by the rectum. It responds to the menstrual cycle, the effects of hormones produced by the pituitary gland, and the ovaries, which cause ovulation. During pregnancy, the uterus, often referred to as the womb, grows from a relatively small pelvic organ into the largest abdominal organ. It displaces the intestines, stomach, and heart and puts pressure on the bladder, rectum, and abdominal wall. Total capacity of the uterus at the end of pregnancy is 500 to 1,000 times greater than in the nonpregnant state.

The uterus has three layers: an outer covering called the perimetrium, a thick muscular layer called the myometrium, and an inner layer called the endometrium. The myometrium has three layers of muscle. The outer layer has fibers that run longitudinally. The thick middle layer has interweaving strands, and the inner layer has muscle fibers that run circularly, around the entire organ. The endrometrial layer thickens and is shed during menstruation.

The uterus is the center of the reproductive tract (Figure 3.4). On either side are the ovaries and the fallopian tubes. The ovaries are small, almond-shaped organs that play a crucial role in the timing and changes of the reproductive cycle. The ovaries contain the cells that eventually produce oocytes, or eggs, that will mature during a woman's reproductive life. In the middle of each menstrual cycle an egg is released from one of the ovaries. This is called ovulation. After ovulation the egg floats into the fan-shaped funnel that forms the entrance to the fallopian tube. The fallopian tubes are the oviducts through which the egg, or ovum, travels. Fertilization usually takes place within one of the fallopian tubes. The fertilized ovum travels the remainder of the way down the fallopian tube and implants itself into the endometrial lining of the uterus. A successful implantation is called a pregnancy. The corpus luteum, the site at which the egg erupts and is released by the ovary, produces the hormones that initially cause the lining of the uterus to become enriched and to thicken. If no pregnancy occurs, the corpus luteum dissolves. If fertilization leads to a successful implantation, the corpus luteum continues to function for several weeks, until the placenta begins to secrete its hormones.

The uterus is divided into three sections. The fundus is the top of the organ. It is easily palpated and its height is a fairly dependable measurement of fetal growth. The body, or corpus, is the main part of the uterus. It is thick walled and is the main contractile portion of the organ. The isthmus is a small narrow section of the uterus that lies above the internal os of the cervix. The cervix is composed of an internal os (opening), a cervical canal, and an external os. The cervix is composed of muscle and connective tissue. The external cervical os can be seen during an internal exam. It softens and dilates during labor and can be examined manually. The tip of the uterus, where it meets the vagina, is called the fornix.

During pregnancy the cervical os is covered with a film called the mucous plug. In the nonpregnant state the cervix is also bathed in mucous. However, after fertilization, the mucous thickens and completely closes the opening of the cervix to prevent bacteria or other foreign matter from entering the uterus.

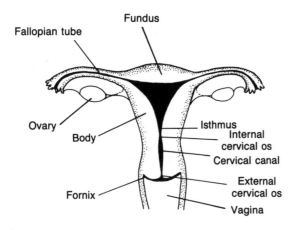

Figure 3.4. The uterus is the center of the reproductive tract. On either side are the ovaries and fallopian tubes. *Note.* From *Human Labor and Birth* (p. 19) by H. Oxorn, 1986, Norwalk, CT: Appleton, Century Crofts. Copyright 1986 by Appleton, Century Crofts. Adapted by permission.

Support for the Expanding Uterus

In addition to support from the levatore ani, the uterus is supported by the uterosacral ligaments, the broad ligaments, and the round ligaments. This support system is somewhat inadequate for the upright posture of the Homo sapiens, and I have often wondered why there was not a uterine ligament that stretched up over the shoulder. If we were quadrupedal, that is, if we still walked on four legs instead of two, as other mammals, or if we used our hands for support as pregnant primates do, our uteruses would be adequately supported and would hang down and swing freely. As most pregnant women would agree, pregnancy would be much more comfortable in the all-fours position!

Immediately after pregnancy, the deeply stretched uterine support ligaments should not be strained. It takes 6 to 16 weeks for the softened, stretched ligaments to regain their pre-pregnancy elasticity, and excessive and strenuous activities can hurt and possibly interfere with recovery.

The Vagina

The vagina is the canal that leads from the uterus to the external orifice of the genital canal. The vagina is capable of great elasticity. A woman may insert her finger into the vagina to feel how its walls mold to its shape. The vaginal walls respond in the same way to the insertion of a tampon or to penetration during intercourse. They are capable of stretching very far to allow the passage of the baby down and through the birth canal.

During pregnancy the walls of the vagina thicken. There is increased mucosity and increased vascular circulation. The increased mucosity is similar to that which occurs after ovulation. Women who feel that vaginal secretions are excessive may want to wear a minipad during exercise routines. Vaginal secretions that have an odor or that are irritating or discolored may be signs of an infection and should receive treatment. Late in pregnancy vaginal mucosity usually increases and shortly before delivery may be pink or somewhat bloody. This indicates that the cervix is softening and ripening for labor and that the mucous plug, which covers the cervical opening of the uterus during pregnancy, has begun to separate. Women who have had a pinkish or blood-stained discharge should not participate in exercise classes.

Women's health and fitness education must include a study of the reproductive tract and the organs we have discussed. Self-awareness and the pleasure of understanding one's own anatomy are the elements of pride and self-esteem, often sadly lacking in women who have never been encouraged to know and appreciate their own bodies.

Structure and Muscles of the Torso

In addition to having a general understanding of the anatomy of the pelvis and the reproductive tract, the exercise instructor should be aware of the other structures and muscles of the torso. Most women study their torsos with a critical eye. As the uterus grows, the appearance of the torso is radically changed.

The bony structures of the torso include the spinal column, the thorax, and the pelvis. The vertebral column that we call the spine is made up of 33 vertebrae, which are the intricate bones that form the system of flexible support for the torso. The spinal vertebrae house the spinal cord, which is the relay system for the entire central nervous system.

Twelve pairs of ribs make up the bony structure of the thorax or rib cage. The first 10 pairs articulate with the sternum, and when the sternum is lifted, the thoracic cavity is lifted, giving the impression of excellent posture. However, simply lifting the rib cage in an exaggerated military stance is not really an example of good posture. The remaining two pairs of ribs are called floating ribs. It is this area of the thorax that widens late in pregnancy, flaring out to accommodate the enlarging uterus and angled diaphragm. The manubrium (the bony upper portion of the sternum), the body of the sternum, and the xyphoid process (the tip of the sternum) make up the other bones of the thorax.

All of the muscles of the torso can be strengthened during pregnancy. Even the abdominal muscles, which must stretch as the uterus grows, can be strengthened. Exercise routines should be planned carefully to avoid strain. After performing strengthening exercises, which include contraction of a muscle group, women should follow with a gentle relaxed stretching of those muscles.

Before beginning any exercise class or routine, you should be aware of a fairly benign condition called diastasis recti. Diastasis recti is a separation of the rectus abdominus at the midline of the belly. Multiple pregnancies coupled with being overweight tend to be factors in this condition. A woman with diastasis recti may palpate her abdomen and feel the separation. To do this she should lie on her back with her knees bent and her feet flat on the floor. She should lift her head and shoulders so that she is just beginning to work the abdominals. It may be wise to begin each new exercise session with this procedure. If she can feel any opening (i.e., from a quarter of an inch to several inches) between the muscles from the belly button down the midline of the belly to the symphysis pubis, she should discuss her exercise routines with you and her care giver. She can support a mild separation during exercises, but she should be careful to avoid straining the abdominals. An opening of an inch or more may prevent a woman from engaging in vigorous routines but should not prevent her from engaging in milder forms of exercise.

Kinesiology

Before we begin our study of the muscles of the body, I would like to introduce you to the term *kinesiology*. Kinesiology is the study of movement, including the anatomical and mechanical aspects of movement and the systematic analysis of that movement. It is a fascinating field and beyond this introductory material there is an abundance of excellent resources available for study. We will discuss many concepts related to kinesiology but first, there are two that I would like to introduce at this time because of their relevance to our perspective on healing and becoming whole through learning.

The first is the concept of synergy, which was used earlier to describe the interactive and interdependent nature of the body's systems and of the maternal-fetal system. The word synergistic is used to describe the combined actions of groups of muscles that contribute to a movement or prevent undesirable movements. The muscles of the body all work in groups, with no one muscle's ever being completely responsible for movement. When movement is initiated, muscles on both sides of the bones work together. The agonist muscles pull on the bones to create the movement whereas the antagonist muscles stabilize the movement and prevent unwanted actions. The agonists are those muscle groups that are directly responsible for a movement. They are considered movers when they are contracting. The antagonist muscles are on the opposite side of a joint being moved by an agonist. They stretch when the agonists contract, and if they were to contract they would produce the opposite effect of the agonists. Some muscles act to neutralize others; other muscles act to stabilize a bone or a body part. All movements occur because of the synergistic and cooperative actions of the muscles.

The second idea that comes from kinesiology is that there are two types of motion: linear motion from place to place and angular motion, which rotates around an axis or turns around while staying in one place. In chapter 1, we referred to the traditional model of health and healing as a linear model. That is, it moves from one assumption to another assumption in a straight and logical line, often ignoring or leaving out information that does not follow logically or in a systematic manner. A more holistic model of healing has been described as being somewhat spiral, much like a double helix. The spiral model suggests that healing and living are a moving process, going around, sometimes coming back to the starting point, but always moving through a gentle curvilinear pattern.

If you combine the linear descriptor of movement with the angular descriptor, you will find that you are describing a moving, spiraling process that in fact can be seen as a holistic spiral of life and health.

Now let's look at the body and its muscles. Figures 3.5, 3.6, and 3.7 show you the major muscles of the trunk and upper legs. Being able to refer to these muscles by name enhances your ability to

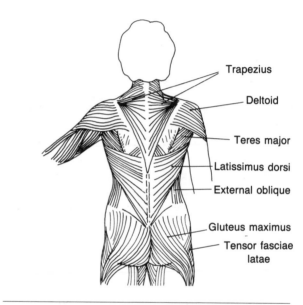

Figure 3.5. The major muscles of the posterior trunk and upper legs in the nonpregnant female.

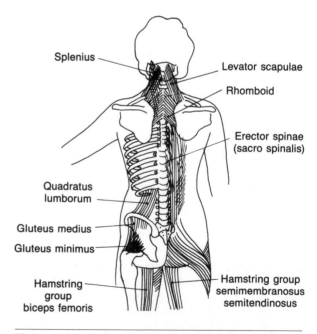

Figure 3.6. Further detail of posterior muscles.

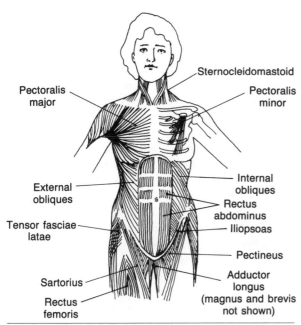

Pectoralis major

Sternocleidomastoid

Pectoralis minor

External obliques

Internal obliques

Rectus abdominus

Tensor fasciae latae

Iliopsoas

Pectineus

Sartorius

Adductor longus (magnus and brevis not shown)

Rectus femoris

Figure 3.7. Anterior view of the muscles in the nonpregnant female.

instruct women about exercise, posture, and the efficient use of their bodies during pregnancy.

Look at the function of the muscles in the diagram, remembering that, although there are many more muscles of the body, we are now focusing quite specifically on those that affect a woman's ability to carry her pregnancy in relative comfort and to use her body efficiently during childbirth.

Terminology of Muscle Action

The muscles of the body act to create the force necessary for movement. The location of each muscle determines its action. Muscles work together and are often referred to as members of muscle groups acting on bones to create movement. Those movements include the following:

- Flexion: the bending of a joint that decreases the angle between the two bones that meet at that joint.
- Extension: the unbending that increases the angle of two bones meeting at a joint.
- Hyperextension: movement beyond the neutral position.
- Abduction: movement away from the midline of the body.
- Adduction: movement towards the midline of the body.
- Rotation: either inward or outward turning of the bone at the joint.
- Circumduction: rolling or circular motion.

Many muscles are capable of producing several actions, and, in most cases, the location of a muscle determines the action it can produce. Muscles on the anterior (front) of a joint produce flexion. Muscles on the posterior (back) of a joint produce extension. Muscles on the medial (inner) side of a joint produce adduction. Muscles on the lateral (outer) side of a joint produce abduction.

The Muscles of the Neck

If you pay attention to your neck for a moment and allow your head to move you will discover that the structure of the neck and the muscles that support it allow for a great deal of flexibility. The neck can rotate, flex, extend, and hyperextend. It can also flex laterally. Seven muscles actually contribute to this range of movement, and they surround the neck anteriorly, laterally, and posteriorly. The lateral and posterior muscles of the neck and shoulder are easily strained during nursing and while carrying infants and their equipment, and it is wise to strengthen them during pregnancy to avoid discomfort later on. The splenius (posterior) helps to keep the head erect by maintaining proper postural position of the neck. The sternocleidomastoid (anterior and lateral) flexes the head and rotates it. Exercises that promote flexibility of the neck and avoid hyperextension are recommended during pregnancy. The use of light weights and performance of exercises on Nautilus machines or Universal gyms that strengthen the upper back and the upper arms also contribute to strengthening the neck. Bridging, in which the weight of the body is supported by the head and neck, is not recommended. It is not necessary for most pregnant women to use head harnesses or resistance training to strengthen their necks.

The Muscles of the Shoulder

The muscles of the shoulder girdle directly affect posture and appearance. The shoulder girdle itself consists of the clavicle and the scapula. The shoulder girdle is identical on both sides of the body. The very strong, long bone of the upper arm, called the humerus is included in this discussion of the shoulder girdle.

The shoulder girdle can move up, which is the hunching of the shoulders called elevation, and down, which is the return to normal position called depression. The rolling motion of the shoulder girdle is called circumduction and it can also flex, adduct, abduct, and rotate.

The shoulder joint, referred to as the glenohumeral joint, occurs where the head of the humerus meets the scapula at the glenoid cavity. It is a shallow ball-and-socket joint. The shoulder joint is very flexible with a wide range of motion. Range of motion is determined by several factors. One is the shape of the joint itself and the bones that articulate it. The second factor is the restraining effect of the ligaments and tissues that surround the joint, and the third is the bulk of those tissues. Range of motion is also called flexibility. The movements of the shoulder joint include flexion, hyperflexion (flexion beyond 180 degrees), extension, hyperextension (swinging backwards beyond the anatomical position), adduction, abduction, outward and inward rotation, and circumduction (swinging the arms in a circle). Like the hip joint, the shoulder joint is well supported by bands of ligaments. Unlike the hip joint, the shoulder joint has no weight-bearing function except when an individual assumes an inverted posture.

The structure of the joint and the muscles that surround it allow for the great movement and strength of the arm. The muscle groups that flex the shoulder joint lie on the anterior side of the joint. They also contribute to outward rotation of the arm. Those muscles that are superior, or above the joint, move the arm up and away from the body, whereas those on the inferior side of the shoulder joint draw the arm down and in toward the body. Muscles on the posterior side of the joint extend the arm.

The anterior muscles of the shoulder girdle cover the chest. The pectoralis major is a fan-shaped muscle that provides support for the breast while working to flex and medially rotate the arm and draw it towards the body. It is assisted by the pectoralis minor, which lies beneath it and helps to lift the rib cage and improve posture. The women in your classes can strengthen these two muscles by performing modified push-ups throughout pregnancy and using light weights or pulleys.

The trapezius muscle contributes to the stability of the shoulder girdle and promotes the movement of the deltoid muscle, which flexes and rotates the arm. The levator scapulae acts with the trapezius when the shoulders are hunched up and works during lateral flexion of the neck. It is important for the maintenance of good posture. Exercises that promote flexion, elevation, depression, and rotation of the shoulder girdle increase the strength of the trapezius and levator scapulae muscles.

The rhomboids act with the trapezius muscles to depress the shoulders. These can be exercised by doing the front crawl stroke when swimming. Weakened rhomboid muscles lead to forward rotation of the shoulders. The latissimus dorsi, a broad sheath of muscle that covers a large portion of the back, is also considered part of the posterior shoulder group. It acts to draw the arm in towards the body, rotate it, and move it from front extension to the side. The teres major assists the latissimus dorsi in all of its actions.

The deltoid muscle, on the superior side of the shoulder joint, is a very complex muscle that contributes to flexion, extension, and complete range of motion of the shoulder. It works with the trapezius. Rowing, throwing, shoulder presses, and a range of arm lifts strengthen the deltoid muscle.

The biceps brachii and brachialis cover the front of the upper arm. These muscles flex the arm. The biceps works to turn the forearm outward, supinating the hand. The triceps, on the back of the upper arm, extends the forearm. These muscles should also be strengthened through a wide range of exercises, calisthenics, and weight training, in preparation for the hard work of mothering.

The Muscles of the Abdomen

The muscles of the abdomen are layered longitudinally, horizontally, and diagonally. They stretch during pregnancy and can be used very effectively during the bearing-down portion of delivery. They are also the cause of much postpartum frustration as many women try to regain their flat tummies. Weak abdominals allow the pelvis to rotate forward, aggravating the curve in the lumbar portion of the spine. Exercises to strengthen but not strain the muscles of the abdomen are appropriate during pregnancy.

The rectus abdominus is a long, broad muscle that runs longitudinally from the front of the pubic bone to the ribs. It controls the tilt of the pelvis, and, by holding the pelvis up in front, it helps to flatten the back, reducing the curve in the lower back. It acts to flex the lumbar and thoracic portions of the spine. When only one side contracts, it produces lateral flexion to the same side. A strengthened rectus abdominus muscle makes the erector spinae more effective as an extensor of the spine, causing the hip flexors, especially the iliopsoas muscle, to be more effective in raising the leg. Modified situps are excellent for strengthening the rectus abdominus.

The external oblique is a broad muscle that runs diagonally from the ribs to the anterior portion of the iliac crest. It contributes to forward and lateral flexion when both sides are acting together and to twisting to the opposite side when both sides are acting singly. The external oblique muscles work independently or with the rectus abdominus. The internal oblique muscles are also diagonal sheaths that lie below the external obliques and pull in the abdominal wall. When working on one side, they produce lateral flexion to the same side and when working together, they produce flexion of the lumbar and thoracic spine.

The transverse abdominus (not illustrated in Figure 3.6) lies beneath the rectus. In the non-pregnant state, it helps to keep the abdomen flat, along with the obliques and the rectus abdominus muscles. Pregnant women can exercise the transverse abdominus by pulling in and attempting to draw the belly back toward the spine.

Exercises that strengthen the muscles of the anterior of the torso enhance a woman's ability to participate in a variety of sports and activities in addition to helping her play an active role in the delivery of a baby. Weakness in the abdominal muscles leads to poor posture, backache, and inferior performance in a wide variety of activities. Modified sit-ups and curl-ups with variations in the placement of the hands and arms (i.e., crossed over the chest, on top of the head, reaching through the legs) are recommended. Lifting the head and shoulders forward as well as diagonally during a modified sit-up is permissible during pregnancy. Knees should always be bent. Some women enjoy rocking curl-ups, which lift the feet and buttocks from the floor. Straight, back-lying double leg lifts should be avoided. After sit-ups, women should roll to their left side and gently stretch their arms up and overhead to relax the abdominal muscles.

The muscle of the posterior side of the abdomen is the quadratus lumborum, which originates on the inner lip of the iliac crest and inserts at the two lower ribs on the back. This important muscle works during extension of the lower back and in lateral flexion.

The Muscles of the Back

It is essential to work on posture, postural awareness, and posture improvement by strengthening the muscles of the abdomen and the back throughout pregnancy. Proper postural alignment assures that the body is stable. Though it is difficult to strengthen the extensors of the back and spine directly during pregnancy, because those exercises frequently require one to lie prone on the belly, many exercises that strengthen the anterior and lateral muscles of the torso will contribute to the strength of the back muscles. The careful use of light, hand-held weights may increase the effectiveness of those exercises.

A large group of muscles previously called the sacrospinalis, and now referred to as the erector spinae, covers the entire back, from the base of the skull to the posterior crest of the ilium and down to the sacrum. This group has many insertion points and functions best when the pelvis is held up in front. You can easily observe that the abdominals work most effectively at holding the pelvis up in front when the back is straight and the ribs are held up.

The Muscles of the Hip and Thigh

We have already discussed the bony structures of the pelvis and the hip joint. Like the shoulder joint, the hip joint is a ball-and-socket joint that has considerable flexibility. However, because of its weight-bearing function, it is more stable than the shoulder. The deep cavity of the joint provides this structural stability. The muscles of the hip and thigh are called into action in all sports, many dance and yoga exercises, the martial arts, and, of course, childbearing.

The muscles of the hip and thigh can be divided into groups by their action and location. Many of the muscles perform several functions. This is due to the sizes and different fibers of the muscles themselves.

The Hip Flexors

The hip flexors contribute to the efficient placement of the body and use of strength during the birth of the baby, referred to as the expulsion of the fetus. The iliopsoas, on the interior of the upper thigh, is a strong hip flexor. It assists with flexion of the hip and, when the thigh is fixed, forward flexion of the trunk. It works to raise the leg when an individual is supine. It can be strengthened by performing V-sit exercises, flexing and extending the legs while supine, running, and performing standing leg-raises at the ballet barre. The pectineus on the front of the pubis, works in flexion, adduction, and slight rotation of the thigh. The sartorius runs from the ilium to the inside of the thigh and is the longest muscle of the body. It works during flexion and rotation outwards. When a woman sits in a cross-legged, tailor position, the sartorius contributes to the abduction and outward rotation of the hip. The rectus femoris is a powerful flexor running from the iliac to the patella. It flexes the thigh and extends the knee. The second phase of a sit-up, in which the trunk curls forward, also strengthens the hip flexors.

The Hip Extensors

The extensor group includes the gluteus maximus, the biceps femoris, and the hamstring muscles. The gluteus maximus originates across the back of the ilium and along the sacrum and inserts on the back of the upper portion of the femur. It is the largest and most powerful of the three muscles of the buttocks. It works to extend the thigh and rotate it outward. Depending on the work required of it, the gluteus maximus may adduct or abduct. This powerful muscle gives shape and firmness to the buttocks area when it is strong, and there are significant fatty deposits surrounding it in most women. Using the stationary bicycle is a good way to strengthen the gluteus maximus during pregnancy.

There are three extensor muscles included in the group called hamstrings. The hamstrings support the body as it accelerates through movements. The biceps femoris originates at the tuberosity of the ischium and extends down the back of the thigh to below the knee. It works during extension of the thigh, flexion of the knee, and outward rotation of the lower leg. The semitendinosus and semimembranosus also extend the thigh, rotate the thigh inward, and flex the knee. Strengthened hip extensors decrease the forward tilt of the pelvis.

The Hip Abductors and Rotators

The hip abductors include the other two gluteus muscles that lie close to and below the surface of the gluteus maximus. The gluteus medius originates on the outside of the hip on the ilium and inserts on the outside of the thigh. It works in abduction and rotation of the femur inward. Tension in the muscle stabilizes the pelvis during walking. The gluteus minimus lies beneath the medius. Its primary function is inward rotation of the femur and it helps with abduction. The medius and minimus muscles work together during many activities to prevent the standing hip from sagging.

If the gluteal muscles are weak the pregnancy waddle is even more pronounced. The tensor fasciae latae contribute to flexion, slight abduction and inward rotation of the thigh. Strengthening the hip abductors while stretching the adductors allows a woman to function efficiently during the expulsion phase of labor.

The adductor group (i.e., longus, magnus, and brevis; not shown in Figure 3.6) contributes to adduction and flexion of the thigh. Placing a beach ball between the feet or legs and squeezing it strengthens the hip adductor group.

There are six deep outward rotators of the thigh that rotate the hip outwards and assist in stabilizing the femur. They are strengthened through practice of many dance and athletic activities and through the healing exercises described in chapter 11.

Summary

Cultivating strength in the muscles of the torso, abdomen, pelvis, perineum, and the hips is extremely important for pregnant women. These muscles work synergistically to align the body and allow it to move. It is important to help women understand that weakness in one area can lead to strain and overcompensation in another area. This imbalance can predispose women to a variety of pregnancy-related discomforts and injury. Firm, toned, strengthened muscles allow a woman to carry her pregnancy in relative comfort. Delivery of the fetus is facilitated by strength in the abdominals, perineum, and thighs, and recovery from childbirth is speedier and happier for a woman in good physical condition.

In chapter 4 we will introduce and discuss guidelines for exercise during pregnancy. In 1985 the first exercise guidelines for pregnant women were published by ACOG. ACOG was established in 1951 and has been providing continuing educational services, setting guidelines for improved health care, and developing prenatal care programs for over 30 years. In our search for balance and integration of information, it is important to evaluate guidelines with a careful and objective eye. Doctrines regarding women's health and fitness have, over the years, been unnecessarily restrictive. However, these materials are vitally important to our professional practice and to the health and safety of the women in our classes. In the next chapter, we will examine the guidelines, their implications for exercise, and their impact on instruction.

Chapter 4

Pregnancy Exercise Guidelines

Childbirth educators and fitness instructors should be aware of the guidelines for exercise during pregnancy and postpartum recommended by the ACOG (1985). These guidelines can help you to establish screening processes for your students. Understanding the language of the guidelines will make it possible for you to determine the safety of your routines and the accuracy of the advice you offer to students regarding many different kinds of exercise.

Implications for the careful scrutiny of these guidelines are far-reaching. Because no other widely accepted guidelines exist for pregnancy and exercise, your understanding and willingness to explain the content of these guidelines help to establish your credibility and the credibility of all prenatal and postnatal exercise specialists. I do not mean to suggest that you must adopt these exercise guidelines as absolute law. Rather, you should look at the guidelines as parameters within which we can safely work as well as a baseline for professional reference. As research confirms or alters the guidelines our teaching techniques will stand the test of time and professional responsibility. Much of the material in the guidelines can also be found in Artal and Wiswell (1986, chapter 17). The ACOG guidelines are available by writing to the American College of Obstetricians and Gynecologists in Washington, DC.

In the first three chapters we examined many of the changes in anatomy and physiology that occur during pregnancy. As many authors have pointed out, many of these changes are predictable and well understood, whereas the causes and effects of others remain mysterious. Those that we do not understand have become the most important fac-

tors in research and in developing recommendations on and about prenatal exercise.

Until very recently there were no definitive exercise guidelines for pregnant women or those who had recently given birth, and most women were advised to exercise or not based on common sense (which can be reliable or not) and a variety of old wives' tales. Recent overviews of research and recommendations for prenatal exercise have advised caution and a conservative approach to exercise. Concern for fetal well-being and prevention of low birth weight prevails in most studies. Exercise guidelines from work by Morton, Paul, Campos, Hart, and Metcalfe (1985) and Snyder and Carruth (1984) are similar to and consistent with those published by the ACOG (1985).

Guidelines for Exercise During Pregnancy

The ACOG guidelines emerged from extensive research findings on maternal and fetal well-being during exercise and fetal condition at birth. Over the past dozen years, physicians and other medical researchers have conducted research and collected results of laboratory experiments conducted on women, sheep, pigs, and various rodents in an effort to determine the effects of maternal exercise. The animal research has been far more intrusive than that done on the humans. The information on the effects of exercise on pregnant quadrupedal mammals, therefore, is far more complete than it is for humans. It is also somewhat contradictory; for example, the degree of decrease in uterine blood flow varies considerably in different research studies on pregnant ewes, though it appears that uterine blood flow returns to normal shortly after cessation of activity. Questions regarding the redistribution of blood flow to the uterus and the amount of oxygen available to the human fetus remain unanswered. However, though pregnant human subjects have not been manipulated in the laboratory to the same extent as the other pregnant mammals, they have been carefully monitored, and the guidelines seem, at the present time, to offer a sound, if somewhat conservative, basis for exercise prescription.

The ACOG publication recommends that before enrolling in any exercise class, a pregnant woman should have a complete physical. Prenatal care is one of the most vital components of maternal/fetal health. A woman may choose a clinic, a private obstetrician, or a midwife; however, the model of health care that a woman chooses should be of less concern than the importance of making the choice to seek the best care possible for herself and her child.

Most women receive a thorough physical when they initiate prenatal care. Care givers should now routinely discuss exercise with their pregnant clients. Women who participate in regular exercise or who plan to participate in exercise activities during their pregnancies should receive specific information about pulmonary and cardiovascular rates. Individual rates should be measured and suggestions for target heart rates and limits should be explained. Refer to chapter 5 for more detailed information on heart rates.

A prenatal exercise program for women in the general population should specify the type, intensity, and duration of all activities. Safety for both mother and fetus should be of primary concern (Artal & Wiswell, 1986, p. 226). Artal and Wiswell identify these as the most serious risks for mother:

- the potential for musculoskeletal injury,
- cardiovascular complications,
- premature labor, and
- hypoglycemia.

The most serious risks for the fetus include

- possible fetal distress,
- intrauterine growth retardation,
- fetal malformations, and
- prematurity.

Though some of these risks sound extreme, research in this area is not yet complete. It seems wise to advise cautious moderation of exercise intensity. Careful monitoring of intensity, length, and frequency of exercise should become routine in your classes or exercise facility.

Guidelines for Exercise Intensity

When women ask about how far they should run or how much they can do, they are asking about exercise intensity. The ACOG guidelines (1985) suggest that cardiovascular peak heart rate should be kept to 140 beats per minute (bpm). For most women, this means a reduction in exercise intensity. In their discussion of applications for exercise stress testing, Artal and Wiswell (1986) suggested that exercise intensity be lowered at least 25% because of reduced cardiac reserve. This must be understood, however, in the context of the women in the general population. The range and gradations of age and fitness of pregnant women who participate in fitness activities will be represented in your classes. It will be important to take into account the 49-year-old multigravida (a woman who has had more than two children) for whom a heart rate of 140 bpm would be much too high, or the long-distance runner who may be able to tolerate a much higher rate of cardiovascular stress. Therefore, it is extremely important for you to stress individualized heart rate tracking in your classes. By teaching women to monitor carefully their own responses to exercise intensity, you can significantly reduce the risks to both mother and fetus.

The ACOG Exercise Guidelines

In this section, a synopsis of the exercise guidelines is provided for your use. I have paraphrased and elaborated on each of the ACOG exercise guidelines where appropriate and provided definitions to enhance their clarity.

- Pregnant women should engage in regular exercise, at least three times a week.

    Sporadic, inadequate, or overly strenuous activities do little for fitness and can lead to injury. Regular aerobic exercise, at least three times a week, has been shown to improve cardiovascular functioning in pregnant and nonpregnant individuals. Exercise sessions should include a warm-up, a combination of stretches and strength-building exercises, and a cool-down.

- Competitive activities should be discouraged.

    Because maternal pulmonary function does not necessarily compensate for increases in oxygen demand during high levels of aerobic activity (ACOG, 1985, p. 2), this guideline is designed to protect both mother and fetus from the effects of overexertion, hyperventilation, hyperthermia, and fatigue. In addition, cardiac output, which increases during pregnancy, usually cannot increase in the event of excessive demand. Many athletes have competed successfully throughout pregnancy; several women have won medals at the Olympics (1952 and 1956) and others have participated in marathons. Performance is not automatically affected adversely by pregnancy, however, concerns for their health and safety have led many athletes to withdraw from competition by the third or fourth month. Obviously, each individual, with her care givers, must determine her own competitive destiny.

- Vigorous exercise should not be encouraged when it is hot and humid or when the mother has a fever.

   As discussed earlier, pregnant women have more difficulty dissipating excess heat and may become overheated, dehydrated, or seriously ill during exercise if it is excessively hot or if she has a fever.

- Women should avoid ballistic movements (e.g., rapid, propulsive jumping or pounding), and twisting, jerky movements to protect maternal joints and ligaments.

   Ballistic is a term applied to stretching techniques that involve repeated contraction and release of muscles to stretch the antagonists while the agonists work. Most prenatal instructors prefer static stretching to increase flexibility. In a static stretch, the muscles are passively moved into their longest position. Research has shown that this method is less likely to produce injury or muscle soreness.

- Women should perform exercise on a carpeted floor, a wood floor, or an exercise pad.

   Avoid a bare tile or concrete floor at all costs.

- They should avoid deep, unsupported flexion to protect the joints.

   Maternal hip and knee joints are particularly vulnerable. Stretches should not be taken to the maximum point of resistance.

- Sudden changes in direction, level, or speed should be avoided.

   This guideline has three implications. First, it is meant to help prevent injury to joints or

strain of the supportive ligaments. Second, it helps to prevent orthostatic hypotension, which refers to a drop in blood pressure due to changes in postural position. Many pregnant women experience a moment of dizziness or slight nausea when they move quickly from the supine position to sitting or from sitting to standing. Gradual shifts in position and level help to avoid orthostatic hypotension. And third, it addresses the problem of the pregnant woman's changing center of gravity and the difficulty that she may have in maintaining her balance when suddenly shifting positions.

- Instructors should begin exercise sessions with a 5-min warm-up and end them with a cool-down of similar length.

   Most reports of injury in an exercise program seem to include the admission that the warm-up was superficial or totally lacking. Warming up increases blood flow as well as oxygen uptake while raising the body's temperature. A warm-up can be related or unrelated to the activity or skill to be performed. Thus a walk, a slow jog, or a few minutes on the stationary cycle may be a warm-up just as easily as stretches or calisthenics. The warm-up should not be of such long duration that it causes the body to get too hot or induces fatigue. Although the guidelines recommend a 5-minute warm-up, most instructors feel that the length of the warm-up should correspond to the length of a class. I usually lead 5 to 15 minutes of warm-up activities for large groups where there are many individuals at different levels of fitness. Intensity and duration of the warm-up, as well as the cool-down, should be adjusted to each individual, her level of fitness, and the length of her exercise period.

- Heart rate should be measured at peak activity level.

   Use the 140 bpm as a baseline but work closely with women whose physical condition may warrant additional monitoring. Remember that some women may feel they are working too hard before their heart rate reaches 140 bpm. Always ask women how they are feeling, if the workout feels too strenuous, or if they need a break.

- Women who have led a sedentary life-style should begin exercise at a very low level of intensity.

You should not discourage women who have not participated in regular fitness activities from participating during pregnancy. Review fitness, smoking habits, and any physical limitations of the sedentary woman and develop an individualized program for her.

- Activity should be stopped and the care giver contacted if any unusual symptoms appear.

  We will discuss these symptoms and some of their possible causes and implications shortly.

- Strenuous activities should not exceed 15 min in duration.

  Rest periods during which maternal heart rate returns to normal should be part of your program. Until research proves that longer aerobic exercise sessions are safe, you should guarantee the safety of your students and protect yourself from possible liability. Weight-bearing aerobic exercise should be alternated with non-weight-bearing activities to protect joints and ligaments.

- Women should avoid exercises in the supine position after 16 weeks gestation to avoid hypotension caused by pressure on the inferior vena cava.

  This recommendation has aroused much discussion. There are some exercises that simply cannot be performed if a woman is not permitted to lie on her back. Adaptations to this guideline include doing a few repetitions of an exercise and then rolling onto the left side for recovery or limiting the period of the time on the back and alternating back-lying with side-lying exercises. Instruct your students to roll into the left lateral position immediately if back-lying exercises cause discomfort, a feeling of suffocating, or dizziness. Remember that in the advanced stages of pregnancy, lying in the supine position may reduce kidney output.

- Breath-holding and the Valsalva's maneuver should be avoided.

  This means that a pregnant woman should not hold her breath while exercising or hold her nose and blow hard to puff out the cheeks and pop her ears.

- Caloric intake should meet the extra needs of pregnancy and exercise.

  Pregnant women should not exercise to lose weight or control weight gain. In fact, women who exercise should eat more to insure that they continue to gain weight at a steady and reasonable pace throughout their pregnancies.

- Maternal core temperature, which rises during extended periods of exercise stress, should not exceed 39 °C.

  Most women are not able to take their temperatures while exercising. Cautions include not exercising when feverish, or when it is especially warm or humid, always dressing in cotton or other exercise clothing that breathes, avoiding exercising in rooms with poor ventilation, and avoiding overheating.

- Liquids should be taken before and after exercise and, if necessary, during class. This is to avoid dehydration (ACOG, 1985, p. 4; Artal & Wiswell, 1986, p. 227).

The guidelines recommend that prenatal exercise focus on strengthening muscle groups, avoiding strain on the ligaments of the abdomen and torso, and correcting postural shifts that frequently accompany pregnancy. It is important to remember that rest and relaxation during and after exercise periods, as well as exercise of varying tempos, are components of a well-balanced program.

Reasons for Restricting or Terminating Exercise

In most cases, women whose current physical condition is described by the categories below should be advised to avoid vigorous exercise. Portions of this list appear in ACOG (1985) and Artal and Wiswell (1986, p. 226). I have added definitions and commentary.

- Active myocardial disease (disease of the inner muscular wall of the heart)
- Congestive heart failure (failure of the heart to maintain adequate circulation of the blood)
- Rheumatic heart disease and/or other heart and blood pressure problems
- Thrombophlebitis (inflammation of a vein with the existence of a blood clot)
- Recent pulmonary embolism (blood clot in the lungs)
- Severe isoimmunization (a pregnant woman with the Rh factor in her blood who is at risk for becoming sensitized to the fetal Rh factor and may produce antibodies that can cause serious disabilities in her baby)

- Those at risk for premature labor due to obstetrical history, multiple gestation, or an incompetent cervix (i.e., a cervix that is malformed or incomplete or that is effacing or dilating too early)
- Any signs of vaginal bleeding or ruptured membranes (vaginal discharge of either blood or the amniotic fluid that surrounds the fetus)
- Evidence of intrauterine growth retardation (as measured by sonogram or fundal height)
- Suspected fetal distress (as documented by reduced fetal movements, fetal monitoring, measurements of intrauterine growth retardation, or sonogram)

Women who fall into any of these categories should be well informed about the seriousness of their physical condition, its treatment, and potential risks of the treatment. These women are considered high-risk obstetrical patients, and they compose a small but critical number of pregnant women.

Reasons for Restricted or Closely Monitored Exercise

Other women whose pregnancies are in high-risk categories may experience conditions that are not immediately life-threatening but do call for carefully restricted or closely monitored physical activity. The risks and benefits of exercise during pregnancy for these women should be carefully evaluated by all of those involved with their care. Reasons for carefully monitoring or restricting exercise include the following:

- Hypertension
- Anemia or other blood disorders
- Thyroid disease
- Diabetes mellitus
- Breech presentation during third trimester
- Excessive obesity or extreme underweight
- History of extremely sedentary life-style (ACOG, 1985; Artal & Wiswell, 1986, p. 226)

These health conditions sometimes lead to complications that mandate the avoidance of exercise for pregnant women. In these situations careful maternal and fetal monitoring is essential. If you are working with women who fall into this category you will have to work closely with a medical care giver to assure that exercise is not placing the mother or fetus in jeopardy.

When to Stop Exercising

Occasionally, the onset of symptoms that signal a woman to stop exercising are quite sudden. Dizziness, nausea, or pain are signs to stop exercising. Other symptoms may be more gradual or go unnoticed until they become serious. The following symptoms should signal the exercising woman and her instructor that she should stop exercising. In all cases a medical care giver should be contacted immediately (ACOG, 1985; Artal & Wiswell, 1986).

- Onset of sudden or severe chest pain
- Onset of a sudden and severe headache
- Onset of uterine contractions

  If a woman thinks that she is in labor and is experiencing contractions at 20-min or shorter intervals she should not be exercising, although walking is probably safe. A woman experiencing persistent Braxton Hicks contractions, the normal tightening of the muscular uterus that occurs throughout pregnancy, during class should stop exercising. She should be advised to change her level of activity and see if they go away. Persistent Braxton Hicks contractions late in pregnancy may indicate an irritable uterus that may precipitate labor. Persistent Braxton Hicks contractions themselves may be interpreted as labor but are usually diagnosed as false labor and do not lead to delivery.

- Vaginal bleeding

  Vaginal bleeding at any stage of pregnancy usually, but not always, indicates that the pregnancy is in serious jeopardy.

- Leaking of amniotic fluid

  The amniotic fluid surrounds the fetus in utero. If the amniotic sac has ruptured a woman should stop exercising and expect the onset of labor.

- Fainting, dizziness, confusion
- Palpitations (rapid fluttering heart beats) or tachycardia (rapid heart rate)

  Any irregular or rapid heart beat should be cause to stop exercising.

- Shortness of breath
- Onset of nausea or vomiting
- Back, pubic, or hip pain
- Difficulty walking

  Any severe pain or unusual symptoms related to foot pain, a sprain, or injury to the symphysis pubis may cause difficulty in walking.

- Sudden onset of edema or blotchiness of skin surface

    Edema, fluid retention, is swelling of hands, face, extremities, or torso. Blotchiness of skin surface may indicate circulatory problems. Either symptom may indicate a negative change in maternal condition.

- Decreased fetal activity

    A mother can learn to check regular fetal activity by having a light meal that is high in carbohydrates and then lying down. After about half an hour the metabolized nutrients will begin to reach the fetus. The woman can then count fetal movements in response to the meal. There should be a minimum of 12 movements per hour. Fewer than that may indicate an inadequate activity level and call for consultation with a care giver.

You should provide this information to your students early in the class. Women should learn to be aware of their bodies and to monitor their own reactions to exercise. Most pregnant women want to be careful. They don't want to hurt themselves or their babies. It is your responsibility to empower them with the information they need to exercise moderately and confidently.

Applying Exercise Guidelines

The information in these guidelines is vitally important. Yet, many instructors have raised the question, How can I be sure that I am creating the safest routines possible? This section describes simple measures you can take to make certain that your classes fall within the suggested exercise parameters.

First of all, always remember that moderation is the key to a successful exercise program. Maternal pulse and blood pressure rates tend to rise much more quickly during exercise, and oxygen consumption does not always rise to meet the increased demands of vigorous activities. Indeed, pregnant women feel fatigue much more quickly as a result of this moderate oxygen debt. Sudden bursts of high-energy activities or prolonged workouts are not appropriate. Tell your students that the adage "no pain, no gain" does not apply during pregnancy; rather, they should follow this rule: If it hurts do not do it.

Advise women to eat a nutritious snack about an hour before exercise and a well-balanced meal after their routines. Dieting, limiting food intake,

and thus burning the body's own stores is absolutely inappropriate. The effects of inadequate caloric intake can be detrimental to fetal development.

It is your responsibility to eliminate all dangerous or questionable movements from your class or instructional repertoire. If you are teaching prenatal classes or meeting pregnant women in your regular programs, use the following guidelines:

- Rechoreograph any routines that include rapid twisting movements; jumps; high-impact dance steps; and rapid shifts in direction, level, or speed.
- Do not include any exercises that cause hyperextension of any joint or flexion taken to the maximum point of resistance. Do not allow the participants' backs to sag or arch, do not practice gymnastic-style splits, and do not do full head circles.
- Eliminate exercises that require a woman to stand with her feet close together and then flex forward at the hip with a straight back, or to reach for her toes with feet close together and knees locked. These exercises are too stressful on the back and may crowd the uterus in women past 20 weeks gestation. If both feet are on the floor, forward flexion should always be accompanied by flexion of the knees.

Aerobic means using oxygen. If a woman is interested in aerobic exercise options she can get plenty of aerobic exercise by walking, using a stationary bicycle, jogging, swimming, or dancing. Aerobic exercise routines should be kept to the 15-min maximum suggested by ACOG. Although some women may feel that this is a very short workout, the time limit protects the body's joints and ligaments and prevents overheating. Until research proves otherwise, it may also prevent the reduction of blood flow to the uterus as a result of increased maternal blood pressure, pulse rate, or the shunting of blood out to the exercising extremities. After 15 min, mothers should rest and allow their heart rates to return to normal before beginning another session.

Before each class have women check for diastasis recti. I do this in class for four reasons. First, women must be encouraged to touch their own bodies, to feel their bellies and know that it is okay to do so. Second, by palpating their own abdomens regularly they can take note of any slight changes in or the appearance of the diastasis recti. Third, any major changes can be noted and examined more carefully by the health care specialist and fourth, any modifications in exercise can be discussed and instituted quickly and efficiently.

Emphasize that exercise should make a woman feel good, not sick. She should stop exercising if she begins to perspire profusely or feels dizzy or sick to her stomach. Women should not be encouraged to come to class if they have any signs of illness, congestion, or fever. If a woman doesn't want to exercise or if she finds a particular activity unpleasant or uncomfortable she should feel free to give it up. Your role is to support her in that decision.

Slow down your routines and help women tune in to their own bodies. Talk about body signals. Ask them if they can feel the baby reacting to the exercises or the music. Make exercise safe, fun, and personal. Each woman in your class should understand that she is responsible for herself and for her baby. Her body is her best guide, and she knows it better than anyone else.

Student Permissions and Waivers

At this point, we must carefully consider the professional performance responsibilities and potential liabilities of prenatal exercise instructors. There is no doubt that this is a potential arena for litigation. It is imperative that you purchase malpractice insurance that covers you in the routine performance of your profession. Some instructors work for athletic facilities or health care centers that act as their insurance umbrellas. Independent instructors do not have this security. Those of you who fall into the latter category may want to look carefully for coverage before you begin teaching.

It is your responsibility to screen the women who wish to enroll in your classes. The materials from the ACOG (1985) guidelines should be very helpful. In addition, as consumers and participants, women must be informed of the potential risks of prenatal exercise discussed in this chapter. You should be prepared to provide your professional credentials and a list of references to any women who request such information.

You would be wise to require every woman you are supervising to have written permission to exercise from her attending physician or midwife. Women who have had more than two miscarriages, a history of precipitous labor, uterine cramping, spotting or bleeding, or who are carrying twins may be advised not to exercise. The ACOG guidelines (1985) advise women who have had two or more abortions not to exercise.

As an instructor, you should be familiar with each student's age, general health, number of previous pregnancies, and previous exercise levels. You should ask your students to provide this information on their registration forms. You should then adjust the pace and technique of your class to its various members at their different stages of pregnancy. You should be aware of the responses to exercise that are particular to pregnancy.

You should screen women for postural or anatomical problems that can contribute to discomfort or injury. Women with scoliosis, a condition in which there is a mild to severe sideways curving of the spine; bow legs; knock knees; or extremely flat or high arched feet may have problems that require special consideration during prenatal exercise.

You would be wise to have each class participant sign a waiver of responsibility and a disclaimer that relieves you of any legal or financial responsibility in case of an accident or injury. You should definitely seek legal advice regarding the wording of your release form. I have included examples of the registration information (Appendix 4.1) and waiver (Appendix 4.2) forms I have used in my program to give you some direction in creating your own forms.

Summary

Deciding to conduct prenatal exercises means that you are willing to take on the responsibility for other women's health and well-being. I have tried to make the research and recommendations in the first four chapters of this book as clear and meaningful as possible so that they are helpful to you. It is important that you evaluate your own qualifications for teaching such classes. Have you attended any special workshops for exercise instructors or studied the physiology of pregnancy, labor, and delivery? If a woman came into your class and asked you specific questions about exercise during pregnancy, could you provide well-informed answers or refer her to another recognized authority? Your answers to these questions will give you a good idea how competent and comfortable you feel about working with pregnant women.

I think it it essential for instructors to work in cooperation with other professionals who are specialists in prenatal care. Your classes should be observed by these professionals, and, as a team, you should develop a philosophy about exercise, education, and safety. No one should ever work in a vacuum. Feedback and the exchange of information and ideas are essential to professional growth.

As the research specialists and physiologists proceed with their work, we will all learn more about the effects of exercise on the maternal-fetal unit. It remains our responsibility to keep abreast of all new developments and keep all systems open to new information.

In Part II of this text we look at ways to modify popular fitness activities for pregnant women. The information should help you to adjust your teaching and expectations about pregnant participants. Women who are participating in these activities will ask you whether they are safe and how they should be modified during pregnancy. Careful consideration of the structural and functional changes of pregnancy, as discussed throughout the first part of this text, should contribute to your understanding of the modifications suggested.

Pregnancy Exercise and Education Registration Information

Today's date _____   Your due date _____

Name _____ Age _____

Address _____ City and zip _____

Phone _____ Emergency phone _____

Work phone _____

Care giver's name _____

Are you aware of any health/risk factors that may affect your freedom to exercise? _____

  If yes, please indicate. _____

Do you have diabetes? _____ High blood pressure? _____ History of miscarriage? _____

Are you experiencing leg cramps? _____ Side aches? _____ Backaches? _____

  Heartburn? _____ Any other pregnancy-related discomforts? _____

Don't be shy, how about varicose veins or hemorrhoids? _____

My general physical condition is

  Excellent _____ Good _____ Fair _____ Poor _____

I am especially interested in learning more about

  Education for childbirth _____

  Exercises for pregnancy _____

  How to maintain strength and stamina _____

  Expected and adequate weight gain _____

  Relaxation and breathing for labor and delivery _____

  Sexuality and self-image _____

  The anatomy and physiology of pregnancy _____

Any other areas of special interest? _____

Number of previous pregnancies _____

Number of previous live births _____

May we use pictures of you taken during class for seminars or workshops? _____

Prenatal Exercise Waiver

Please read this form carefully and discuss it with your medical care giver.

I, _____ , have enrolled in (<u>class title</u>) pregnancy exercise and education classes of my own free will and with the permission of my doctor, _____ .
I am not considered a high-risk pregnancy and have no physical problems that would put me or my baby in jeopardy during an exercise class.

I hereby release and forever discharge _____ and (<u>class title</u>) and any of its instructors of and from all claims of action, suits, manner of actions, and causes of actions whatsoever, for or by reasons of any cause or matter arising out of my participation in this program.

Signed _____ Date _____

If you have any questions, please feel free to call me.

Part II

Modifying Popular Fitness Activities

When a women chooses to participate in exercise, she makes a choice that is an active and positive decision to mobilize the body, stimulate its metabolic functions, and encounter self as an active and dynamic force. When a woman chooses to participate in exercise during pregnancy, she is choosing to be an active agent in the establishment and maintenance of her own health. Her choice means that she is willing to assume more responsibility for her own health, her baby's health, and the health of her family. She is learning, changing, and growing through exercise, and all of her choices fit into the holistic approach to prenatal health education.

It is important to keep in mind that almost all women, even if they are single parents, are members of families. Fitness activities are chosen on an individual basis, but they can contribute to the whole family's health and enrichment. The health and wellness of each family member affects the others, and individual as well as family health fluctuates depending on the individuals and the environment. The health of the family ecosystem depends on the health of its individual members.

I believe that during pregnancy, the body is on a journey to an unknown, inborn peak. During pregnancy a woman will have to modify her activities for the maintenance of both physical fitness and self-esteem. Although she does not need to train her body to carry a pregnancy, she can train herself to be strong and to carry her pregnancy in relative comfort. Experiencing the balance between personal fitness, family wellness, and self-esteem is a fluid, joyful experience. As maternal health and fitness educators we can promote this positive experience by modifying exercise programs to meet the needs of our class participants.

Chapter 5

Exercise Programs: Objectives and Precautions

Exercise has been classified in many ways. In this chapter we look at the traditional objectives of exercise. This information will be helpful as you integrate traditional and holistic concepts about fitness.

Depending on the activity and its purpose, participation may or may not contribute to maternal well-being during pregnancy. You need to know which activities are safe for pregnant women and which should be avoided. You should be able to evaluate the goals of activities and their relative safety for the pregnant participant.

Carrying a child is probably the most dynamic experience a human being can have. The transformation of the physical body is a mere fraction of the greater cognitive and emotional transformations that occur during the creation of life. During this time, many women are interested in developing a sense of belonging to their changing bulk and of coping with their changing body boundaries. It is important for you to initiate discussions about exercise objectives with your students so that decisions about participation can be made on a shared basis. Consider each woman's skills, needs, interests, and limitations in this process.

Classifying Exercise by Objectives and Goals

According to ACOG (1985), "the goals of exercise during pregnancy and the post-partum period should be to maintain the highest level of fitness consistent with maximum safety" (p. 3). Exercise includes a wide range of activities, and there are many ways to classify exercise. According to Cooper and Cooper (1972), exercise can be classified as having the following objectives: improved cardiopulmonary stamina, weight loss, body building and contouring, and sheer enjoyment and play. Let's look at these objectives in terms of the pregnant woman and her specific needs.

The first objective is improving cardiovascular fitness, which is an appropriate exercise objective during pregnancy. The American College of Sports Medicine (ACSM, 1978) and ACOG (1985) have both issued guidelines on the quality and quantity of cardiovascular exercise. Though the ACSM guidelines apply to the general population, they suggest that to build cardiovascular stamina the healthy adult should participate in regular exercise, three to five times a week, with a duration of 15-60 min. Though pregnant women have been advised to reduce the length of standing aerobic sessions to 15 min per session, they may repeat their workouts after heart rates return to normal as often as desired as long as signs of exhaustion and overwork do not appear. Pregnant women should never complain of stress fractures.

Weight loss, the second objective of exercise, is rarely advisable during pregnancy. Dieting and exercising to lose weight tend to reduce the calories available to the growing fetus and may create a situation that is harmful to the fetus if body fat is burned.

The Coopers' third objective is body contouring, which is one of the goals of weight lifting. Body sculpting or body contouring is not an appropriate goal of prenatal exercise because the female form sculpts itself during pregnancy. The widening girth of the abdomen, hips, buttocks, and thighs is the body's natural adaptation to maternity. Muscles can be toned during pregnancy, however, and muscle toning is certainly advisable.

Finally, the fourth objective is that exercise should be fun. This is very important for prenatal classes because it motivates students and puts them at ease about exercise. Exercise classes, tapes, books, and records are all designed to promote the enjoyable qualities of exercise.

Fitness Components for Pregnant Women

The ACOG (1986) Safety Guidelines for Women Who Exercise describes fitness as having three major components: aerobic endurance, muscular strength, and joint flexibility. All three of these are appropriate objectives for the healthy pregnant woman. Each is dealt with in turn in the following sections.

Building Endurance During Pregnancy

Many women train seriously for athletic competition. They work to increase their performance speed and endurance and to strengthen their muscles. Many pregnant athletes and dancers have been known to perform very well. However, as we have discussed earlier, pregnancy puts most women at a disadvantage in competitive sports because of the increased demands on the cardiopulmonary system and changes in the center of gravity.

A pregnant woman may train to improve endurance by increasing the repetitions of an exercise and participating in activities during which the pace is held at an even rate over the entire length of the program. Sustained activity improves the ability of the body's circulatory and respiratory systems to function efficiently, supplying the body with oxygen and nutrients and tolerating the build-up of lactic acid. Lactic acid is the waste material produced by the cells during exercise. Both the disposal and the tolerance of lactic acid directly affect endurance. Pregnant women should not dramatically increase the speed or intensity of their activities to improve endurance. Intensity in weight lifting usually refers to the amount of the weight that is moved. Intensity in movement refers to the amount of energy expended or to speed. Building endurance requires consistent practice. Cardiovascular training less than twice a week, at less than 50% of maximum heart rate, for less than 10 min at a time does not improve endurance.

Building Strength During Pregnancy

Strength is defined in a variety of ways and is affected by the kind of muscular contraction involved as well as the speed of those contractions. Strength building usually involves moving increasingly heavy loads. During pregnancy strength can be built if the level and length of performance are extended very gradually. Extremely careful supervision of those increases is mandatory during pregnancy.

Strength-building exercises can be classified by the kind of muscular action they require. Isometrics involve contracting muscles without moving a joint. There is tension but no movement in an isometric exercise. Pushing both palms together or contracting muscles of the body to induce tension are isometric exercises. Women with hypertension should not engage in isometric exercise. Isotonics are the contraction of muscles to perform within a range of movement. The muscles shorten while working a consistent load. Weight lifting, some calisthenics, dance exercise, aerobics, and bowling are isotonic exercises. Isokinetic contractions are exercises performed with an even amount of tension throughout the full range of motion. The use of equipment helps the individual control the speed of muscular contractions in many isokinetic exercises. Some aspects of weight lifting, the arm stroke in the crawl, and some ballet exercises are considered isokinetic exercises.

The terms concentric, static, and eccentric are also used in discussions of strength building. Concentric contractions of muscles occur when there is the development of tension and a corresponding shortening of the agonist muscles, which flex the joint. Static contractions occur when a weight is placed in the hand, for example, and the muscles tighten but no movement takes place. The shortening of a muscle is considered a static contraction; thus, when a pregnant woman with a large belly is standing, the shortening of the extensor muscles of the back is a static contraction. Eccentric contractions of the muscles occur upon return from the concentric contraction, when the antagonist muscles shorten and the agonists lengthen to return the weight or resistance to the starting point.

The term overload is used in strength training when resistance is gradually increased so that a group of synergistic muscles—that is, a group of muscles that works to promote, support, and deter certain movements—is working against a greater resistance or weight than previously possible. True strength training, complete with visions of bar bells and bulging muscles, involves increasingly higher levels of resistance using weights or machines and is not appropriate for the average woman during pregnancy. Light weights or hand pressure add to the exercise load and should be applied with care during prenatal exercise.

Increasing Flexibility During Pregnancy

Flexibility is related to many factors, including the kind of joint involved, the tissues and muscles that surround it, and even the skin that covers it (chapter 3). It is an appropriate component and goal of prenatal exercise.

Flexibility of a joint is related to the ability of the surrounding muscles to stretch and then to relax. Because muscles tend to shorten when they are not used or when they are compensating for postural imbalance, cultivating strength and cultivating flexibility go hand in hand.

Each woman has her own unique range of motion at any given joint. As we age, postural habits, reduced activity levels, accidents, and injuries reduce our flexibility. During pregnancy the hormones estrogen and relaxin act on the body's connective tissues, bringing about an un-usual but necessary improvement in the level of adult flexibility. In exercise class we often hear women wonder aloud about being able to open their legs wide enough to allow for birth. It is important to explain that strengthening the hip flexors and outward rotators and stretching the hip extensors and inward rotators will contribute to successful body positioning during birth.

After a preliminary warm-up, stretches that elongate the muscles improve flexibility. Self-stretching, in which the individual woman controls the length of time during which she is stretching, is safe for pregnancy. Gravity-assisted stretching, which uses swinging motions to begin a stretch, is fine. Any stretches that cause pain or that are taken to the maximum are contraindicated. Assisted stretches, passive stretches, or stretches using

apparatus may be advisable for some women, especially those involved with physical therapy; however, because of the potential for injury to the joints, great care should be taken to avoid excessive pressure.

Improved Posture as a Distinct Goal of Prenatal Exercise

Posture affects breathing, balance, and body comfort. Years of incorrect posture as a result of being nagged to keep one's chest up and one's stomach in forces us into shallow breathing patterns. How can anyone breathe deeply when the torso is supposed to be rigid? Round-shouldered, kyphotic posture that depresses the chest and shortens the pectoralis muscles is equally detrimental. During pregnancy, the expanding uterus encroaches on the diaphragm and lungs, and posture can directly affect the depth and comfort of respiration.

Correct posture reduces the possibility of injuries and serves as a starting point from which all movements can be initiated. In the ideal posture, all of the body segments, head and neck, shoulder girdle, thorax, spine, pelvic girdle, legs, and feet would be evenly balanced, aligned on top of one another (see Figure 5.1).

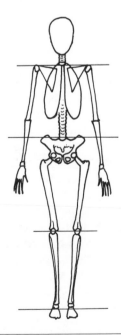

Figure 5.1. In the ideal posture, all of the body segments, head and neck, shoulder girdle, thorax, spine, pelvic girdle, legs, and feet, would be evenly balanced and aligned.

This ideal is easier to describe and to illustrate than it is to achieve, and you must remember that no one will achieve this absolutely perfect alignment, especially during pregnancy. Therefore, you should be alert to individual differences in body structure and postural alignment. By using a full-length mirror you can teach women about their body segments and experiment with how pregnancy affects their bodies' balance, stability, and alignment.

Posture, Balance, and Stability

Balance is a critical problem as pregnancy progresses. As you will recall, quick changes in direction, level, or speed are contraindicated during prenatal exercise. One of the reasons for this is that the pregnant woman experiences a change in her center of gravity. The center of gravity is a theoretical point at which the body weight is evenly distributed and thus the point at which the body is most stable. Every segment of the body has its own center of gravity, and the common center of gravity refers to the entire body and is the reference point for this discussion. The center of gravity is usually lower in women than in men, and, in fact, its location changes with every movement and in every position. External loads—or in this case, the weight of the uterus—alter the center of gravity. A new balance point must be established for movement from each new position and care must be taken as the woman continuously readjusts to the new load level. Some women compensate for the shifting center of gravity caused by the weight of the uterus by widening their stance and placing their feet further apart to form a more stable base and to reduce lumbar stress. They may also adapt their gait to what is referred to as the pregnancy waddle. The waddle is actually a healthy adaptation as long as the woman does not allow the feet to roll in or out or develop an exaggerated duck walk, which can create problems for the knees and feet.

Posture also affects stability. Stability refers to the relative ability of the body to resist being upset. The degree of stability afforded a woman in any given position will be affected by her ability to maintain the alignment of body segments and to have a wide enough base of support. High heels and a pregnant belly create a highly unstable combination. A widened stance and flat-heeled shoes increase the base of support and a woman's stability.

Proprioception is a sensory process that monitors posture, balance, and position in space. It is a feedback mechanism supported by the semicircular canals of the ear that monitor balance and structures called muscle spindles, which help maintain body position and posture by responding to muscular activity. A woman's proprioceptive system usually helps her keep her balance even as her center of gravity changes, but she may lose her balance and fall if movement is too rapid or if she is not strong enough to adjust quickly to a new or demanding movement.

Balance also means equilibrium. At term, maintaining her equilibrium may be a real balancing act for the expectant woman! The term static balance describes the individual's ability to maintain her balance in a stationary position. Strong muscles help a woman to maintain her static balance. Dynamic balance is the ability to maintain control of movement during performance. Dynamic balance may become increasingly difficult for the pregnant dancer, skater, or skier. The muscles that are the most active during standing, static balance are the iliopsoas; the soleus on the back of the leg; the hamstrings; the gluteus medius and tensor fascia latae, which prevent lateral sway; and the erector spinae, which counteract the force of gravity that pulls the torso forward. The lower abdominal muscles (the internal obliques) are active during quiet, stable standing. The trapezius, the upper fibers of the deltoids, and the serratus anterior are also active during static, balanced standing.

Balance, Stability, and Movement

As pregnancy progresses, women tend to move more slowly, being careful to maintain alignment and balance. However, occasionally a pregnant woman will have to move quickly, especially if she is caring for other small children. You should work with women to improve their ability to move quickly and directly by presenting them with skills that help them plan and anticipate how they may need to move. Some suggestions include the following:

- When she must move quickly from a lowered position to standing she should keep her body segments in the best possible alignment and use the strength of her muscles as equally as possible. Strengthening the hip extensors is essential and can help avoid back strain.
- When she must move quickly from one location to another, she should make certain that she has her balance before she begins to move. A missed step, a fall, or a strain can often be prevented.

- When she must stop quickly, she should widen her stance, bend her knees, and lower her center of gravity.

Postural Deviations and Reeducation

Women with poor posture are prone to a number of serious postural deviations, including lordosis (see Figure 5.2a), kyphosis (see Figure 5.2b), and, occasionally, scoliosis. If a deviation is severe in one area, there will be a reactive deviation in another area. Pregnant women tend to suffer from backache, pubic pain, and muscle spasms, and are vulnerable to injury because of maladaptive postural adjustments. Overall body strengthening and awareness of postural alignment are the best treatments for postural dysfunction. For an example of correct posture, see Figure 5.2c.

Postural work, including postural awareness, movement training, and muscle strengthening, is an essential component of a balanced, prenatal exercise program. Awareness of posture and the muscular strength to maintain correct posture directly affect one's appearance as well as one's self-image. Posture tells a great deal about self-

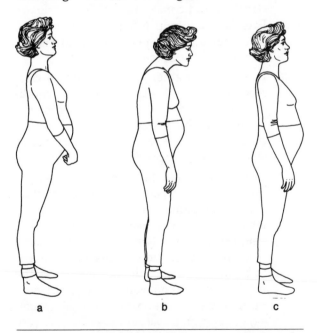

Figure 5.2(a). Lordosis leads to an exaggeration of the curve in the lumbar spine, hyperextension of the knees, and an awkward backwards lean. **(b)** Kyphosis leads to an unattractive round-shouldered appearance. Frequently the neck appears to poke forward. **(c)** Comfortable relaxed posture. The knees are relaxed, pelvis is lifted, and the shoulders are relaxed and above the pelvis, neither rounded forward nor thrust back. The ear is just above the shoulder.

esteem and reveals a great deal through silent but meaningful body language. What we do with our bodies while standing, sitting, talking, or even resting communicates volumes that never require words. Postural reeducation is almost always a positive experience. Learning that improved posture is a healthy change can be very motivating.

Summary of Prenatal Exercise Goals

The goals of prenatal exercise will be different for each woman. For some, the purpose of exercise is to relieve stress and to be able to achieve a level of relaxation after an exercise regime. Others approach exercise from a more pragmatic position, feeling that it is a safeguard against postpartum flabbiness. You will also find that some women have thoroughly integrated the goals of holistic health and exercise into their lives. In the most direct terms, the goals of exercise that are most appropriate for pregnant women to work towards include:

- maintaining muscle strength,
- improving or maintaining cardiovascular fitness,
- improving flexibility,
- improving posture,
- having fun,
- improving general health, and
- experiencing the positive integration of mind and body through movement.

For a quick guide to identifying appropriate and inappropriate exercise goals during pregnancy, see Table 5.1.

The safety guidelines we have discussed thus far put some limitations on the kinds of exercise activities that you would want to teach to pregnant women. Pregnant women should be advised to use intelligent judgment when performing any exercise routines, to avoid straining, and to avoid those activities during whose performance she could incur a severe fall. Activities should *always* be evaluated and selected on the basis of safety.

Why Women Should Exercise During Pregnancy

Exercise is important for everyone and it is especially important for pregnant women. Unless a

Table 5.1 Exercise Objectives

Objective	Recommended	Not recommended
Cardiopulmonary stamina and endurance	X	
Body contouring		X
Having fun	X	
Weight loss		X
Increasing performance speed		X
Increasing intensity		X
Maintaining strength	X	
Building strength	X[a]	
Training for competition		X
Improving flexibility	X	
Improving body/mind integration	X	
Improving posture	X	

[a]Strength building in most sports typically requires significant increases in intensity and endurance. Strength increases can be made during pregnancy but should not be undertaken without careful consideration of the pregnant woman's changing capacity for exertion. Women who wish to improve upper arm, neck, abdominal, or upper leg strength should do so gradually under careful instruction and supervision.

woman has a history of miscarriage or spontaneous abortions, is experiencing vaginal bleeding, or has some other serious medical condition, exercise should become routine from the beginning of pregnancy. Exercise can be a real bonus for pregnant women: It contributes to a sense of control, comfort, and overall health and well-being. Exercise reduces some of the common discomforts of pregnancy, helps prepare a mother for birth, and makes the postpartum experience easier. The following is a list of some of the other benefits of exercise for pregnant women.

1. Exercise leads to improved circulation, which in turn may reduce the severity of varicosities. Varicose veins can be a real problem during pregnancy. They occur when the veins lose their elasticity. Blood tends to pool, especially in the legs and vulva, causing deep purply veins that can be quite painful. Building muscular strength may help women reduce the discomfort of varicose veins.

2. Exercise can enhance muscular balance and strength. Backaches are one of the most frequent discomforts of pregnancy. Learning proper posture and how to cope with the postural shifts of pregnancy are essential to guarding against muscle and joint soreness.

3. Exercise may help reduce the edema of pregnancy and return mobility to swollen joints.

4. Exercise may ease gastrointestinal discomforts and constipation.

5. Exercise may help to reduce leg cramps. (Exercises should be performed with a flexed foot and not a pointed toe.)

6. Exercise strengthens abdominal muscles. Abdominal muscles that are in good condition and strong, stable support from the adductor/abductor muscles of the thighs contribute to the efficiency of the second stage of labor (expulsion of the baby).

7. Exercise that maintains or builds strength may create an advantage for a woman who wishes to assume an alternative position for labor or birth. In the past, women who delivered their babies lying flat on their backs with their feet up in stirrups did not have to be strong because the doctors did all the work. Women who want to give birth in an upright position, use a birthing chair, squat, sit, or kneel on hands and knees for delivery will benefit considerably from exercise.

8. Postpartum recovery can be easier and swifter for women who exercise. Firm abdominals contract much more readily after childbirth and speed the figure/weight recovery period. The postpartum section of this book describes a complete return to exercise format. In addition to aiding physical recovery, exercise may help a woman to

cope with the baby blues, which are a very common form of postpartum depression.

9. Exercise gives a woman access to her body. As her body grows bigger and heavier, she can experience those changes with grace. She learn to know herself, which can be a joyous and important experience.

10. Exercises that include the physical practice of the birth positions and breathing techniques for birth are very important for women who wish to be active participants during birth.

There is no conclusive research indicating that women in good shape have shorter or easier labors. However, they may require fewer medical interventions because they are generally in better health, are better nourished, and have more strength and stamina. The real benefits of exercise may be felt after the birth when a strong, healthy woman is able to get up, walk around, and enjoy her baby.

All pregnant women who wish to engage in prenatal exercise activities should have permission of their medical care givers to do so. Open and honest discussions about exercise intensity and frequency are a vital component of good prenatal care. A potential student should have a complete description of the type of program in which she is enrolling. Its length, the kinds of activities, and the purposes of the exercises routines should be made absolutely clear.

It may be advisable for some women to have an electrocardiogram (EKG) to determine whether there are any potential cardiac risks. An EKG taken during exercise, while the woman is on a stationary bike or a treadmill, is most informative. Blood pressure levels will be determined by a woman's care giver and monitored throughout pregnancy. If the chosen exercise program is aerobic, that is, intended to build cardiovascular stamina, a woman must learn to monitor her heart rate. She should know her normal resting pulse and be aware of the action and changes of the cardiopulmonary system if she is going to pursue an active exercise regime.

Monitoring Cardiovascular Response to Exercise

Cardiovascular fitness is considered one of the most important components of physical fitness. Monitoring one's heart rate is part of the aerobic fitness regime because the cardiovascular training effect is based on purposeful elevation of the heart rate over an extended length of time.

A simple and important lesson in learning to be responsible for one's own health is learning to monitor one's own heart rate. To begin, women should be encouraged to determine their own resting heart rates when they first wake up in the morning or after they have been sitting quietly for 10 or 15 min. Follow these steps to monitor heart rate (HR):

1. Locate pulse either on the wrist, palm up, or in the carotid artery between the Adam's apple and the side of the neck.
2. Count pulse rate (HR) for 10 seconds.
3. Multiply that number by 6.

For example, to identify resting heart rate:

Pulse rate = 12   12 x 6 = 72 = the heart rate

Cardiovascular training also works according to the overload principle. The theory is that if you gradually increase the demand placed on the cardiovascular system during exercise, the system will respond by growing stronger and more capable of performing at the required levels. As training continues, the system grows even stronger. The gradual increase in demand is important. Too much demand too soon results in exhaustion rather than training. The conditioning effects occur when exercise is neither too hard nor too easy.

Calculating Target Heart Rate

As mentioned previously, women can measure their resting heart rates before getting up in the morning or after sitting quietly for 10 to 15 min. Maximal heart rate is the theoretical limit to the number of times the heart can beat per minute. Two hundred beats per minute is the standard maximum heart rate. It is a level of extreme stress, and reaching it should never be a goal of prenatal exercise.

Monitoring aerobic exercise includes learning about maximum and minimum heart rates and target heart rate ranges. The maximum working heart rate is the upper end of the target range. The minimum working heart rate is the lower end at which an individual can work and yet still experience the cardiovascular training effect.

The target heart rate range falls between the maximum and minimum rates. Pregnant women pursuing cardiovascular training should not work within the standard target ranges. They should calculate their target ranges and work from no lower than 50% to no higher than 65% of maximum.

To determine target heart rate range, use the calculation described here. Usually target ranges are calculated to show a range within which it is safe to work. In the nonpregnant population that range is 60-90% of maximum. The first set of calculations is for a nonpregnant, 20-year-old woman who has a resting HR of 72 bpm.

$$
\begin{array}{rl}
220 \ (\text{max HR}) & \\
- \ 20 \ (\text{age}) & \\
\hline
= \ 200 & \\
- \ 72 \ (\text{resting HR}) & \\
\hline
= \ 128 & \\
\times \ .60 & \\
\hline
= \ 76.8 & \\
+ \ 72 \ (\text{resting HR}) & \\
\hline
= \ 148.8 &
\end{array}
\qquad
\begin{array}{rl}
200 \ (\text{max HR}) & \\
- \ 20 \ (\text{age}) & \\
\hline
= \ 200 & \\
- \ 72 \ (\text{resting HR}) & \\
\hline
= \ 128 & \\
\times \ .90 & \\
\hline
= \ 115.2 & \\
+ \ 72 \ (\text{resting HR}) & \\
\hline
= \ 187.2 &
\end{array}
$$

In a nonpregnant person, the cardiovascular training range would be between 148.8 and 187.2: 148.8 is the lowest rate at which training could be achieved, or the threshold rate; 187.2 is the peak of the target range, beyond which exercise would not improve fitness. In accordance with the ACOG recommendations, the pregnant woman should calculate her heart rate and plan to work between 50% and 65% of her normal target range.

$$
\begin{array}{rl}
200 \ (\text{max HR}) & \\
- \ 20 \ (\text{age}) & \\
\hline
= \ 200 & \\
- \ 72 \ (\text{resting HR}) & \\
\hline
= \ 128 & \\
\times \ .5 \ (\text{max HR}) & \\
\hline
= \ 64 & \\
+ \ 72 \ (\text{resting HR}) & \\
\hline
= \ 136 &
\end{array}
\qquad
\begin{array}{rl}
200 \ (\text{max HR}) & \\
- \ 20 \ (\text{age}) & \\
\hline
= \ 200 & \\
- \ 72 \ (\text{resting HR}) & \\
\hline
= \ 128 & \\
\times \ .65 \ (\% \ \text{max HR}) & \\
\hline
= \ 83.2 & \\
+ \ 72 \ (\text{resting HR}) & \\
\hline
= \ 155.2 &
\end{array}
$$

In this case, the target heart range for a 20-year-old pregnant woman with a resting heart rate of 72 would be between 136 and 155.2. Fifty percent of maximum, or 136 bpm would be the threshold of training, whereas a heart rate over 155 bpm would probably be too strenuous as pregnancy progressed. I highly recommend that you work with each woman to determine her individual pregnancy target range. There are also several other pretest calculations that should be done before one undertakes a serious, competitive, cardiovascular

fitness program; however, they involve using the calculated recovery heart rate. A pregnant woman who does not know her recovery heart rate should not attempt to calculate it. Such a calculation involves exercising to maximum stress levels and could be harmful to mother or fetus under these circumstances.

Monitoring Perceived Rate of Exertion

Because of the changes in the cardiovascular system, heart rate monitoring for the prevention of overexertion is not nearly as accurate as a measure of oxygen consumption would be. Calculations which determine oxygen uptake and energy expenditure, however, are not methods that are accessible to the average classroom teacher. Therefore, in addition to heart rate monitoring, I have begun using the Rating of Perceived Exertion Scale (RPE), which is based on the individual's ability to rate her own level of perceived exertion. Introduced in the 1960s by Swedish psychologist, Gunnar Borg, RPE is a numbered rating scale. Each number in the scale corresponds to descriptions of the perceived rate of exercise intensity: 7 stands for very, very light; 9 is very light, 11 is fairly light; 13 is somewhat hard; 15 is hard; 17 is very hard, and 19 is very, very hard (see Table 5.2). The original claim regarding this scale was that it seemed to correspond, if one added a zero to the end of the individual's RPE, to measured heart rates of exercisers. It is doubtful whether these results could be replicated in the general population, and I am certain they do not apply in pregnancy.

If you choose to use the RPE system, instruct your students on the use of the chart and teach them to describe how they feel during exercise in terms of the scale. During pregnancy the perceived rate of exertion will climb; that is, it will feel harder to perform at lower levels. The training zone is between 11 and 15. Although a woman may feel she is working harder at exercises that she previously considered easy, she should be reminded not to compete with her former fitness levels. Pregnant women should monitor how exercise feels and not work above the 13-15 range for more than 15 min. Pregnant women should not continue exercising above 15 on the RPE scale. Another part of learning how exercise feels includes determining whether exercise is causing uterine cramping or a decrease in fetal activity. Both are signs to reduce exercise intensity.

Table 5.2 Perceived Exertion

How does the exercise feel?	Rating[a]
	6
Very, very light	7
	8
Very light	9
	10
Fairly light	11
	12
Somewhat hard	13
	14
Hard	15
	16
Very hard	17
	18
Very, very hard	19
	20

Note. From ''Perceived Exertion: A Note on History and Methods'' by G. Borg, 1973, *Medicine and Science in Sports,* **5**, pp. 90-93. Copyright 1973 by the American College of Sports Medicine. Reprinted by permission.

[a]The rating multiplied by 10 is approximately equal to the heart rate. For example, ''Fairly light'' = 11 x 10 = a heart rate of 110.

Summary

If you are working with women who are seriously interested in pursuing or maintaining aerobic fitness you should encourage them to choose care givers who are knowledgeable about the physiology of prenatal exercise. A team approach will be necessary to monitor both fetal health and the intensity of the maternal exercise program.

The active woman, for whom pregnancy may appear to interfere with fitness objectives, should be pleased to learn how much she *can* do rather than how much is prohibited. Those who are less active should be encouraged to start slowly and enjoy! In the next chapter, pregnancy is reviewed by trimester and we will examine the relationship between fetal growth and the changes in maternal activity.

Chapter 6

Fetal Growth and Maternal Activity

In this chapter we will discuss some of the changes that occur throughout gestation and how these changes affect a woman's experience of exercise. The growth of the fetus is felt on many levels and the physical and emotional experiences intertwine, creating an extraordinary opportunity for learning. If you are interested in a full account of fetal development, refer to *The First Nine Months of Life* (Flanagan 1962).

First Trimester Fetal Development

During the first 3 months of pregnancy the embryo grows from an undifferentiated cluster of cells into a tiny, human fetus. The conceptus grows rapidly and, within a week of fertilization in the fallopian tube, implants itself into the wall of the uterus. Some women experience implantation bleeding and assume that they have had a light menstrual flow; however, this is not the case if the woman is pregnant.

Between the 26th and 28th days, buds of arms and legs appear, and during the next month the embryo continues to develop very rapidly. Even during these early weeks it moves. Its organs begin to work and its brain begins to function. These functions are, of course, extremely rudimentary.

During these critical weeks, when a woman may not even know that she is pregnant, the embryo may be particularly vulnerable to alcohol, drugs, chemicals, and the potential adverse effects of maternal disease. It is imperative that all women be alert to the negative consequences of excessive alcohol consumption, and the use of marijuana, cocaine, heroin, or other drugs that may seriously affect the developing embryo. Smoking cigarettes, drinking ginseng tea (a stimulant), and consuming excessive amounts of caffeine are also potentially harmful. All prescription medications should be evaluated by an attending care giver or pharmacist to determine their safety during pregnancy. Even aspirin should be avoided because medications for pain, convulsions, or any other maternal condition may directly affect the embryo. Urge your students to discuss the use of all over-the-counter medications with their physicians.

The potential negative effects on fetal growth due to maternal hyperthermia are unclear, but during these early weeks activities to avoid include very hot whirlpool baths, saunas, and steam baths.

Participation in athletics needn't come to an end when a woman becomes pregnant, and, for the active woman, any sport in which she is currently engaging is probably safe during the first trimester of pregnancy. However, once a pregnancy has been determined, a woman should not dramatically increase the level or intensity of her exercise regime.

There are certain activities that a woman should avoid if she thinks she is pregnant: skydiving, hang gliding, high diving, deep-sea diving, playing football or rugby, or jumping feetfirst into the water. For women who are inactive, pregnancy is not the time to initiate vigorous aerobic exercise programs. However, women whose lives have been fairly sedentary may certainly engage in sports at this time and should be encouraged to begin a gentle exercise regime (walking is highly recommended). Fatigue is a very common symptom of early pregnancy. Strenuous activities often produce significant fatigue in the trained or untrained woman. All women should know that excessive fatigue, pain, cramping, and bleeding are indicators to stop exercising.

Exercise During the First Trimester

During the first several weeks of gestation the only signs or symptoms of conception may be a missed menstrual period or the unexplained nausea or fatigue that is so common in the first trimester. Both nausea and fatigue are transient and are usually diminished by the end of the first trimester. For women experiencing fatigue, routines should be slowed and expectations for performance similarly reduced. This can cause some maternal anxiety about weight gain; mothers need to be reassured that slowing down is normal and should be expected.

Mild to moderate nausea, commonly referred to as morning sickness, occurs as a result of fluctuating hormone levels and can affect a woman's interest in exercise. Contrary to popular belief, it may occur at any time of day. Mothers should eat small, frequent meals if they are experiencing pregnancy-related nausea. Severe vomiting can be dangerous, leading to dehydration and exhaustion. Excellent nutrition is important even during periods of morning sickness, and because anemia can be a problem, mothers should take vitamins with iron to assure that the oxygen-carrying potential of the bloodstream remains optimal.

Other changes will occur in the early months of pregnancy. Many women notice tingling sensations in their breasts. This usually has no affect on exercise, though a comfortable brassiere is important.

The pear-shaped uterus expands in the first 12 weeks and soon becomes more globular. By Week 12 it can be palpated above the pubic bone. Its increased size puts pressure on the bladder, and urinary frequency is common.

Table 6.1 summarizes the symptoms or changes experienced during the first trimester and the effects of those changes on exercise. Other changes can and do occur for different women.

Table 6.1 Changes in the First Trimester

Symptoms or changes	Effects on exercise
Mood swings, fatigue.	Mother may not have the energy to exercise.
Uterus begins to enlarge.	Pressure leads to increased need to urinate. Mother should go to the bathroom before, during, and after exercise.
Bowel changes; gastrointestinal system slows down.	Increase fruit, bran, and liquid intake. Establish a regular exercise time each day. Purgatives and mineral oil are prohibited.
Morning sickness may be mild to severe.	Mom may feel too tired to exercise, but light to moderate workouts should be encouraged. Frequent light meals should be encouraged.
Breasts enlarge, causing some tenderness.	Purchase good exercise bra.
Slight vaginal discharge (luekorrhea).	Consult care giver, but slight discharge is normal. Mother may want to wear a minipad or panty liner.
Headaches.	Exercise and activity may provide relief. Relaxation and meditation may reduce stress-related headaches.
Vaginal bleeding.	Consult physician; mother should not exercise.

Second Trimester Fetal Development

Rapid fetal growth continues through the second trimester. Between 16 and 20 weeks the mother becomes aware of the fetus as it moves about, feeling a bit like butterflies or tiny tickles. The growth of the fetus is sustained by the functioning of the placenta. The placenta begins to function several weeks after conception. It is rich in blood vessels and is attached to the upper portion of the uterus. The placenta acts as a lung, a kidney, a liver, and a hormone-producing organ. The baby is connected to the placenta by the umbilical cord, which carries nutrients to and waste products from the fetus.

During the second trimester mothers should avoid dieting. Crash diets, fad diets, high-protein diets, nondairy vegetarian diets, macrobiotic diets, and even low-sodium diets (unless prescribed by a knowledgeable care giver) are not appropriate for pregnancy. Dietary plans should be developed with a nutritionist or care giver who is fully informed about prenatal physiology and who understands the caloric needs of the pregnant woman who exercises.

Women should continue to avoid using drugs of any kind. This includes diuretics; appetite-suppressants; antibiotics; certain teas, particularly ginseng; alcohol; and caffeine.

Women should feel well enough to participate in a variety of activities during the middle weeks of pregnancy. Most professional athletes give up the more competitive aspects of their sports, though skilled performance of a variety of sports is still possible. In general, slowing the pace of any game or event will help to prevent accidents. Pregnant women should avoid doing any sports or activities that involve kicks to the abdomen and lying prone on the belly or pose the potential of injury to the abdomen. Sports to be avoided while pregnancy progresses include kick boxing, high diving, fencing, deep-sea diving, hang gliding, skydiving, ice hockey, field hockey, race car driving, competitive running, and marathons.

During midpregnancy, those with or without experience may enjoy social dancing, ballet (not *en pointe*), modern dance, low-impact aerobic dance, walking, certain forms of the martial arts, swimming, working on Nautilus machines, biking, hiking, baseball, tennis, volleyball, golf, bowling, calisthenics, paddle ball, Ping-Pong, yoga, and archery. Some women continue to cross-country ski, play basketball and racquetball, ride their surfboards, and go mountain climbing!

Exercise During the Second Trimester

The second trimester begins at the 12th week and lasts until Week 24. By this time in the pregnancy, the uterus can be felt above the level of the mother's umbilicus. Many women feel the baby moving within them by 16 weeks. By the end of the 5th lunar month, or 20 weeks, even the strongest abdominal muscles will allow for a noticeable forward bulge. The crowding of the intestines and

colon, resulting from the expanding uterus, can cause constipation, but generally mothers feel relatively comfortable.

By midpoint in a woman's pregnancy, her interest in learning about pregnancy may heighten. At this time her body is working most efficiently, and any of the unpleasant side-effects of early pregnancy have probably disappeared, sometimes overnight! During these middle months a mother is most likely to join a pregnancy exercise class. In fact, by 20 weeks, it is important for her to do so to learn the many exercises that are particularly helpful for facilitating the final months of her pregnancy and the birth of her child.

Minor symptoms of heartburn or acid indigestion may be caused by the displacement of the stomach and duodenum by the enlarging uterus or by a hiatal hernia, which is the protrusion of the stomach upwards into the esophageal opening in the diaphragm. Both conditions are relieved after childbirth.

Pregnancy-induced hypertension may first be diagnosed midpoint in a woman's pregnancy. Although a small rise in blood pressure should not mandate the cessation of exercise, routines should be carefully evaluated and stress levels reduced where appropriate. Activities that require intense contractions of muscles, such as weight lifting, should be avoided. It has been shown that practice of relaxation skills can contribute to the reduction of blood pressure in some individuals with hypertension. Although research on pregnant women with hypertension is in its early stages, it has suggested that relaxation may contribute to improved maternal condition.

It is essential for women to monitor their pulse rates during any exercise. Those women who are swimming, biking, jogging, or participating in aerobic dance classes should be careful to take rest periods every 15 min and to avoid overheating.

There may be women in prenatal exercise classes who have never exercised along with those who are still playing tennis, jogging, or working out with weights on a daily basis. Those who are used to a strenuous personal workout may, as long as there are no contraindications, continue their own exercise regimes while using a prenatal exercise class as a check point. Those who are beginning to exercise for the first time should be carefully monitored.

Table 6.2 summarizes the changes that occur during the second trimester, maternal responses to those changes, and their possible effects on exercise.

Table 6.2 Changes in the Second Trimester

Physical changes	Maternal responses	Effects on exercise
Body is usually working at top efficiency.	Mothers often feel exceptionally well; tend to join exercise classes and pay attention to nutrition.	Positive.
Mother looks pregnant.	Mother enjoys maternity clothes and comraderie of other expectant women.	May experience shift in center of gravity. Should avoid exercises that hurt, leave her breathless, or require sudden changes in direction, level, or speed.
Weight gain.	Should be steady and moderate. Mother should not diet or try to inhibit weight gain.	Routines should focus on maintaining present level of fitness.
Blood pressure.	Slight decrease is normal. An increase may indicate the onset of pregnancy-induced hypertension.	Mothers with high blood pressure should not exercise unless under extremely careful supervision. Relaxation exercises and changes in diet or behavior may help reduce blood pressure.
Appearance of varicose veins.	Discomfort, tired legs.	Elevate legs when possible; wear elastic stockings for support. Avoid standing or sitting on the commode for long periods.
Constipation or heartburn.	Examine diet: Add fiber and avoid irritating foods.	May feel indigestion while doing some exercises. Movement is helpful and stimulates the digestive system.

Third Trimester Fetal Development

During the final 12 weeks of gestation, the fetus gains most of its birthweight. At term, 266 days after conception, the baby will usually weigh between 6 and 8 lb. During the final weeks of gestation, its movements remain strong but its range is limited in the crowded uterus. By the middle of the 8th month, the baby usually settles into a head-down position in the uterus. Poor nutrition, poor health, or overwork may cause a woman to give birth to her baby prematurely. A baby born too early, before complete gestation, has a diminished chance of survival. At birth the baby begins its rapid and miraculous adjustment to life outside of the womb.

During the last trimester, women should avoid exercises that compromise circulation through compression of the vena cava. Lying in a supine position (on the back) or in the right lateral recumbent position may cause hypotension, with its symptoms of nausea or dizziness. Women should continue to eat nutritious, well-balanced diets even though meals are usually smaller due to the pressure of the uterus on the stomach.

Activities that require great agility or quick changes in direction, level, or speed should be saved for after pregnancy. Women should avoid performing double leg-lifts, which should not be done even in the nonpregnant state, and working on certain pieces of Nautilus equipment (I will cover this in more detail when I discuss weight training). Inverted yoga postures are of questionable value. Activities that drive maternal pulse rate up over 140 bpm; prolonged squatting; passive, assisted, and ballistic stretching; or activities that cause hyperextension of the joints are not recommended. Again, pregnant women should not be encouraged to participate in overly strenuous workouts.

During the final weeks of gestation, women should feel free to enjoy any activity that does not cause discomfort and during which she is not jeopardizing her life or the life of her child. The pace should be modified as needed. Women should not feel compelled to compete with others or their former selves. Activities that bring on cramping, breathlessness, pain, dizziness, or nausea should be discontinued.

Common sense is the key. Careful, sensible reduction of pace and intensity will allow a woman to continue to be active throughout her pregnancy. Most women who jog will find that they reduce their speed and distance as pregnancy progresses. Those who enjoy racquetball will play an easier, less aggressive game, being careful to avoid being hit by the ball. Skaters and skiers may choose to give up their sports until their center of balance returns to normal. Carefully adjusting the competitive spirit to the realities of a changing center of gravity and reduced agility makes most sports safe and enjoyable.

Exercise During the Third Trimester

The final 12 weeks of pregnancy are frequently the most exciting for the mother and those around her. As delivery grows near, feelings of excitement, anxiety, and anticipation may preoccupy the mother as she grows increasingly aware of the baby within her and of the events soon to come. The size and forward thrust of the uterus is now quite pronounced. Exercises that threaten balance or stability should be avoided. Even mild bouncing can cause strain on the supporting uterine ligaments. Lower backache is common due to the weight of the uterus and the strain on the uterosacral ligaments. Attention to posture is essential. The pelvic tilt exercise, performed on all fours, is usually effective for reducing backache.

The change in the position of the heart and the upward pressure of the uterus on the diaphragm contribute to the breathless, heavy, almost smothered feeling some women describe late in pregnancy. This sensation is relieved somewhat when the baby begins to settle down into the pelvic cavity. This is called lightening, or dropping, and its onset indicates the nearing of the delivery day. Some women do not experience lightening until the day of delivery, whereas others notice it a week to several weeks before labor begins.

Late in pregnancy the pressure of the baby's head and the weight of the expanded uterus may create achiness and discomfort deep in the pelvis. Pressure in the perineal area and an increased need

to urinate are quite common. For some women, even walking can create considerable pressure. Women should perform the kegal exercise routinely and wear a minipad if leakage of urine is a problem.

There is a normal increase in vaginal mucosity late in pregnancy. However, any discharge that is heavier and slightly tinged with blood is referred to as a bloody show and could indicate the beginning of labor. If a woman suspects that she has either lost her mucous plug or had a bloody show, she should contact her care giver and should not engage in active exercise.

Increased Braxton Hicks contractions are normal late in pregnancy; however, any woman who finds that these contractions increase markedly during or after exercise should be advised to reduce exercise intensity. Some women have an irritable uterus, which may put them at risk for premature labor if strenuous exercise continues. If the contractions do not go away with a change in activity or posture and if they grow longer, stronger, and closer together, they are probably real labor contractions. Braxton Hicks contractions that continue at the same intensity and do not grow longer or closer together are frequently called false labor. Women who suspect that they are in labor should not exercise vigorously. Using up strength at the onset of labor means reduced reserves for later on.

Table 6.3 on page 62 reviews some of the major changes of the final trimester, the variations of responses to those changes, and their effects on exercise during the final weeks before birth.

Bleeding During Pregnancy

Bleeding during pregnancy has been identified as a reason to stop exercising and contact the care giver. Early in pregnancy, bleeding from the vagina can indicate only a minor event, such as implantation bleeding when the fertilized egg nestles into the wall of the uterus, or it can indicate the beginning of a miscarriage. A miscarriage is the spontaneous end to an early pregnancy. This kind of bleeding is usually accompanied by some cramping and a flow of blood as well as tissue from the vagina.

Another problem that can cause bleeding in early pregnancy is called an ectopic pregnancy. An ectopic pregnancy occurs when the egg is fertilized outside the womb and attaches to the fallopian tube. Eventually this will cause bleeding, and the

Table 6.3 Changes in the Third Trimester

Physical changes	Maternal responses	Effects on exercise
Mother experiences excitement and some anxiety as delivery grows near. May focus inward and seem very calm.	May need more contact with other pregnant women and more support and assurance than before.	Resigned to her enlarged silhouette, she may stop exercising now if not encouraged to continue. May be very tired after workouts; or, may be very proud to be in class until the day she delivers!
Increased size of the uterus may cause shortness of breath, which is relived somewhat by lightening.	Mothers may feel awkward and embarrassed as the size of the uterus interferes with exercises. May feel increased discomfort in lower abdomen, pressure in groin, and increased need to urinate.	Routines should be slowed, and those that uncomfortable or cause pain should be avoided. Mothers should be encouraged to go to the bathroom frequently. May want to wear a minipad if leakage of urine is a problem. Exercises should include awareness of breathing patterns.
Ankle swelling or mild general edema.	Swelling may be due to sodium and water retention and increased venous pressure.	Mother should elevate legs, avoid knee stockings, and continue exercise if there is no discomfort.
Sudden swelling, presistent headache.	Mother should not exercise because these changes may be signs of high blood pressure.	She should be advised to seek immediate consultation with care giver.
Mucous discharge may increase.	This is normal. If mother suspects that the mucous plug is being discharged, she should see her care giver.	Mother may want to wear a minipad. If mucous plug has begun to come away from the cervix, mother should not exercise.
Increased softening of cartilage of pelvis and hips.	More pronounced waddle. Increased discomfort in lower back or hips.	Emphasis on posture and body placement. Avoid unsupported flexion.
Increased Braxton Hicks contractions.	Time them. Change activity to see if they will disappear.	If Braxton Hicks contractions increase considerably after exercise, reduce exercise intensity. Goal should be to prevent premature labor.
Gush of water from vagina.	Check color: Amniotic fluid should be clear or milky white. Discolorations may indicate fetal distress. Onset of labor imminent. Call care giver.	Discontinue exercise. If this occurs during exercise class, call an ambulance.

tube itself may rupture. Pain, bleeding, cramping, and even shock can occur.

Any woman who experiences a flow of blood from the vagina during early pregnancy should avoid exercise and contact her care giver immediately. She should not wear tampons. Pads are safer and if necessary can be examined for fetal tissue.

Bleeding in early pregnancy may indicate a miscarriage. Later in pregnancy, bleeding can indicate several possible conditions. First of all, a woman may be in labor. The blood may be part of the bloody show that may occur as the mucous plug at the opening of the cervix is discharged. A woman with a bloody show should avoid exercise and might want to make preparations for childbirth!

A heavier flow of blood can indicate a serious problem. Occasionally, the placenta will begin to pull away from the uterine wall, causing abdominal pain and bleeding. This is called abruptio placentae. In the case of abruptio placentae, the fetus is put in considerable jeopardy due to reduced circulation and oxygen supply. Placenta previa may also cause bleeding late in pregnancy. It occurs when the placenta has attached to the uterine wall in a much lower position than normal. The placenta may in fact cover the opening of the cervix, which makes a normal birth almost impossible. As the cervix begins to efface and dilate, bleeding may indicate a serious medical emergency. Sometimes bleeding in pregnancy is not serious at all. Other times it is of great concern. Women who are bleeding should be advised to seek immediate medical care.

Summary

The material presented in this chapter is meant to help you integrate the information about the changing symptoms of pregnancy with their practical effects on exercise. As pregnancy progresses, the magnitude of the physical changes have an increasing impact on a woman's physical and emotional experience. Sensitive teaching will help ease the anxiety that these changes can create. Communication between you and the women you teach cannot be underrated. Throughout the exercise regime women need to share with you how exercise feels and how their bodies are responding. You cannot lead a good class without this feedback. The isolation between group leader and class members that occurs when there is no feedback is detrimental to everyone. Be sure to ask women how they are feeling and offer information about the effects of exercise so they can tune in to their own tolerance for activity.

Now we are ready to look at a wide range of fitness activities and determine how they can be modified for pregnant participants.

Chapter 7

Adapting Physical Activities During Pregnancy

In this chapter we look at selected activities and sports and determine the modifications that make them suitable for prenatal exercise. These materials will be especially helpful if you are working in a health spa or fitness center.

Most people are surprised to learn that physical fitness and athletics for women were unheard of until the turn of the century. Until recently the myth of female frailty and belief in the necessity of confinement during gestation pervaded the social and medical attitudes about women's health during pregnancy. In the last 80 years, great strides for women have been made in sport and medicine. As prenatal educators we have an opportunity previously unheard of to base our programs on the concepts of a holistic approach to physical fitness. Information, social support, prenatal care, and good nutrition are now part of the total fitness picture. It is vitally important that we address the need to provide safe and suitable activity adaptations for pregnant women.

Aerobic Dance

Aerobic training means that exercise is being performed to increase oxygen uptake and improve the body's efficient use of that oxygen. Most people enjoy aerobic exercise. It burns calories, contributes to improved endurance, and keeps the body toned. Low-impact, gentle aerobic dance is considered safe for pregnancy if done with careful adaptation to the woman's changing needs. Certain elements of aerobic training should be understood by both the instructor and the participant.

Continuous training, during which aerobic movements are arranged to keep the student moving and the heart rate in the appropriate target range for a specific length of time, is appropriate for pregnancy. Continuous training means that the movements remain at a steady pace and that the student keeps moving for the entire aerobic phase.

Interval training, during which there are short bursts of intense anaerobic exercise, is not appropriate during pregnancy. During interval training the heart rate is raised quickly to high levels, and the demand may be too intense for the pregnant woman.

It is important to remind pregnant aerobic dance participants to increase caloric intake to compensate for burned calories and to make certain that acceptable levels of prenatal weight gain are maintained. In the following section I will discuss what you and the pregnant woman should be aware of in terms of her participation in a regular aerobic dance class.

The Regular Aerobic Dance Class

Many women are taking aerobic dance classes now, and we can assume that they would want to continue to do so if and when they become pregnant. I usually recommend that pregnant women enroll in special prenatal aerobics classes because they are slower paced, are mild impact only, and follow all the recommendations suggested in the guidelines presented in chapter 4. Ideally, every facility and every community would offer supervised prenatal exercise classes. In the case that is less than ideal, however, it is not difficult to integrate pregnant women into an aerobic dance class. The following suggestions may help you guide the pregnant participant. Pregnant women in a regular aerobics class should do the following:

- Pay close attention to how they feel.

  Are they working too hard? Are they getting too hot? You might find it especially useful to use the RPE scale (chapter 5) to help women determine how their bodies are responding to exercise.

- Avoid the faster paced routines.

  Substitute walking or a gentle jog during the most vigorous routines. Jumping and twisting threaten balance and create potential for injury. This includes jumping jacks and heel jacks.

- Avoid exercising on their backs for more than a few minutes at a time.

  The pressure of the uterus on the vena cava can cause dizziness or nausea and may affect fetal circulation. Some women will not be affected by this and others will feel uncomfortable very quickly. Thirty seconds may be too long for some women, whereas others may be able to tolerate the back-lying position for several minutes or longer. I advise doing one set of exercises and then, before continuing, rolling into the left lateral position to recover.

Women should also be reminded that at different stages of pregnancy they will find themselves easily fatigued by familiar routines that once caused no difficulty at all. They must learn to accept their changing bodies and work with the realities of pregnancy. Again, they should never feel as if they are competing with the others and with their own previous performance.

Each woman is going to respond to pregnancy differently. If you can provide the reasons and explain the adjustments and modifications of activities that are appropriate for prenatal exercise, you will be helping each woman to participate at a level that meets her needs and fits her personal fitness model.

Additionally, you must be able to advise women of the risks of excessive or incorrect exercise, which include the possibilities of damage to maternal joints and ligaments and, in severe cases, poses risks to the fetus. Those risks, though highly unusual, may include intrauterine growth retardation and premature delivery. All of the material from the ACOG (1985) guidelines (see chapter 4) will be useful when you discuss how to adapt exercise to suit the changing needs of the pregnant woman.

If you create a comfortable, safe exercise environment, women will trust you with their bodies and follow your instructions. You must be clear about the safety and structure of your program. Regardless of how much experience you have, you will be considered an expert. You should be well aware of the responsibilities and obligations of good teaching. These obligations apply to any exercise program.

The Prenatal Aerobic Dance Class

Prenatal aerobic dance classes will have many of the standard features of regular aerobics classes. One of the most important features of any movement program is the warm-up. The warm-up increases the pulse and warms up the muscles by producing heat. The warm-up should include gentle, full range of movement at the major joints that encourages the release of synovial fluid. Synovial fluid lubricates and protects the joints. Avoid bouncy, jerky movements and concentrate on warming up all of the body's major muscle groups by starting at the top of the head and working all the way down the body.

The warmed-up temperature of exercising muscles is over 102 °F. Although this warmed-up temperature does not affect the body's core temperature, it is very important to remember that pregnant women should avoid vigorous exercise when they are feverish or if the exercise room itself is overly warm. Normally, pregnant women have a slightly elevated body temperature. They tend to perspire more readily than nonpregnant women, and their bodies work harder to maintain a homeostatic temperature. If you are working in a warm room, or if the humidity level is high, your students may be extremely uncomfortable.

The toning section of the class expands the movements introduced during the warm-up and includes flexibility and strength building exercises. Movements are bigger, and repetitions may be increased. Control (rather than flailing movements), awareness of body mechanics, balance, and good breathing techniques are important here. Women should pay attention to breathing as movements grow bigger. Lunges, bends and reaches, torso stretches, and exercises for the legs and calves are important.

The cardiovascular training section of the class builds strength and endurance. In a prenatal aerobics program, you can increase the repetitions and speed of exercises but should avoid leading advanced high-intensity routines and those with lots of bouncing and jarring movements. Rapid changes in direction and level can be particularly dangerous and may cause painful abdominal strains or threaten a woman's balance. Most aerobic dance classes have an active 15- to 30-min cardiovascular segment. According to ACOG (1985) guidelines, pregnant women should keep their standing aerobic activities to a 15-min maximum. You may want to reduce this level even further and intersperse 5- or 6-min cardiovascular training routines with slower, less strenuous routines. Women should take their heart rates several times during the aerobic segments and moderate activity accordingly. They should be encouraged to stop and slow down if they become red in the face or breathless.

The aerobic training segment could include a 2- to 3-min gentle aerobic warm-up to raise the heart rate, an active aerobic phase (7-9 min) of continous rhythmic movements designed to keep the heart rate in the designed target range, and an aerobic cool-down phase (2-3 min) that includes walking and gentle patterns that shift the weight and gradually bring the heart rate back down. Rocking, swinging the legs and arms, and doing knee bends help to prevent the blood from pooling in the lower extremities.

The floor work during prenatal aerobics classes may be specifically focused on training the body to assume and maintain good mechanics during labor and delivery. In this way, the floor work serves a dual purpose: toning muscles and preparing women for the physical demands of childbirth. I will discuss this in greater detail when I cover exercises to prepare for birth.

The relaxation portion of the class follows the floor work. This is probably the most important part of your class. When you are working with pregnant women, it is essential to use the relaxation time as a teaching experience. I leave a full 15-20 min for relaxing, during which I lead the class through conscious release of muscle tension, visualization, and breathing for labor.

You may want to refer to Table 7.1 when you are designing your low-impact prenatal aerobic dance class or when you are consulting with a woman who is participating in an aerobics program designed for the general population.

Keep in mind that prenatal target heart rates

Table 7.1 Prenatal Participant Recommendations: Aerobic Dance

Activity	Recommended	Not recommended
Mild impact dance	X	
Continuous training	X	
Interval training		X
High-intensity routines		X
Exercising on the back		X
Full range of motion movement	X	
Bouncy, jerky movements; rapid changes in direction, level, or speed		X
Heart rate monitoring before, during, and after exercise	X	
Fifteen min of aerobic exercise per session	X	
Becoming breathless		X
Maintaining balanced diet	X	

are significantly lower than for those in the nonpregnant population. Don't be surprised if pregnant women reach their target rate range very quickly.

Dance Exercise: Jazz, Ballet, Modern, and Improvisational

Traditionally, dance exercise referred to those movements that prepared the dancer for performance. They are the positions and exercises of ballet and modern and jazz dance. *Dance exercise* is a term currently being used to refer to any aerobic exercise done to music. It includes a variety of styles and techniques. In this text, dance exercise refers to exercises that come from the tradition of dance instruction and do not specifically claim to build cardiovascular fitness. Participation in a dance exercise class, however, can promote aerobic endurance, muscle strength, and flexibility.

Most women are not professional dancers, yet many enjoy participating in adult-level dance classes in the community. A woman who has enjoyed dance exercise classes may continue to do so during pregnancy. The ACOG (1985) guidelines provide a solid and sensible basis for exercise; refer to them with any further questions.

If you are working in the dance studio with women who are professional or semiprofessional dancers, you will be aware of their superior muscle tone and control over their balance while standing or moving. Control of the torso, flexibility, strength, and an intuitive awareness of body placement and position are all second nature to the dancer. Practice of the techniques of dance, including the mechanics and techniques of elevation (*relevé*) enhance a woman's sense of balance and control of her body through strengthening of the hips, knees, and ankles. Practice of the opposite action (*plié*), flexion and extension of the hips and knees by the quadriceps, gluteus maximus, and hamstrings, is also strengthening and contributes to the efficiency of the second stage of labor. The guidelines below will promote additional safety for both the dancer and her baby.

- Stretches should not be taken to the maximum point of resistance.

- Beyond mid-pregnancy, exercises that compress the vena cava should be either avoided or performed for only brief periods of time.

- Barre work that requires the leg to be raised above hip level should be avoided. This activity may compress the abdomen or put too much stress on the acetabulum and should be done with great care, if at all.

- Exercises that require the dancer to lie flat on her belly, to arch her back, or to jump, leap, or tumble should be avoided.

- Fatigue may play an important role in the dancer's activity level. Rest is more important than work if fatigue is significant.

- Dieting should be avoided. Most dancers eat very well but are extremely careful about gaining weight. Dieting during pregnancy to slow weight gain or to prevent the natural expansion of the body should be strictly prohibited.

- Tilting the pelvis forward to attain a maximum turn out should be discouraged.

The Dance Exercise Class for Pregnant Women

Dance exercise works well with pregnant women because so many women have had some ballet or modern dance training. The movements come directly from that early training and include many familiar standing, barre, and floor exercises.

When discussing activities with your class, impress upon them that the word *dance* should not scare off any nondancers. When you are working in an adult education format, not aiming at fancy choreography or dance production, no one should feel they have to learn complicated dance steps or compete to star in a performance. The essence of the experience should be the range of the style and the quality of movement. The pleasure of graceful motion is undeniable; this should be your main emphasis.

A dance exercise class for pregnant women can retain all of the qualities of dance that are pleasing and comfortable, while eliminating those that require sudden changes in speed, direction, or level. The quality therefore will be more gentle, the changes in direction slower and evenly paced, and the changes in level carefully executed. You won't see pregnant women leaping, hopping, and tumbling about on the floor.

An interesting facet of these limitations is that they require both group leader and student to spend time exploring the qualities of movement that we might ordinarily take for granted. By using sustained and rhythmic movement, and by exploring different qualities, sizes, and shapes of movement, women are able to enjoy the varieties of dance movement that lead to a positive impression of the body's capabilities. Instead of the cancan, which leaves the class breathless and uncomfortable, a more gentle triplet with some variations can be extraordinarily pleasing.

The most important difference between dance exercise classes and aerobic dance classes is that dance exercise tends to focus on the isolation and strengthening of different muscle groups. This is done so that the dancer may eventually move with strength, coordination, and agility. Therefore, there are many dance exercises that specifically involve the leg to strengthen the muscles of the hip and thigh. This kind of training can be an advantage during birth. However, if the external and internal obliques are ignored, the pelvis tilts forward, the iliopsoas tightens, and there is an arching in the small of the back. Dance exercise classes for pregnancy must include modified sit-ups (with legs bent, feet flat on the floor) and standing side bends for toning the obliques and abdominals. The biceps femoris, which is one of the long muscles on the back of the thigh, is one of the three muscles of the hamstrings. This muscle must be carefully stretched while sitting or standing to prevent injury when more vigorous movements are required.

All dance exercise classes should include exercises for all the muscle groups. This enables the student to develop control and coordination of movement in a systematic manner and to develop strength in all muscles. Classes might include a warm-up, which is usually a standing series of exercises; floor work; barre work; dance making; a cool-down; and a relaxation period.

Movement Activities

In this section I include several movement activities for dance making. Each is different and reflects a different style and objective. Every instructor has her own method and preferred approach to dance making. Please feel free to use these suggestions selectively, depending on your own style.

From time to time I have had the pleasure of working closely with women who are interested in improvisational movement. This form of dance movement is the organic essence of modern dance, and it has a remarkable history in the modern, creative, and self-expressive schools of dance. Because pregnancy creates so many fascinating changes, a woman who is inclined to dance will be captivated by the changes and their effects upon movement. She will enjoy exploring how her pregnant body moves, how movement changes, and how it feels to live and dance within that changing and cumbersome body.

Some women enjoy moving their bodies in ways that relieve tension or explore feelings. In some of my past classes, the group has decided which topics to explore through dance. In other classes, I have made suggestions that have become major dance themes. We have used themes like growing old, encountering change, and experiencing fatigue. We have danced to themes of love and hate, fear and joy, as well as giving birth, passion, fear of loss, and dying. Of course, we have created many humorous dances about coping with a big belly! At this level, your choice of music is important. Classical, jazz, and more modern instrumental music lend a creative, free-form atmosphere to the experience.

I often suggest that we form human cluster sculptures that reflect our dance themes. I ask the women involved to explore how it feels to be part of a living, breathing, moving sculpture; how it feels to be so close to other women; and how they feel about touching one another. Creative use of words as images allows for the creative use of the body. I enjoy working with imagery and exploring how we move by using words to create feelings. For example, I may begin our dance by telling the women that we are going to explore different ways that the body forms itself in space. I instruct them as follows:

Allow the body to make a shape. (*Pause.*) Feel it growing, rising upward, and unfolding. (*Pause.*) Feel it advancing into space. (*Pause.*) Allow it to widen, opening out and away. (*Pause.*) Allow your shape to move to one side. (*Pause.*) And now, to the other. (*Pause.*) Feel it move across and around the room. (*Pause.*) Now, feel it narrowing and shrinking. (*Pause.*) Feel it closing in and folding. (*Pause.*) Feel yourself retreating (*pause*), sinking downward and backward until you are small.

You might want to try using other words, like stretching, fluttering, expanding, undulating, curving, circling, extending, and releasing.

Dance class is an excellent time to work on posture. During pregnancy we often see lumpy, sequential walking, duck walking, penguin walking, or even torpedo walking, which is a gait described by the forward poke of the head. Try a waltz step or a triplet to see how differently the women are able to move when you are guiding them. I often encourage women to think about the word *lightness* and to allow that word to describe how it feels to walk across the room. Then we compare that to how it feels to be *sluggish* or *heavy*.

Notice how important it is to give good body cues. If an exercise or movement sequence has several parts to it, you should be able to describe each part. You must know the exercise and be able to separate it into its different components in order to teach it. Because you are working with pregnant women who are probably not professional dancers, you must be careful to avoid placing unreasonable or unnecessary demands on them. Avoid criticizing the students except by way of suggestion; be careful not to embarrass anyone. Table 7.2 will help you to determine what kinds of changes you may have to make to create a safe and enjoyable dance class for pregnant women.

Women enjoy talking about how they feel as they move, what feelings the movements evoke,

Table 7.2 Prenatal Participant Recommendations: Dance Exercise

Activity	Recommended	Not recommended
Dance exercise	X	
Maximum static or ballistic stretch at barre or on floor		X
Fast-paced routines		X
Strenuous *en pointe* routines		X
Leaping, tumbling		X
Exercises done while lying on the belly		X
Exercises done while lying on the back		X
Balanced diet	X	
Wearing comfortable clothing	X	
Exploration of movement potential	X	
Maintaining full range of motion	X	
Using evenly paced routines	X	

and what images come to mind as they dance. The choreography can be serious, thematic, or funny, depending on your style and sense of humor. Many women are willing to experiment with improvisational dance, so enjoy this special opportunity to share feelings and ideas through movement and music.

Jogging

Jogging is an amazingly popular fitness activity. It's the kind of activity one can do alone, with a friend, or on a team. Coupled with a mild weight training program and moderate flexibility exercises, jogging is an excellent form of exercise: It's relatively easy, cheap, and great for the cardiovascular system. Running, jogging, and walking are aerobic isotonic exercises. Sprinting, which is

not recommended for pregnant women, is running as fast as you can for brief periods of time. Sprinting is anaerobic because it uses up more oxygen than the body takes in.

One of the questions I hear all the time is, Can I still jog during pregnancy? Yes, a woman can still jog during pregnancy. Many women do! Although the physical changes of pregnancy may be cause for any woman to give up her jogging temporarily in favor of less strenuous exercise, many women jog throughout pregnancy without serious consequences.

There are some concerns about jogging during pregnancy that we should address at this time. The effects of jogging are not all predictable, and the long-range impact of running during pregnancy is not clearly understood. Some women report feeling very tired after running. Current research findings show that many female runners become particularly fatigued during their menstrual cycles, and that iron loss may be caused by the repetitive pounding of the feet during running. Pregnant women who decide to continue jogging should be especially careful to monitor fatigue and to pay attention to the potential effects of anemia.

Women with hypertension or asthma or who smoke cigarettes should avoid jogging unless supervised by a specialist who is familiar with the effects of exercise on high-risk prenatal physiology. Very little research is currently available on the effects of running during high-risk pregnancies. Women who experience irregular heart beats, chest pains, or allergies, or who have any orthopedic problems of the hip, knee, foot, ankle, or back should check with their care givers if they plan to jog during pregnancy.

Concern over the effects of jogging on the fetus are legitimate. It is already known that in most cases the fetal heart rate rises during strenuous maternal exercise and returns to normal more slowly than the maternal heart rate. Fetal breathing movements also appear to increase during periods of maternal exercise stress. Whether these are indicators of potentially dangerous situations is not yet clear. Clearly, the care-giving team should participate in a decision about jogging during pregnancy.

Thus far, researchers have disagreed about whether maternal exercise reduces the level of blood flow to the uterus. In research cited by Jarrett and Spellacy (1983), shunting of blood away from the internal organs and out towards the exercising muscles results in significant changes in internal blood flow. If this change also effects the uterus, inadequate fetal oxygenation may occur.

Another possible concern is the potential of fetal hyperthermia, which occurs when the fetus is unable to dissipate enough heat due to increased maternal core temperature. However, moderate maternal jogging (about 1.5 mi) does not lead to fetal distress or increased maternal core temperature.

Another consideration is the length of workout time. Considerable research on sheep, goats, and pigs has shown that animals who are exercised to exhaustion on a treadmill show significant decreases in uterine blood flow when pushed with workouts ranging from 20-45 min. Vigorous maternal exercise routines should be limited to 15 min as suggested by ACOG in 1985. Though human physiology is certainly different from that of the experimental animals, I advise caution until more is known about human pregnancy (Artal & Wiswell, 1986).

Animal research has also shown that regular exercise during pregnancy is tolerated well by both mother and fetus. Fetal birth weights in guinea pigs born to exercising mothers were normal; however, increased incidences of spontaneous abortion have been noted in some cases. In human research, no significant increases in prematurity or lowered birth weight have been noted. Whereas some physicians feel that strenuous exercise may put mothers at risk for premature dilation of the cervix, research by Berkowitz et al. (1983) indicated that women who continued to participate in moderate fitness activities had a significantly decreased risk of premature delivery. The main concern is safety. Women need to pay attention to body signals and be prepared to stop jogging if their health or the health of the baby is in jeopardy.

Jogging Safety

Joggers should wear well-fitted shoes. Good shoes protect the feet, ankles, and legs from the impact of running, and are especially important during pregnancy. Pain at the knees, hips, back, or symphysis pubis may be a direct result of improperly protected impact. Good support also means choosing a good exercise bra. As breast size and weight increase, the bouncing associated with jogging may be very uncomfortable. I do not recommend that a pregnant woman strap up her belly to run, even though it might feel better. If the belly needs support and if it hurts without it, perhaps the runner should choose a less strenuous workout—remember, if it hurts, don't do it.

Joggers should drink plenty of water and continue to eat a well-balanced diet with the required quantities of protein for pregnant women and more carbohydrates than nonrunners.

A woman should stop running if these or other signs of stress appear: foot, ankle, leg, knee, or pubic pain; abdominal pain, shortness of breath; dizziness; nausea or excessive fatigue; bleeding; prolonged rapid heart beat; or sudden or severe headache or fainting. The jogger must learn to take her pulse and work only within her target heart rate range.

The pregnant jogger should keep distances short. Depending on her speed, the woman should jog from 1 to 2 mi per workout, or a maximum of 15 min.

Joggers should always dress for the weather. In cold weather it is best to wear layered clothing and to be careful to avoid hypothermia. Pregnant joggers should avoid running on ice. In hot, humid weather, most runners should try the pool. I always suggest that pregnant joggers try running with a friend. Most important, your role as an instructor is to encourage a woman to pay attention to her body, listen to her care givers, and be prepared for lots of anxious looks from passersby! Table 7.3 on page 72 lists the major recommendations for pregnant joggers.

If a runner decides that she wants to give up her routine during pregnancy, then you need to support her decision and help her to choose a fitness activity that she will enjoy for the remainder of her pregnancy. A friend of mine (who is a devoted runner) approached me when she was 7 months pregnant and asked me what she should do about her passion for running. Although she felt physically strong, her husband was worried about her daily running and the possible harmful effects on their baby. She had agreed to stop running but now felt anxious and physically more uncomfortable than she had while she was running. We talked about the possibility of substituting walking for running. I recommended that she read the *Taoist Health Exercise Book* by Da Liu (1974), which instructs the student in the art of meditative walking.

This form of walking is done in gentle coordination with breathing. Although the speed of the walk may alter, the rhythm of both the walk and the breath should remain consistent and calm. Weight should be transferred from one foot to another in an even pattern; the feet should roll from heel to toe, and the hips should remain level as shifts in the body's weight are almost imperceptible. For meditation, Da Liu recommends that the walker concentrate on a place 2 in. below the naval, which is a delightful focal point for many pregnant

Table 7.3 Prenatal Participant Recommendations: Jogging

Activity	Recommended	Not recommended
Walking	X	
Jogging	X	
Wearing appropriate running shoes	X	
Wearing a maternity bra	X	
Drinking plenty of water	X	
Eating a well-balanced diet	X	
Running when ill		X
Running when in pain		X
Running with any signs that pregnancy may be in jeopardy		X
Running in very hot weather		X
Running for longer than 15 min		X
Strapping up the belly to run		X

women. The breathing cycles should be synchronized with walking rhythms. Head and shoulders should be erect, eyes forward, and tongue forward against the palate to promote salivation. My pregnant friend took up this form of meditative walking and breezed through the last 8 weeks of pregnancy.

Swimming

Swimming is another wonderful form of prenatal exercise. It provides aerobic exercise, strengthens and tones the entire body, and can be performed throughout the pregnancy. It is relaxing and yet invigorating and a perfect choice for prenatal exercise.

Swimming is one of the most adaptable fitness activities available. Water sports range, of course, from mild to wild, but there is almost always room in the pool for a pregnant woman who wants to exercise. As pregnancy progresses swimming remains one of the few really versatile, adaptable forms of exercise. It is a non-weight-bearing aerobic activity that requires no dangerous twists or turns; no ballistics; and no sudden changes in direction, level, or speed. In many ways, it is an ideal form of exercise.

During early pregnancy when the changes in the body are least dramatic, the swimmer experiences little change in stroke or efficiency. She should remember, however, that stroke is most efficient when the hand comes in continuous contact with the water for as long as possible. Fatigue may be a problem, and a swimmer should be prepared to slow her pace or shorten her workout if necessary. As pregnancy progresses, increasing buoyancy may cause her to surface more rapidly after push-off, but the adaptations in her stroke and kick are unlikely to lead to injury.

Pregnant swimmers should be made aware of the importance of resting and allowing the heart rate to return to normal every 15 min. Instruct these women to take pulse readings before, during, and after swimming to determine stress levels and to avoid swimming until they are breathless or exhausted.

The dynamics of swimming efficiently require the swimmer to use the least amount of energy to propel the body through the water. *Drag* is the effect of inefficient mechanics. The pregnant swimmer, by virtue of her changing body shape, will experience more drag as the trimesters pass, and this may affect her kick. However, as a dear friend commented to me, ''When I was in the water, it was the only time I felt normal.''

Because the belly of a pregnant woman may change the effect of the kick, a woman may be inclined to kick too hard. This uses up a great deal of energy. If, as pregnancy progresses, a woman finds herself getting too tired during a workout, suggest that she use flippers and try a less propulsive kick.

The regular breathing pattern and the slow, steady stroke of a relaxed swimmer combine to create an excellent form of cardiovascular exercise as well as training for the regular breathing patterns for childbirth. Whether the pregnant swimmer chooses to use regular or bilateral breathing is not important. However, *hypoxic* breathing, which is a form of breath-holding for racing, is not recommended.

Table 7.4 Prenatal Participant Recommendations: Swimming

Activity	Recommended	Not recommended
Swimming	X	
Frequent rest periods	X	
Monitoring pulse	X	
Using flippers	X	
Wearing goggles	X	
Regular breathing patterns	X	
Hypoxic racing breathing		X
Strokes that cause discomfort		X
Calisthenics in the pool	X	
Treading water	X	
Snorkeling	X	
Jumping into the water		X
Springboard diving		X
Scuba diving		X
Using hot Jacuzzis/whirlpools		X

Swimming can be adapted to almost anyone's strengths or style. If a woman feels abdominal pulling, she should avoid the back crawl stroke and the elementary backstroke. If her back hurts, she might want to try the sidestroke. The butterfly, properly executed, requires a strong combination of dolphin kicking and upper body strength. The kick and the body alignment of the butterfly are probably unnecessarily strenuous for the average pregnant swimmer, but until it becomes too tiring, a woman who is strong enough can continue to do it. The breaststroke is a gentle and adaptable stroke, and the sidestroke is a favorite of many. Knowing one's own body and its signals is the best way to monitor proper levels of intensity.

The water is also a fine place for calisthenics or other forms of aerobic exercise. Walking across the pool is an excellent form of exercise that uses the water as resistance. Gentle bobbing, sculling, and treading water are fine exercise activities. A pregnant woman can do jumping jacks or even jog in the pool without fear of the jarring effects of such an activity. Leg lifts, arm circles, and a wide variety of stretching exercises can be performed safely in the pool.

Snorkeling is relatively safe and can be done without extra concern. It is probably wise to avoid jumping feet first into the water because of a small possibility that water could be forced up into the vagina. However, the old myths about not swimming during pregnancy or menstruation, for fear that water could leak into the uterus, are unfounded.

High diving and scuba diving are not generally recommended during pregnancy. A missed springboard dive could cause a potentially dangerous blow to the abdomen, causing the placenta to separate from the inner wall of the uterus. It is uncertain how the changes in pressure would affect a fetus during deep-sea diving; however, scuba diving to a depth of more than 60 or 80 ft may affect the oxygen/nitrogen levels in the mother's bloodstream. Decompression sickness (the bends) would probably be harmful to the fetus. Recommendations for pregnant swimmers are provided in Table 7.4.

Expectant women are generally being advised to avoid hot Jacuzzis or whirlpool baths based on concerns regarding fetal hyperthermia.

Yoga

In this section we look at the ancient art of yoga and how it can be adapted to suit the needs of pregnant women. Yoga classes designed especially for pregnant women are very popular in some communities. If a specialized class is not available, yoga postures and exercises can easily be integrated into a prenatal dance exercise program.

Preparation for childbirth is a journey into the unknown. Birth is both the joyous arrival of the child and the experience of a great physical and emotional event. Many women have found that yoga, with its gentle stretching and concentrated breathing exercises, is the perfect form of prenatal exercise and preparation for birth. The integration of mind and body through yoga has been praised by yoga instructor Judi Thompson (1977): "Concentration and self-control are enhanced through regular practice of Yoga as body and mind are integrated and better able to function under full power" (p. 1).

Yoga is a form of exercise that originated in India. Properly used, it relieves tension, tones muscles, and enhances flexibility. Hatha-yoga consists of exercises called *asanas* that concentrate on exercising the body in a gentle, pleasant way, stimulating the circulation, and awakening sensory perception. The *asanas* include many static self-stretches for the torso and limbs. The gentle, careful practice of yoga is particularly well suited to pregnancy.

In western culture yoga has come in and gone out of style many times over the years. Many of the traditional poses are considered too stressful for pregnancy by the current standards of ACOG and the International Dance Exercise Association (IDEA). However, yoga is an ancient tradition and careful study and practice allow for its continued use throughout pregnancy.

The philosophy of yoga does not have a mechanistic view of the human body. In yoga science, the physical body exists together with the mental and spiritual bodies in the human system. The goal of yoga is to ensure that all the body systems function together on a healthy, integrated plane.

There are many different forms of yoga, its study and its practice. In the form I recommend for pregnancy, all of the exercises should be done slowly and systematically. All postures involve breathing techniques that are not unlike the breathing practice we encourage in childbirth classes. Generally speaking, movements that bring the limbs in, towards the body, or that shrink the torso, are accompanied by exhalation. Movements that expand the body space and reach the limbs outwards are accompanied by inhalation. All movements have a rhythm and a pace that allows for the conscious release of the breath. When practicing yoga, women should wear comfortable, soft clothing that is neither too tight nor too loose; bare feet are best.

Judi Thompson (1977) recommends that during pregnancy, women should avoid strenuous upwards or backwards stretches or any bending seated positions that put pressure on the uterus. Face-down postures that require lying on the belly should be eliminated after the first trimester. Some yoga instructors feel that the inverted postures are safe during pregnancy. Most western instructors feel that shoulder stands and headstands should not be included in prenatal routines. This is a matter of individual philosophy and practice, and you must decide how to approach this issue in your own classes. Whatever you decide, always consider individual safety first.

Avoid teaching the forms of yoga that include vigorous abdominal contractions. Mild forms of *uddiyana-bandha*, which is the taking in and out of the stomach, can be performed, but forceful abdominal work is definitely not recommended.

There are many things I particularly like about teaching yoga. Classes are usually small and are held in rooms with carpeted floors. Women usually bring their own exercise mats, which comfortably define the individual's exercise space. The music is soft and relaxing, and the entire class can be incredibly peaceful.

When providing instructions, you should give directions slowly and explain the variations of all postures. This encourages individualized teaching, which is very important. You will encounter a wide range of experience and skill in your students. Some will have had no yoga at all whereas others will be already quite familiar with various postures. Your being able to provide alternatives and variations of poses will encourage everyone to participate and feel that they are working in a range that is safe and comfortable.

There are several misunderstandings about yoga. The first concerns diet and yoga. The practice of yoga does not require a person to eat a vegetarian or macrobiotic diet. The yoga philosophy includes a concern for nutrition and for common sense about eating habits. Although it certainly advises restricting the intake of nonnutritious foods and practicing traditional cleansing and purifying rituals, yoga does not require individuals to participate in them.

A second misunderstanding concerns yoga's relationship to religion. The practice of yoga does not require a person to give up his or her present religion. Rather, it can be practiced as mere exercise, it can be used for health benefits and relaxation techniques, and it can be the basis of a spiritual awakening. These are totally individualized experiences and not prerequisites for enrollment. Yoga is not mind control. Some spiritual practitioners seek a level of moral perfection and control of the senses, but this is not the general purpose of our prenatal practice of yoga.

Yoga is a particularly gentle form of exercise that is especially adaptable to pregnancy. Women who are comfortable with the lotus position (a cross-legged position that requires great flexibility) or a modified lotus position (the American tailor sit), and who can relax their bodies deeply, as taught through the exercises and meditations of yoga, may have a significant degree of success at natural childbirth, although research has yet to verify this relationship.

According to Judi Thompson (1977), pregnant women especially enjoy yoga because it emphasizes common sense about comfort and the length of exercise periods. Students compete with no one and practice their yoga postures to learn about their own bodies.

Yoga exercises for pregnancy are gentle, graceful, stretching movements. Many exercises you perform and teach in your classes have their origins in Indian hatha-yoga. Yoga positions are easily integrated into any exercise program as part of the warm-up, cool-down, or floor work.

Yoga Positions for Pregnancy

Yoga has many kinds of positions and poses, the most difficult of which require sufficient experience and flexibility to perform. I will introduce several of the most basic poses. From these basic postures, you can lead your classes in the performance of other simple and complex movements. Instruct your students to accomplish poses and the movements initiated from them slowly, with steady, rhythmic breathing.

The Half-Moon Pose. This is an excellent starting position for stretching. Standing erect, slowly raise the arm sideways and then up overhead, placing palms together (see Figure 7.1). Exercise from this pose: Gently stretch over to the side without twisting. Elbows and ears should be parallel. Return to

center and repeat to the other side. Hold each position for a count of 10. Variations include interlocking the fingers and turning palms upwards with a twist of the wrists. This exercise firms and tones the entire body and improves posture and breathing.

Current exercise safety for pregnant women requires that you do not permit side bends with both arms extended overhead. An alternative is to extend only one arm overhead at a time or to perform a minimal stretch as you bend to the side.

Varjrasana Pose. This pose is also referred to as the firm, or fixed, pose. It is a kneeling pose, excellent for calming and centering or for doing the pelvic tilt. Women should be encouraged to straighten their backs and flatten their feet behind them thereby distributing their weight evenly along their shins (Figure 7.2a). Remember that hyperextension of the neck during any exercise may cause damage to the cervical vetebrae and should be avoided (Figures 7.2b and c).

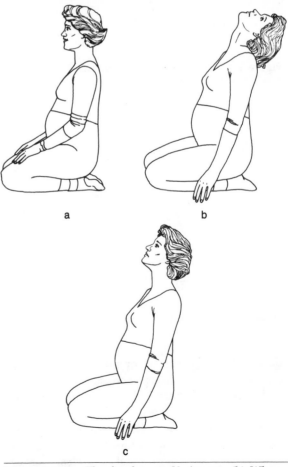

a　　　　b

c

Figure 7.2(a). The fixed pose: *Varjrasana.* **(b)** When exercising the head and neck, women should avoid hyperextending the cervical vertebrae. This pose exhibits *incorrect* positioning. **(c)** This pose exhibits *correct* positioning.

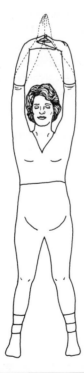

Figure 7.1. The half-moon pose: Remind women to bend their knees and inhale as they lift their arms.

Samasana. *Samasana* and its variations are seated exercises in the tailor position (see Figure 7.3). *Padmasana* is the lotus position, which some women find very comfortable (see Figure 7.4). *Konasana* finds you seated with the soles of the feet together. These are particularly beneficial for relaxing the upper thigh and widening the pelvic outlet. Instruct women never to put pressure on the inside of their thighs in an effort to touch their knees to the floor.

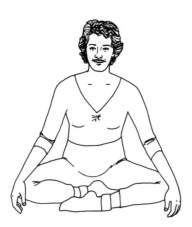

Figure 7.3. The tailor-sit pose: *samasana.*

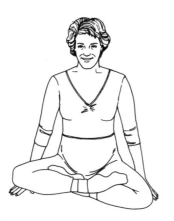

Figure 7.4. The lotus pose: *padmasana.*

Bidalasana. *Bidalasana*, or the cat pose, closely resembles the pelvic tilt exercise done on hands and knees (see Figure 7.5). In the yoga tradition, this pose exercises the upper back. Adapted for pregnancy, the *bidalasana* concentrates on developing flexibility in the hips, reducing lower backache, and toning the abdominal muscles. Remind women not to allow the back to sag (Figure 7.6).

To begin, while on all fours with the back as flat as possible, visualize pulling the pubic bone towards you. As you pull in on the abdominal

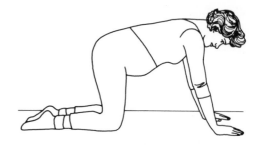

Figure 7.5. The cat pose: *bidalasana.* This is the same position used for a variation of the pelvic tilt exercise. The cat exercises the upper back. Adapted for pregnancy, the pelvic tilt works on the lower back.

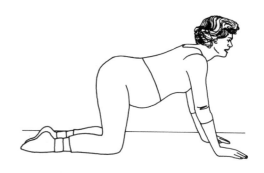

Figure 7.6. Incorrect *bidalasana.* Do not allow the back to sag.

muscles, exhale. Release and inhale. Please avoid letting your back sag when the cat is resting!

From the cat, it is easy to move to the inverted-V position (see Figure 7.7). This is a wonderful pose that stretches the backs of the calves, lifts the uterus out of the pelvic basin, and relieves pelvic pressure. It also strengthens the arms and opens the armpit as elbows and ears are parallel, back is flat, and knees are straight.

The Salaam Pose. This pose is also referred to as the *praying to Mecca* position (see Figure 7.8). The

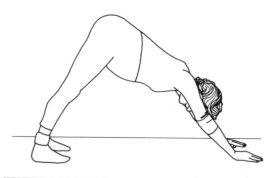

Figure 7.7. The inverted-V pose: Move from the cat into this stretch. Keep arms straight and elbows and ears parallel.

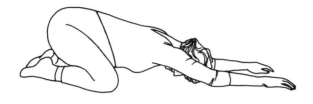

Figure 7.8. The *salaam* pose. Open the knees as wide as necessary and allow the uterus to hang down. Reach the fingertips as far out in front of you as possible. Keep the head and neck completely relaxed.

salaam pose is the resting position used after many exercises. Women should open their knees as wide as necessary to accommodate the pregnant belly. Fingertips should stretch forward, and the spine should be as long as possible. Encourage your students to practice deep and relaxed breathing in this position.

The Awkward Sitting Pose. This pose is basically a second position *plié* with feet placed forward. Traditionally, it is done standing without support. Adapted for pregnancy, it can be performed against a wall, much like the invisible chair exercise skiers perform to strengthen the extensors of the knee (see Figure 7.9).

Place the back firmly against the wall, bend the knees as deeply as possible without allowing the buttocks to pull the body weight down, and hold the position with feet flat on the floor for a count of 10. Slowly return to standing. A variation is to

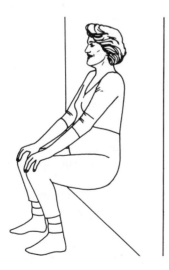

Figure 7.9. Adaptation of the awkward sitting pose, often called the wall-sit or the skier's squat. Press lower back against the wall. Make sure to keep breathing! Hold for 10 to 30 seconds and return to standing.

move the feet and adjust their position slightly on each descent.

The Balancing Stick Pose. I often teach this pose as an alternative to backwards leg lifts, which can strain the lower back (see Figure 7.10). Adapted for pregnancy, stand upright and use the barre for support. Bend forward from the hip, keeping the body straight, and lift one leg straight behind the body; flex the foot and imagine that the body is one straight line. Extend one arm (use the other one for support) straight out to the front. Look down and reach forward with your fingertips. Slowly return to standing.

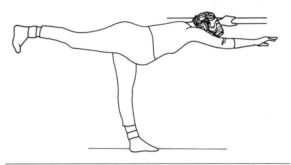

Figure 7.10. Adaptation of the balancing stick pose requires support. Flex the extended foot. Keep the back as flat as possible.

Aswini-Mudra. This is the Indian version of the kegel exercise and can be performed sitting, in the fixed pose, or supine (lying down). In the yoga version, it is performed in conjunction with a slight pelvic tilt. Encourage supine women to tighten and release alternately the muscles of the buttocks and those of the thighs. Remember, however, that pregnant women should not spend more than a few minutes in the supine position. (ACOG [1985] guidelines include no exercises in the supine position.)

Maha-Mudra. This is a stretch many dancers do. Seated, with the legs comfortably apart, bend one leg so that the heel of the foot is placed at the symphysis pubis. As you exhale, stretch to the side, reaching for calf or toe with both hands. The stretch to the toe is called the *janushirasana*. Adapted for pregnancy, the pose is performed with one arm raised to avoid crowding the uterus (see Figure 7.11).

Sun Salutation. The sun salutation is a series of movements that is done slowly as a greeting to the opening of the day. You can use it at the beginning of class as a greeting or at the end of class as a closing. If you wish to teach a sun salutation you will

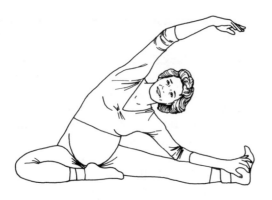

Figure 7.11. Adaptation of *maha-mudra* for pregnancy. Perform with one arm raised to avoid crowding the uterus.

Table 7.5 Prenatal Participation Recommendations: Yoga

Activity	Recommended	Not recommended
Yoga	X	
Breathing techniques	X	
Vigorous upwards or backwards stretches		X
Face-down postures		X
Inverted postures		X
Vigorous abdominal exercises		X
Wearing loose, comfortable clothing	X	
Maximum static or ballistic stretches		X
Any position that hurts		X
Postures that compress the abdomen		X
Forward flexion with twist		X

have to adapt some of the positions for pregnant women. The following steps are a modified sun salutation:

1. Stand erect with palms together at the chest-line, elbows down, and thumbs touching the breast bone (manubrium) very lightly.
2. Inhale deeply and lift the arms up over the head with feet slightly apart.
3. Slowly bend down at the waist, knees bent and head down, until you place your palms on the floor. Do not bend down with locked knees.
4. Extend one leg back behind you.
5. Extend the other leg behind you. This is called the wheelbarrow posture. Women in advanced pregnancy who have not performed this position regularly should not attempt it. It looks very much like the starting position for a push-up.
6. Push back into the inverted-V pose.
7. Sit back into the *salaam* pose.
8. Come to the fixed pose. Palms together as in starting position.

Table 7.5 should help you to plan prenatal yoga classes or incorporate yoga exercises into regular prenatal exercise classes.

Yoga is a peaceful, centering activity. It emphasizes the individual and encourages self-awareness through exploration of movement.

Weight Training and Nautilus

More and more women are using the weight room. It used to be that free weights and barbells were the equipment of male weight lifters. Since 1971 and the introduction of the Universal Gym and Nautilus machines, however, weight training has emerged as a very popular activity for both men and women. This is due, in part, to the fact that its vigor and intensity can be adjusted to the age, sex, and physical condition of the participant.

A well-designed weight training program can meet the goals of prenatal exercise for women who are experienced in weight training. However, pregnancy is not the time to begin a weight training program. Weight lifting is also not recommended for any woman with cardiovascular disease or high blood pressure.

Weight training is a sophisticated and fairly complicated form of exercise. Although it is not particularly effective as an aerobic or cardiovascular exercise, it may be of real benefit to women who suffer from varicose veins because the movement of the blood through the vessels is enhanced by the squeezing effect of the working muscles.

The benefits of weight training during pregnancy include increased strength and a sense of relaxation and well-being, which are the results of regular workouts. As long as the pregnant woman avoids overworking and straining, the consistent strengthening of the body's muscles, tendons, and ligaments will improve joint stability. Improved strength will be most beneficial during labor, delivery and the postpartum recovery.

Weight Lifting and Injury Prevention

Injuries during weight lifting are not as common as one might think. Pregnant women, whose joints are particularly susceptible to injury, should be careful to avoid careless use of the weights or machines. If women wish to build strength, rather than just maintain the development they have already achieved, a very gradual increase in the amount of weight being lifted is imperative. Slow, smooth movements are by far the safest and most beneficial.

During pregnancy, it is especially important to avoid maximum static lifting (suddenly lifting a maximum amount of weight). The rise in blood pressure during intense lifts and the differences in pressures on the vessels caused by the swelling of the large muscles during an all-out effort could create serious problems for a pregnant woman.

Some specialists advise against the use of free weights by pregnant women. The chances of dropping a weight on the uterus are slim but the outcome of such an accident could be quite serious. A pregnant lifter should stop working out if she is tired. Fatigue is the diminished capacity of the muscles to perform their work. In many respects it is a protective mechanism that occurs when the effort of exercise exceeds the body's capacity to bring oxygen to the muscles. Fatigue may affect pregnant lifters sooner and more profoundly than nonpregnant lifters.

Body sculpting is not recommended during pregnancy. The systematic use of the weights results in the development and shaping of the body's musculature; thus the term body sculpting has become synonomous with weight training. Though the nonpregnant lifter can enhance muscle mass and reduce body fat significantly if she adheres to dieting and training guidelines, the pregnant lifter's attempts to achieve muscular contouring will be confounded by the pregnancy itself.

Lifters should be aware of the recommended breathing techniques. The lifter should exhale on exertion and inhale on recovery. When a woman pushes out on the weights she should blow the breath out. As she returns the weight to her starting position she should inhale. Women should avoid breath-holding and the Valsalva's maneuver during pregnancy.

Weight Lifting Terms and Guidelines

Weight lifting involves the contraction of muscles against resistance. Increasing the length of the contractions and the weight of the resistance builds and strengthens muscles. Weight lifting has its own vocabulary; some of these terms are listed below. Instructors should use these weight lifting terms properly and be able to demonstrate the correct execution of exercises.

1. A *curl* is any movement involving flexion. It is probably safe during pregnancy as long as it does not hurt or crowd the uterus.
2. A *press* is the slow, continuous lifting of a weight by extension of the arm or leg. It should not strain the abdomen during pregnancy.
3. *Clean* is a slow, continuous movement that is probably safe during pregnancy.
4. A *jerk* is an explosive, rapid movement of the weights. It is *not* recommended during pregnancy.

These are a few suggested guidelines for pregnant women who wish to engage in weight lifting. Incorporate these guidelines into your classes and review them with your students before they begin any weight lifting programs.

- Women should check the weights and equipment before workouts. They should make sure the bars or machines are correctly loaded.
- During a regular workout, the pregnant woman should perform four to six exercises for the lower body and four to eight for the upper body. The routine should be planned carefully with a trainer to make certain that it is well balanced.
- The instructor should help the woman select a resistance that allows her to perform 10-15 repetitions.
- Pregnant women should be instructed to concentrate on flexibility by performing all repetitions slowly through the full range of motion.
- Pregnant women should move slower, never faster.
- Pregnant women should never sacrifice form.
- If a pregnant woman does a full-body workout at each session, she should train no more

Table 7.6 Prenatal Participation Recommendations: Weight Training

Activity	Recommended	Not recommended
Weight lifting	X	
Lifting when fatigued		X
Maximum static lifts		X
Clean lifts	X	
Presses	X	
Curls	X	
Doing jerks		X
Exercising with a partner	X	
Using any machines that require straps on the belly		X
Using any machines that require lying flat on the belly		X
Using any machines that may cause strain		X
Exercising three times a week	X	
Rapidly increasing resistance		X
Increasing speed		X
Increasing repetitions	X	
Practicing correct use of the breath	X	
Body sculpting		X
Relieving varicose veins	X	
Exercising with high blood pressure		X

than three times a week. If she trains only certain areas of the body, she may alternate training days, but remind her to train each area of the body a maximum of three times a week.

- Pregnant lifters should maintain their present level of resistance and increase weights very slowly, if at all. Increasing resistance should not be a priority during pregnancy.
- Pregnant women should never exercise alone.

The following are activities pregnant women should avoid during weight lifting programs. Keep them in mind as you design your classes and review them with your students before they begin to train.

- Any machines that require a belt to be tightened snugly over the abdomen.
- Any exercises that require a woman to lie flat on her belly.
- Hip abductor and adductor machines after 16 weeks of pregnancy to avoid arterial compression.
- Leg extensions on the compound leg machine (CLM) to avoid strain on the abdomen. The CLM is a hip flexor machine but may be too stressful if used improperly.
- The leg curl, which is done while lying on the abdomen.
- The duo hip and back machine, because of the strain on the abdomen and back and the necessary security belt.
- The 10-degree chest machine.

Finally, emphasize that women should avoid straining; during pregnancy, pain means trouble! Table 7.6 summarizes lifting recommendations for pregnant women. Use them as you develop your own program.

The use of free weights during pregnancy remains very controversial. The dangers lie in straining the abdomen, damaging connective tissue, or dropping a weight on the abdomen. An expectant woman lifter needs to assess carefully her strengths and goals. In all cases, however, a woman using free weights should never work alone.

The Martial Arts

The martial arts are self-defense and fitness activities that include t'ai chi, karate, and judo. This section examines karate and assesses its feasibility for the pregnant participant.

Pregnancy is not the time to begin the study of the martial arts. A karate student who finds herself expecting a baby, however, need not abandon her training as long as she is careful and works together with her sensei, her master or teacher, to avoid injury.

There are many forms of martial arts training. Some are quite aggressive, others are more meditative. The more aggressive forms are probably too dangerous to practice during pregnancy, whereas those whose philosophical basis reflects peace of mind and body strength are safer for practice during the prenatal months.

The mental and physical training in the martial arts is both vigorous and demanding. The physical practice of the art form, the required strengthening of the body, the breathing techniques, and the decorum all take many years to perfect. For the woman who studies karate, it is exactly this systematic training of body and mind that can be crucial to her experience of childbirth. Those who choose to continue their studies of karate while pregnant are often in excellent physical and mental condition and remarkably able to cope with the intensity of birth.

An hour-long karate class usually includes a warm-up session, practice of the *katas* (i.e., combinations of movements), performance of the self-defense *katas*, sparring, and a second cool-down workout.

Many of the exercises done in the warm-up and cool-down sessions are of particular value to pregnant women. Two that come well recommended are the modified sit-up and upper-thigh strengthening exercises. Push-ups are popular in karate classes, and a pregnant student may do them unless she experiences any of the following:

- Her tummy gets in the way.
- It hurts her belly. She should not do any exercise that causes pain in the form of excessive strain, pulling, stabbing, or tearing, or causes sharp pain in her abdomen.
- She begins to demonstrate any adverse symptoms after push-ups (e.g., nausea, pain in the abdomen, back, or chest, fainting, erratic breathing or pulse rate, etc.).
- She becomes fatigued.

The warm-up session may include the performance of a great number of side kicks and standing leg circles. A pregnant student of karate should avoid the repetitive side-kicking exercises, which put unnecessary stress on the symphysis pubis and hip sockets.

The *katas* are small movement phrases that are performed not for speed, but for clarity. A series of *katas* is much like a dance, and each tells a story determined by the choices and the order of the movements included. Each of the many schools has its own *katas*, the style and execution of which is determined by the philosophy of the school.

The self-defense *katas* are specific combinations of punches, kicks, jabs, and blocks. These form the basis of the sparring activities. Many self-defense *katas* include jumps and midair twists. Exciting to watch, they are demanding to perform. By mid-pregnancy women should omit those *katas* that require sudden shifts in direction, level, or speed. They should also omit all those that require high kicks to the front, side, or back.

Many women who have studied karate before they conceive have received training in the art of falling. This is another unique benefit to pregnancy from the study of the martial arts. A woman's ability to catch herself in a stumble, in a slip on the ice, or down the basement stairs can be critical. All women should learn to fall away from the center of weight, to avoid landing hard on the buttocks, and to regain the center of balance quickly.

Sparring in the martial arts means practice encounters, or practice fights. During sparring, which typically occurs near the end of a class, students work in pairs, practicing both their offensive and their defensive skills. I strongly discourage pregnant women from sparring, especially after the first trimester. After the first 12 weeks of gestation the uterus has grown and can be palpated above the pelvic bones. At this stage it is essential to avoid kicks or jabs to the abdomen and pelvic regions.

The dynamic tension and focus of the breath is an essential component in the study of most forms of human motion. You will find breathing techniques in all of the martial arts, yoga traditions, and childbirth education techniques. The training of the breath is critical in the advanced study of karate. *San-shin* breathing in *Washin-Ryu*, a school of karate that integrates a wide variety of styles of karate into one hybrid form, is a style of breathing that contains, controls, and releases the breath. The breath is inhaled as a powerful energy source, and the exhalation is a concentrated act of pushing energy out of the body as oxygen is expelled from the abdomen, the solar plexus, and the mouth. The exhalation grunt or shout is a common sound in most *dojos* (karate centers). The fascinating, determined focus on breathing presents an exciting and powerful option to the woman in labor. Unlike the style of breathing that encourages a woman to focus out and to breathe lightly from the chest, a woman using *san-shin* will focus on control and the dynamic interplay of the body and its muscles, tension, and points of release. She inhales through her nose and exhales through her mouth. Different, too, is the alertness of mind characteristic of karate, which contrasts with those relaxation/breathing techniques that encourage a mother to focus on a more meditative, spiritual level.

During birth, *san-shin* breathing may be of particular value. In the traditional breathing techniques for pushing during delivery, women have been encouraged to take two releasing breaths and then to hold their breath, bear down, and push. In contrast, the long, vocal exhalation of dynamic tension breathing is a powerful version of physiological pushing that is now being popularized by childbirth educators.

Karate and the other martial arts are studied for discipline, self-esteem, and inner strength. The more advanced the study, the deeper the focus. It is vital that a pregnant woman avoid the risk of injury during her training and monitor her own fatigue. A careful *sensei* and a well-trained woman may find that continued study of karate is most beneficial. Table 7.7 reviews recommendations for practice during pregnancy.

Table 7.7   Prenatal Participant Recommendations: Martial Arts

Activity	Recommended	Not recommended
Martial arts	X	
Repetitive kicking practice		X
Vigorous self-defense *katas*		X
Sparring		X

Racket Sports

Badminton, tennis, and racquetball are popular across the country. Many women have played a gentle game of tennis or badminton up to the day of delivery. Those who are avid players of racquetball need to observe considerably more caution. The game is faster, requiring far more agility, and the potential for injury is greater as pregnancy progresses. It would be foolhardy to play racquetball competitively after the first trimester. Table 7.8 summarizes the recommendations regarding racket sports.

Exercises that strengthen the body for the racket sports are those that build the muscles of the legs and arms. During pregnancy, when the knee joint is particularly vulnerable, a woman should continue exercises to build or maintain leg strength.

Table 7.8   Prenatal Participant Recommendations: Racket Sports

Activity	Recommended	Not recommended
Racket sports	X	
Competitive racquetball		X
Warm-ups	X	
Moderate strength training	X	

These include using the stationary bicycle and doing variations of toe raises and leg presses for leg strength and performing push-ups and exercises with light hand-held weights for arm strength. A warm-up is important before a game and should include side bends, arm and shoulder shrugs and circles, knee bends, and stretches for the hamstrings. As pregnancy progresses, the crouched, ready stance of a competitive tennis player may crowd the uterus or tire the back. Adjusting the speed of her game, the velocity of her serve, and the timing of her movements will allow a pregnant woman to continue to enjoy her sport.

Home Exercise Routines

Although a pregnant woman may want to exercise with a group or in a class, she may find that the at-home routine fits better into her schedule. In some cases, this is because of a work or child-care schedule, and in other cases, the community in which she lives simply does not offer the kinds of activities or classes she may desire. There are a wide variety of at-home gyms and pieces of exercise equipment from which to choose. Some are worth every penny and others are simply not appropriate or safe. If you are asked for guidelines by women who prefer to exercise at home, you will find these suggestions helpful.

Jump Ropes

Easy to use and cheap, the jump rope is most children's first piece of exercise equipment. Most pregnant women find that bouncing becomes uncomfortable, but some enjoy a moderately paced rope-skipping routine. Women should monitor their pulse rates. Good supportive shoes are essential. A threatened miscarriage, vaginal bleeding, high blood pressure, or other signs of an unstable pregnancy are indicators to discontinue this form of exercise.

Light Weights

There is considerable research being conducted about whether the use of light, hand-held weights (2-4 lb) adds any aerobic effect to a workout. Conclusive evidence is not available at this time. As long as there is no resulting joint pain, however, the use of weights is very effective for building upper arm strength and for toning the muscles of the neck, especially the sternocleidomastoid and splenius; the muscles of the shoulder girdle, including the trapezius and rhomboids; the pectoralis muscles of the chest; and the deltoids, biceps, and triceps. In fact, it may be advisable for some women to use light weights throughout pregnancy to prepare the shoulder girdle for the tasks of carrying and feeding the new baby. A mother who has previously injured her neck or cervical vetebrae should consult a physiotherapist before embarking on a weight training program, but preventive measures to reduce postpartum strain are worth considering. Women who wish to decrease stress on the lower extremities (e.g., hips, knees, and feet) may enjoy the effect that hand-held weights create during exercise.

Advise women to use the hand-held or wrist weights with care. They are so light that their weight is much less of a factor in injury than the length of time that they are worn. Begin with 3-min periods and work up from there. Avoid straining and be aware that overuse can be very stressful to the ball-and-socket joint of the shoulder and the hinge joint of the elbow.

Some women report using ankle weights to strengthen their legs or to get additional aerobic benefit during workouts. Some orthopedists advise the moderate use of ankle weights to strengthen the hinge joint of the knee after surgery. I do not recommend that pregnant women use them. Ankle weights may put considerable strain on the pregnancy-softened joint at the knee. Of course, self-monitoring is the key to avoiding injury. Careful use and handling of all weights is vitally important. Pain, post-workout stiffness, swelling, or weakness in any joint signals the need to discontinue using the weights. Always be careful to avoid dropping a weight on the abdomen.

The following are safe and enjoyable exercises using weights. Instruct pregnant women in their proper use if they intend to work out at home.

- Seated cross-legged on the floor, hold the weights securely and lift one up and over the head. Place the other arm or forearm on the floor to support the body. This stretch lifts the rib cage and improves respiration (see Figure 7.12).

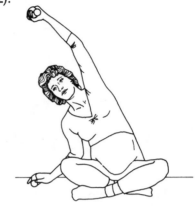

Figure 7.12. Using weights while seated prevents lower back strain. In this exercise inhale as arm lifts up and over the head. Use the lower arm for support. Exhale during the release.

- Seated cross-legged on the floor, extend the arms out to the side. Keeping shoulders down, flex the elbow and work biceps, triceps, and deltoids (see Figures 7.13a and b).

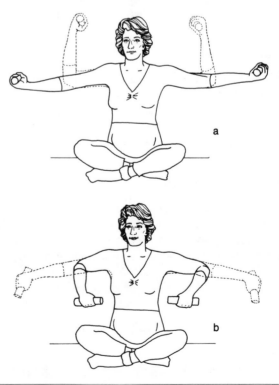

Figure 7.13(a) and (b). Seated exercises using weights for deltoids, biceps brachii, biceps brachialis, and triceps.

- Lying on the floor with knees bent and feet flat on the floor, extend the arms out to the side. Lift the weights and bring them together above the chest (see Figure 7.14). Roll onto the left side if back-lying causes dizziness or nausea.

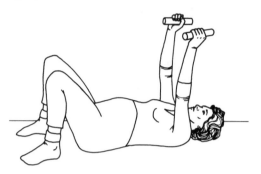

Figure 7.14. Lift the weights and bring them together above the chest.

Because the research on the effects of using light weights during exercise is not confirmed, it is difficult to develop clear and specific safety guidelines. However, it is probably wise to avoid rapid, repeated full extension of the elbow and shoulder joint when working out with light weights. This helps to protect the soft tissue around the joint. Also, when using the weights, women should be reminded not to hyperextend the neck.

Rowing Machines

Women accustomed to using rowing machines may continue to use them as long as they do not develop any abdominal pain, pubic pain, high blood pressure, or uncomfortable shortness of breath or pain when breathing.

Motorized Treadmill

The individual should monitor pulse rate, note any discomfort, and use the treadmill accordingly. A walking workout or moderate jogging pace can be set on an individual basis. Each session should include a warm-up and cool-down period. Each woman should monitor her pulse before, during, and after her workout several times to establish her own baseline. She should avoid overheating and keep her workouts to 15-min sets. A particularly nice feature about the treadmill is that you can avoid the heavy jarring effect of jogging on pavement.

Outdoor Cycling and Stationary Cycling

A stable, well-built bike is important. Workouts should begin slowly and build up to the 15-min maximum. A cool-down period should follow each session.

Collings, Curet, and Mullin (1983) conducted research in which 20 pregnant women exercised on stationary bicycles three times a week. Each session included a 10-min flexibility warm-up and a 10-min cool-down session of light pedaling. After the warm-up, each woman pedaled at her prescribed level (based on the ACSM, 1978, guidelines for heart rate) to achieve a heart rate of about 65% of maximum. Maternal and fetal heart rates were checked before, during, and after exercise. Functional aerobic capacity improved for most women, despite maternal weight gain. Fetal heart rate tended to rise during this type of activity, possibly due to decreased maternal blood flow or increased maternal core temperature. In research on cardiac output, women were able to adjust to exercise stress at lower levels, but high levels of stress put them at a disadvantage. Data from other researchers showed no signs of fetal distress after moderate short-term maternal pedaling (Artal & Wiswell, 1986; Morton, Paul, & Metcalfe, 1985; Pijpers, Wladimiroff, & McGhie, 1984).

Women who enjoy outdoor biking may be encouraged to continue this form of exercise until and unless they feel that they are no longer comfortable or that their center of balance has shifted and they no longer feel safe. They should also discontinue outdoor cycling if they find that the curved-body position puts too much pressure on the uterus or strain on the lower back. The most serious concern is that the unexpected fall or accident might seriously injure mother or baby. As an alternative to outdoor cycling, the pregnant woman might try stationary cycling. A good exercise routine would include pedaling for about 10 min at a rate of about 7 mph. This can be repeated two or three times a day.

Home Exercise Videos

The availability of exercise videotapes has probably had a significant impact on the numbers of women exercising. Now, any woman may exercise in front of her television. This is both a positive and a negative consequence of video technology. I am delighted that women can exercise at home and that they are willing to buy or rent the tapes that they like. Unfortunately, as with computer learning, there is no one to turn to for advice or answers to questions. Performing exercise poorly, using poor body mechanics, or straining to keep up with the movie stars can cause injury. Some prenatal exercise programs on videotape are designed for women who are very fit, whereas those who are exercising at home may not be so agile. An injury from working too hard or frustration at not being able to keep up with the tape may interfere with exercise aspirations.

I usually suggest that women use the videotapes as often as they like but continue to enjoy as many other activities as possible to avoid getting discouraged or bored. This helps them to maintain a wide range of interests and activities. I encourage women to bring their videotapes and their questions to class. There we can show parts of a tape and discuss it, comparing the video routines to our own, adopting things we like, and deciding why certain routines are not appropriate for our group.

Summary

There are many athletic endeavors that I have not covered in this chapter. The activities I chose to discuss have been the most popular among women in my classes and tended to be the ones about which I have received the most inquiries. Please remember that advice can never be standardized. Each woman is unique and each activity program should be individualized. Also, as an instructor you must always be aware of the different needs of the women in your group. From week to week and session to session, your population is going to change. Classes and instructional material must change as the women themselves change.

In Part III of the book we will look at the design and presentation of specialized prenatal exercise classes. These classes take on a remarkable life of their own and offer much more than exercise. They become support groups; prenatal education classes; and forums for sharing, learning, and growing. It is in these classes that your role as an educator and healer emerges.

Part III

The Specialized Prenatal Exercise Class

Maternal health and fitness education is an exciting new field. When I started teaching in Foster City, California, in 1978 we knew of no books, records, videos, or guidelines for prenatal exercise. We were enthusiastic but woefully ignorant. Today, women may choose from a marketplace of exercise options, books, and videotapes in their search for information about exercise and childbirth. That is why your skills in the specialized prenatal class are so important. The information about self, health, and the body is clarified and crystalized through you, your skills as a teacher, and the depth and breadth of your knowledge.

The traditions of women's healing and teaching, different from the traditions of linear mechanistic healing, can guide you. Our traditions come from ancient and primitive people who believed that awareness of the universe came through women and was part of female magic. Women healers believed that the body was good, whole, and perfect, and that the reproductive cycle was natural, healthy, and symbolic.

Today, prenatal educators are able to bridge the gap between what is technical, scientific, and medical, and what is known on many ancient and intuitive levels. As teachers, we are able to bring a blend of healing techniques to the classroom, all the while knowing that learning is a healing, helping process that permits wholeness. Our healing techniques include providing information, experiencing movement, exploring mythology, giving massage, attuning to the breath, and learning to relax. Some teachers/healers bring gems and others bring music. Some bring their voices, the scientific data from the laboratory, or herbs. Common to all teachers is that they bring themselves, as open systems; they are able to be creative by asking new questions, seeking new answers, discovering strengths, and accepting that there have been wounds.

In our culture we no longer consider pregnancy a disease or a condition that requires confinement, though its care and supervision require monthly and then weekly visits to the doctor. This careful monitoring definitely promotes maternal-fetal health and helps to prevent unnecessary disease and disability. The problem arises when women begin to perceive this monitoring as the medicalization and usurption of pregnancy by their care givers. In a series of interviews conducted with women in childbirth education classes I found that women sought warmth and support from their care givers and were disappointed by impersonal care and the lack of information offered to them. They shared with me that the repeated visits to the doctor were both comforting and disturbing because they reinforced the idea that pregnancy was a disease, that at any moment something might go wrong and that they were dependent on their care givers to manage their pregnancies. Many of these women trusted their traditional care givers to provide quality care but admitted that they felt somewhat intimidated by them and often went home feeling foolish for asking questions. They also said they were afraid of hospitals but they preferred hospital births because "something might go wrong." Anxiety about hospital routines, routine episiotomy, caesarean rates, and the intensity of childbirth pain were prevalent in all of the interviews and perpetuate the images of pregnancy as an illness and birth as an overwhelming ordeal.

Our cultural memory of childbirth is filled with negative images and many women find they do not receive the emotional and educational support they desire. Your role as a healing teacher in prenatal health education is vital. As a caring teacher you have the opportunity to support this quest for knowledge and self-esteem. Your classroom can be a source of information and healing, a place where women can be reunited with their bodies and feelings about being women. Let me share with you how I teach so that someday, if we meet, you may share with me how you teach.

Chapter 8

Organizing and Teaching the Prenatal Exercise Class

The activities in my prenatal exercise classes have always been an eclectic blend of dance therapy techniques, dance exercise, aerobics, calisthenics, yoga, and improvisation. I have often drawn materials and movements from the martial arts and from ballet in an effort to explore movement from as many perspectives as possible. Movement activities are designed to be physically pleasing. They are usually steady and evenly paced, aimed at reducing discomforts, improving respiration, and strengthening and toning muscles. They are also designed to be intellectually appropriate. I am consciously aware of and interested in the cognitive response to movement during pregnancy. Many of the movement explorations are designed to help women to focus on their bodies and their feelings about their changing lives, responsibilities, and sexuality. Movements that are too fast, threaten balance, or compromise the comfort of the uterus through crowding or twisting are not included. Movements that promote confidence, strengthen muscles without straining, and prepare the body to meet the demands of pregnancy and delivery are explored in a caring and professional atmosphere.

The weekly or biweekly pregnancy exercise class offers pregnant women the unique opportunity to engage in an informed exchange of ideas, questions, and solutions. Women frequently harbor questions, doubts, worries, and superstitions. Our class becomes a place to share those thoughts and listen carefully to the suggestions and ideas of others. Participants enjoy the companionship and caring of their peers. Questions about lingering fears, concerns about unexpected physical changes, and even decisions about care givers are aired and discussed in a support-group atmosphere.

My agenda is to open the door to discussion. A woman can get a good workout almost anywhere, but a specialized prenatal class focuses specifically on the issues and needs of pregnant women.

Becoming a Well-Informed Instructor

The prenatal exercise class is an excellent forum for discussion. It is also the perfect place to introduce the vocabulary and concepts of childbirth education. If the women in your class indicate that they have not registered for childbirth education classes, it is essential that you recommend that they do so. It is totally inexcusable for a woman to go into childbirth unprepared.

If you are a movement educator working with pregnant women, you may find that your biggest challenge is learning to lead discussions that explore the range of topics appropriate to prenatal education. I highly recommend that you enroll in a regular childbirth education series. These classes often last about 6 weeks and are offered by hospitals, physicians' offices, the International Childbirth Education Association, The American Society for Psychoprophylaxis in Obstetrics, groups that teach the Bradley method, and a variety of other childbirth education groups. Call your own care giver and ask which local organization he or she would recommend.

You should also enroll in a childbirth educator teacher training program. These are also offered by different groups throughout the country. Some carry a hefty fee, others are free. The more that you know, the better you and your students will feel about the class and the direction it takes.

Read! I cannot emphasize how important and helpful it is to understand the physiology of pregnancy, labor, and birth, and to have an understanding of the different medical, social, and cultural traditions that surround birth. My own understanding of and ability to teach the techniques of relaxation and breathing for childbirth have given women in my classes the opportunity to practice these skills for months before their regular prepared childbirth classes. Women who have attended my classes and given birth before they had completed their childbirth education classes have unanimously reported that the relaxation training and breathing techniques they learned with me were the most essential elements in their successfully unmedicated births. One women who gave birth to twin boys, 7 weeks premature, never attended any prepared childbirth classes. She delivered using the relaxation and breathing skills I taught her in exercise class.

If you are a childbirth educator or a nurse who has limited background in movement or exercise, you should definitely take the time to enroll in movement classes in your community. You may choose to take modern dance, stretch and tone classes, or aerobics. Familiarize yourself with the feeling of participating in an exercise class. Learn new exercises and explore how it feels to be a student. Observe how a well-designed program flows together and how the pattern of movements progresses from simple to complex, from general to specific.

It would definitely be appropriate for you to enroll in one of the many fine aerobic teacher training institutes that exist throughout the country. Take the time to determine which programs most thoroughly meet your needs. Some have special prenatal training institutes. There are also training programs specifically for prenatal exercise instructors. Check the credentials of the leaders and philosophy of the program.

When you are choosing a facility for your class, remember that the room should be carpeted. If it isn't, women must wear sneakers or aerobics shoes to protect their feet and provide support. Encourage each woman to bring her own exercise mat. A carpet will provide some cushion, but not much. Make sure that the room is well ventilated. Windows should open, and thermostats should work and be adjustable. The room should also have a door that closes for privacy as well as peace and quiet.

The music you select for class sessions is very important. Many instructors prefer to use records, others like cassette tapes. If you have to carry equipment, make sure it is durable and reliable. When you choose equipment, listen to the kind of sound it produces and remember how much sound you will need in your room. Always carry two copies of your tapes in case one breaks. Remember to bring a watch with you to class; your sense of timing is what makes the class flow! The following section discusses the actual design, organization, and teaching of the prenatal exercise class. I present a number of optional classroom formats. You may find these helpful to use as they are or you may decide to design your own class, reflecting your own talents and the specific needs of your students.

Class Format Options

Depending on your schedule, the organization for which you work, and the season of the year, it will probably be convenient to organize your classes into 6- or 8-week sessions. I have always used a system of rolling admissions, believing that it was acceptable to add new women into the group at any point during the session. Ideally, each class should be 60-90 min long. This allows you plenty of time for activities, discussions, and relaxation. Here are four class options you might consider.

1. **Prenatal Aerobics Class:** Standing warm-up (10 min), light-intensity, low-impact aerobic workout (15 min), cool-down (10 min), C-curve floor work (15 min), discussion (20 min), relaxation (20 min).
2. **Prenatal Dance Exercise Class:** Discussion (20 min), standing warm-up (10 min), ballet or modern dance workout (15 min), cool-down (10 min), C-curve floor work (15 min), Relaxation (20 min).
3. **Prenatal Yoga and Creative Movement Class:** Standing warm-up (10 min), yoga

stretches and karate or t'ai chi *katas* (15 min), dance movement cool-down (10 min), C-curve floor work (15 min), relaxation (20 min).

4. **Extra Light Prenatal Workout:** Seated warm-up (10 min), standing warm-up (10 min), light cardiovascular workout (5 min), barre work (5 min), light cardiovascular workout (10 min), cool-down (10 min), discussion (10 min), C-curve floor work (10 min), relaxation (20 min).

In a 90-min class there is plenty of time for movement, discussion, questions, and sharing. Most of my class time is spent moving. I rarely lecture; I describe, share, question, and explain rather than lecture. Occasionally I present a brief review of information or introduce a concept or an idea, but I prefer to keep the format of the group open and relaxed.

The class outlines that follow reflect my own approach to prenatal exercise and education. The prenatal exercise class is not a substitute for prepared childbirth or natural childbirth classes. You may use and adapt any suggestions or materials as you like. I have included chapter references for topics that I have covered in this manual. Of course, the choice of exercises, discussion topics, and meditations is up to you. These materials are only suggestions and may be adapted to fit your needs and instructional goals.

Class 1

Much of your time during the first class will be spent acquainting the women with you, each other, and the basics of what makes exercising and learning together during pregnancy a special experience.

Introductions and Welcome
Student introductions should include name, due date, exercise restrictions, physical complaints, and specific questions.

Optional Topics for Discussion
Reasons for exercise (chapters 3 and 4)

Exercise safety (chapters 4, 5, 6, and 7)

Suggestions for snacks before class (chapter 2)

How to take your heart rate (chapter 5)

Current guidelines on exercise during pregnancy; introduction of major concepts (chapter 4)

Appropriate clothing: sweatpants or stretchy leotards, a good bra, and a minipad if necessary. Aerobic shoes may be necessary. Bare feet may be

appropriate for some classes. Use your discretion about advising students. Consider how much impact the students will be placing on their feet.

Exercises
Healing Exercises 1 and 2 (chapter 10)

C-curve Exercises 1 and 2 (chapter 10)

Yoga postures (chapter 7)

Progressive relaxation: head to toe self-checking (chapter 11)

Class 2

I like to provide information to women about the changes their bodies are going through as soon as possible. You will notice that most of the suggestions I have for discussion topics pertain to anatomy and physiology.

Welcome
Introductions and names again

Optional Topics for Discussion
Anatomy of the pelvis (chapter 3)

Hormonal adjustment to pregnancy and effects on joints and ligaments (chapter 2)

Anatomy of the uterus (chapter 3)

How exercise can relieve pregnancy-related discomforts (chapter 5)

Good posture and postural reeducation (chapter 5)

How to do the Kegel exercise (chapter 10)

Exercise Options
Healing Exercises 1, 2, and 3 (chapter 10)

C-curve Exercises 3 and 4 (chapter 10)

Yoga postures (chapter 7)

Exercises with weights (chapter 7)

Relaxation
Progressive relaxation and introduction to visualization skills (chapter 11)

Class 3

In Class 2 I talk about anatomy and address some of the things that a woman can do to adapt to her changing body's needs during pregnancy. I now start getting my students to think about the actual birth process and the steps they can take to prepare for this experience.

Welcome
If your class is small enough, try to greet each student as she arrives.

Optional Topics for Discussion
Introduction to breathing for labor and delivery (chapter 10)

Massage during labor (chapter 11)

Exercise Options
Dance exercise routines (chapter 7)

Healing Exercises 1, 2, 3, 4, and 5 (chapter 10)

C-curve Exercises (chapter 10)

Weights (chapter 7)

Relaxation
Breathing patterns for practice contractions and visualizations (chapters 11 and 12)

Class 4

I use this class to talk about fear and pain. Your introduction of these words into discussion can be the beginning of the coping process. Of course, if these issues come up earlier you should be prepared to discuss them. The more thoroughly prepared you are as an instructor, the more easily you can adapt to the spontaneity of your students.

Welcome
Always greet your students with enthusiasm and warmth.

Optional Topics for Discussion
Fear, tension, pain, and time (chapter 11)

Birth plan or birth wish list and the importance of communicating clearly with your care giver (chapter 10)

Further discussion and teaching of breathing techniques (chapters 10 and 11)

Exercise Options
Dance routines or other activities as suggested

Relaxation
Breathing patterns and visualization skills (chapters 10, 11, and 12)

Class 5

I use this session to continue to develop relaxation and breathing techniques that will be helpful throughout pregnancy and during labor and delivery.

Welcome
Encourage your students to ask questions in the early part of your class.

Optional Topics for Discussion
At this time during a session I frequently invite a new mom to come in to share her experience with the group. If no one is available, I focus extensively on the material presented in the next chapter on self-image and body image (chapter 9).

Exercise Options
Dance routines or breathing pattern practice if there is time

Relaxation
Complete relaxation as the immediate response to the releasing breath and practice of breathing patterns

Discussion of mantras (chapter 12)

Class 6

I use this class to be more specific about the actual birth process and the experience of the body in labor.

Welcome
These moments should be relaxing and upbeat, providing an opportunity for transition from outside activities to the activities and discussions of your class.

Optional Topics for Discussion
Positions for delivery (chapter 10)

Breathing patterns for pushing (chapter 11)

Exercise Options
Improvisation, or whatever dance theme you and the class have chosen

Relaxation
Responding to releasing breath

Visualization skills (chapters 11 and 12)

Class 7

During Class 7, I concentrate on why some women have cesarean sections and how a cesarean can affect a woman's recovery from birth.

Welcome
Introduce the discussion topic as the women come in to the class so that they have time to formulate their questions for the discussion period that comes later.

Optional Topics for Discussion
What if you have a cesarean section?

Recovery from vaginal or cesarean childbirth (chapter 14)

Contraception after childbirth (not thoroughly discussed in this text, but I always mention that women must be refitted if they use a diaphragm and should not use the pill if they are nursing)

Exercise during immediate postpartum (chapters 14 and 15)

Exercise Options

All routines and variations including improvisation and individual dance themes

Relaxation

Using visualization, focus on postpartum.

Class 8

I think that you will find that all of your classes are learning experiences for you. This final class can be an even greater opportunity to learn if you encourage your students to share their feelings and ideas regarding their experience in your class.

Welcome

This welcome is actually part of a good-bye as you will be losing the group and exchanging phone numbers and names if you haven't done so already. You can reregister women who are continuing with you.

Optional Topics for Discussion

The group experience: suggestions, ideas, and criticisms

Exercise Options

Routines and variations

Relaxation

Visualization and closing

Exercise Class Problems and Solutions

This section is a troubleshooter's guide to teaching prenatal exercise. It is not designed to answer all questions, complaints, or problems; rather, it should anticipate some of the questions and problems you might hear from the women with whom you work.

Why Do My Feet Hurt?

Ill-fitting shoes are often the culprit when a student complains about tired and aching feet. Aerobics shoes, running shoes, and sneakers can get worn out, stretched out, overwashed, or broken down. Often the arch support is worn out or the heel has worn down, which causes the ankles to turn out. During pregnancy in particular, complaints of tired feet may be the result of poor posture and weight gain. In fact, some women's feet grow during pregnancy and they don't realize that they actually need bigger shoes!

You should recommend that they wear properly fitted shoes with adequate lateral support. Sometimes the arch support is either too high or too firm, so careful fitting is essential. Women should shop for new exercise shoes in stores that permit them to return the shoes if the fit is improper.

Swollen feet may be the result of sitting at a desk all day. Ankles and feet tend to swell if circulation is poor. I recommend elevating the feet as much as possible, walking or exercising during the lunch hour, and taking off the high heels whenever possible! Women who must sit for long periods each day should do ankle circles and alternate pointing and flexing their feet to help prevent stiffness. I always recommend foot massage when I hear complaints of tired or swollen feet. Foot massage is discussed further in chapter 12.

Why Do I Ache Throughout My Shoulders and Upper Back?

Poor posture could be the cause of fatigue in the upper back, the neck, or the cervical vertebrae. An ill-fitting brassiere can also create an aching, tired back as well as sore ribs. The fullness of the pregnant breast requires excellent support. A well-fitted brassiere with a nice wide band of hooks across the back can be a wise investment, but if the band is too wide it can cause soreness from the ribs around to the back.

Advise women to do upper body and neck strengthening exercises to prevent the round-shouldered posture that creates neck strain. Some women benefit from using light hand-held weights to strengthen the muscles of the upper back, neck, and upper arms. Women should remember to breathe evenly and exhale fully during exercise. Occasionally a woman will exercise with her shoulders hunched or with tension in her neck. This will result in post-exercise stiffness. Encourage students to stand with their feet parallel and relax their knees. Shoulders should be relaxed and down while the chest is lifted slightly; chin should be parallel to the floor, jaw relaxed, and the ear should be right above the middle of the shoulder. Teach students to think of the pelvis as a bowl and tilt it forward and backward until it feels comfortable and level.

Women may also want to consider

- using a different mattress or sleeping position,
- adding pillows to support the back and thigh in the side-lying sleep position,
- wearing a bra at night,
- trying a change in footwear,
- massaging sore muscles, and, if necessary,
- buying a maternity girdle for women with extreme lordosis or kyphosis, especially in obesity or multiple pregnancy (it must be fitted carefully).

Why Does My Supporting Knee Hurt When I Exercise on My Hands and Knees?

Most women enjoy the pelvic tilt and hip lift (doggie lift) exercises but some find this position wearisome. Advise women to flatten the front of the ankle on the supporting foot down to the floor. They should not curl or flex their feet. By flattening the ankle, the student allows the entire surface of the leg to support her weight, thus sparing the knee. This reduces tension significantly.

Some women work too hard in this position, lifting their working leg much too high or doing too many repetitions. This strains the hips, lower back, knee, and shoulders. Women should avoid creating a sagging back, which occurs when they lift the working leg too high either to the side or to the back. They may adjust the positions of their arms whenever they shift their weight. I usually have women perform extensions with a flexed foot. I have them hold the leg in the extended position for a count of 8 with a controlled return to the starting position, rather than doing many quick repetitions. Remind them that the head and neck are extensions of the spine and should be straight, with the face looking at the floor. They should not hang their heads down or hyperextend their necks to look up.

Why Does My Hip Hurt?

Hip pain is very common in pregnancy and can be the result of many factors. Often the position of the baby creates pressure that is interpreted as hip pain. Sometimes the baby is nestling against a nerve, occasionally on the sciatic nerve, which sends painful pressure radiating down the back and into the leg. Some hip pain is the result of the softening of the ligaments that support the hip. Too much sitting as well as too much exercising can cause hip discomfort.

You should spend a few moments performing exercises that involve hip movement so you can determine a safe range of movement for a woman complaining of hip pain. She should be advised to avoid painful positions or movements and to exercise to, not beyond, the point of pain. Sometimes massage helps to ease hip pain, and the use of a heating pad for 10-min periods can be comforting. Suggest that the women wear flat-heeled shoes and avoid standing or walking in uncomfortable shoes as a way of reducing joint stress. Of course, improved posture may also help.

Why Does My Lower Back Hurt So Much?

Because of the increased weight of pregnancy and the softening of the pelvic girdle, you cannot overstate the case for good posture! Posture affects balance, breathing, appearance, and performance. Have the women stand with feet placed comfortably apart and parallel, and shoulders and hips level. Examine each for the curve in the lumbar spine. It is advisable to actually place your fingers on the women's hips and spines so that they can feel where the back curves. (Let them know that you are going to place your hands on their bodies.) Then ask them to tilt the pelvis back slightly, pulling in and up on the abdominal muscles. This tiny movement may significantly improve posture and reduce foot pain.

We have discussed techniques for postural education, and you may want to use visualizations of lightness and lengthening of the spine to help women improve their posture. Be aware, however, that late in pregnancy, a woman complaining of a backache *may be in labor*. Advise her to rest and check to see whether the backache changes or goes away.

Occasionally a pregnant woman will suffer from more serious back pain as a result of vertebral pressure on the disks. This woman should be under the supervision of an orthopedic care giver and may have certain exercise restrictions. Any exercise that includes the forward flexion of the back may be contraindicated.

For those women with back pain, recommend the pelvic tilt exercise done on hands and knees, supine, leaning against a wall, or sitting down, or any other exercises for releasing back tension or strengthening the torso and lower back. They should definitely avoid wearing high-heeled shoes.

Why Am I Having Pain Across My Lower Abdomen?

Pain along the sides of the abdomen and along the round ligaments that support the growing uterus is very common. Many women experience twinges of pain that range from minor to stabbing when they roll over in bed at night or otherwise suddenly shift their weight or direction.

Some women feel pain at the symphysis pubis, which is due to the softening of the cartilage that joins the pubic bones. This can be aggravated by vigorous exercise or rapid changes in direction, level, or speed during exercise.

You should be aware that in late pregnancy, a woman who is experiencing pain across her abdomen or down low near the symphysis pubis *may be in labor.* A woman feeling abdominal pain should be advised to rest, to have a glass of water, and to determine whether her pains are in fact labor contractions.

As the instructor, you should avoid leading exercises that require rapid changes in direction, level, or speed. Suggest that women support the uterus with their hands during turns or shifts. Women should always avoid exercises that cause discomfort.

Why Do I Get Headaches After Class? Why Is My Vision Blurry?

Symptoms of hypoglycemia, the result of low blood sugar, may include headaches, fatigue, or blurred vision. These symptoms may also occur in a woman who is dehydrated. Remind students to eat a well-balanced meal 1-2 hr before exercising or to have a light high-carbohydrate snack and a drink of water right before class. They should avoid snacks with sugar, honey, or maple syrup before exercising because foods that are high in sugar are quickly metabolized. The pancreas reacts quickly to the high blood sugar levels and produces insulin, which counters the effect of the sugar. This may cause sudden fatigue or the well-known sugar crash. Even potatoes, whose starch is quickly converted to sugar, can cause this reaction. Remind women to check their pulses routinely to avoid exercising into an inappropriate training range. If symptoms persist, a woman with these complaints should definitely consult her care giver.

Is It Okay for Me to Eat Candy After I Exercise?

Anyone who craves sweets after exercise is looking for quick energy and should probably start eating more food more regularly. You should recommend increasing carbohydrate intake. Women who crave sweets tend to go for chocolate. They should be encouraged to avoid the concentrated sugar and caffeine of chocolate or sugary snacks. A well-balanced diet and snacks of high-fiber complex carbohydrates are far more nutritious.

Why Am I So Hot?

Heat production is a direct by-product of the increased metabolism of pregnancy. Heat is also a by-product of exercise during which calories are burned as fuel. Heat diffusion may be a problem for pregnant women whose body temperatures are naturally slightly elevated.

If a woman complains about perspiring very heavily, consider the possibility of a low blood sugar reaction. Remind women to avoid using skin lotions before exercise class, because the lotion coats the skin, trapping perspiration and preventing evaporation.

Why Am I Breathless After Every Exercise?

Breathlessness is a common response to the increased upward pressure of the uterus on the diaphragm. Women who are easily winded should avoid working too vigorously. Set a pace for them that is slow and even. Encourage awareness of breathing patterns, remind women to keep breathing, and teach a breathing pattern for as many exercises as you can. Include exercises that raise the arms and lift the rib cage. This affords more room in the upper torso for full respiration.

Women who smoke are far more prone to breathlessness than those who do not. Always encourage smokers to kick the habit. Every time a pregnant woman inhales the carbon monoxide of cigarette smoke she is denying her baby the healthy warmth of fully oxygenated blood.

Why Is My Heart Pounding?

Even though the heart works very hard during pregnancy, it can usually increase output if the demand is gradual. However, it cannot always increase its output if the demand is sudden or strenuous; consequently, some women will experience a pounding feeling if exercise is too sudden or too stressful. Sometimes women with hypertension will complain of a pounding feeling or palpitations after exercise. Always have women check their pulse rates and reduce exercise intensity if they report a rate of 140 bpm or higher.

Always include a warm-up and a cool-down in your program. It is probably safe for women to exercise at 140 bpm for 15 min (ACOG, 1985), but it is reasonable to set a slightly lower heart rate standard or a shorter interval in your class.

Why Do My Varicose Veins Hurt So Much?

Varicose veins of the legs and vulva are not unusual during pregnancy. After childbirth many women find that these tender veins shrink and are no longer painful. Others find that with successive pregnancies the varicosities worsen. Exercise may improve this condition by improving circulation, and muscles that are firm are better able to support the body's veins and arteries.

Women with varicose veins should not sit or stand for long periods of time. They should try to elevate their feet as often as possible. This includes placing a lift at the foot of their beds, a foot stool at the kitchen counter, and, if they must sit at a desk, a stool beneath the desk so their feet are as high as possible. They should avoid wearing wooden-soled shoes and standing on cement or tile floors. High heels are ill-advised because of the contraction they cause in the muscles of the calves, which may further impede circulation. Women with varicose veins should wear well-fitted support hose or elastic stockings that do the work of slackened muscles and support the legs' veins and arteries. To put them on in the morning, a woman should lift the leg up for a few minutes, then roll the stocking on from her toes to the top of her leg while the leg is still elevated. Women should not wear support hose during exercise because they prevent the air from cooling the surface of the skin.

Safety Precautions and Emergency Procedures

An exercise leader or medical care giver should always be prepared to deal calmly and competently with the unexpected. This means being informed and ready. The first step in dealing with emergencies is to avoid them. Planning ahead can help you do this.

- Make certain the exercise room is well ventilated. If it is too hot, find another room.
- Have the women get a small drink of water and use the bathroom facilities before exercise begins.

- Have the group check their pulse rates at the beginning, middle, and end of class.
- Remind them to keep breathing during exercise and to abstain from any exercise that hurts.

Vaginal Bleeding

If a woman starts to bleed from her vagina, do the following:

1. Have her lie down on her left side.
2. Check visually to see if the cord has begun to descend (this is very rare).
3. Ask if she is having contractions.
4. Call her care giver and an ambulance immediately.

Water Breaks

If a woman's water breaks, do the following:

1. Have her lie down on her left side.
2. Ask if she is having contractions.
3. Visually check to see if the cord has begun to descend (this is very rare). If it has, call an ambulance. Check the color and smell of the amniotic fluid. Discolored fluid may mean the fetus is in distress.
4. Call her care giver.

Contractions

If a woman says she is having contractions, do the following:

1. Ask her how long they have been going on.
2. Ask if they seem to be getting stronger.
3. Ask her to stop exercising and to have a glass of water.
4. Ask her if she wants to call her care giver.

Dizziness

If a woman feels dizzy or nauseous, do the following:

1. Have her sit down and rest.
2. Get her a cool towel for her forehead.
3. Ask if she has eaten recently.
4. Check her pupils, determine if her skin is clammy, and take her pulse.
5. If she does not recovery quickly, call her care giver.

Falls

If a woman falls and appears to have hurt her wrist or ankle, do the following:

1. Have her sit comfortably.
2. Apply ice to reduce potential swelling.
3. Wrap something snugly around the injured part.
4. Elevate the ankle if possible.
5. Call a care giver who may arrange to meet her in the emergency room.

Emergency Childbirth Procedures

It is highly unlikely that a woman in your class or facility would go into such a precipitous labor that she would give birth before she could either get to the hospital or be reached by an ambulance. In most cases labor begins slowly and takes many hours to progress through effacement and dilation. In the event of a birthing emergency, however, it would be wise for you to be familiar with the following outline of emergency procedures. Be advised that I am neither practicing medicine nor instructing individuals about medical procedures. This is simply a brief outline of information that should be available to anyone who lives with, works with, or otherwise attends to a pregnant woman. In case of an emergency childbirth, follow these procedures:

1. Do not panic.
2. Summon help (a doctor and/or an ambulance).
3. Have the mother lie down. She may complain of having to have a bowel movement. Help her to relax as much as possible.
4. Ask her not to push. Encourage her to feather blow. The urge to push is difficult to control but you want to prevent the birth from being too rapid.
5. As the baby emerges, do not pull on its head. Support it gently. If it is still encased in the amniotic sac, lightly snag the membrane so the baby's first breath is air, not water.
6. When the baby's head is out, check to make sure the cord is not wrapped around its neck. If it is, loosen it with your finger and, if possible, loop it over the baby's shoulder.
7. Clear the baby's mouth of mucus, place it on the mother's belly and keep it warm. If breathing does not occur spontaneously, massage the rib cage, rub its feet, or administer cardiopulmonary resuscitation (CPR).
8. Do not cut the cord. Do not pull it out. The mother should deliver the placenta within half an hour.

Summary

One of the most exciting aspects of teaching a prenatal exercise class is that, as a healing educator, you create a nurturing environment in which to address the special needs of expectant women. The choice to create this kind of atmosphere depends on your objectives. The success of your venture depends on your skills. Those things that contribute to your success are the respect you have for each individual and her wisdom and experiences, and the accuracy and depth of the information you have to share.

The organization of your classes is entirely up to you. The outlines I have included are for you to use as a reference in planning your program. Obviously, everyone has different strengths and interests, and classes that you teach will reflect your own perspectives. Safety, caring, and being well organized from start to finish are essential to the presentation of a professional program. We cannot know all of the answers and should not pretend that we do. Always refer women to other professionals if they present questions you cannot answer.

In the following chapters we will discuss many of the teaching techniques of prenatal exercise and show how these are also healing techniques. I will begin by exploring some of the body image issues that play a part in the dynamics and needs of the pregnant participant. A number of classroom activities are described. These activities encourage discussion and may help to set the tone of a group by opening up the floor to honest and supportive interaction.

Chapter 9

Changes in Body Image and Implications for Prenatal Teaching

Knowledge and understanding of female anatomy and physiology and dependable social and emotional support are the cornerstones of a positive body image during pregnancy. As teachers we must be especially sensitive to the changes in body image as they affect self, sensuality, body boundaries, and self-esteem. In this chapter we will explore some of the body image issues that play a part in the dynamics of the prenatal group. A number of classroom activities are described for you. These activities encourage discussion and help open the class to honest and supportive interaction.

Pregnancy can be a time of magnificent health and well-being. A pregnant woman's body not only adapts to the physical demands of gestation but supports and nourishes a fetus for 9 months. Yet, our society, which particularly values shapeliness and sexuality, offers little support or acknowledgement of the pregnant woman's changing shape or needs. The fact that paid maternity leaves are still the exception rather than the rule is strange evidence of this willingness to ignore the needs of childbearing women.

Exercise classes for pregnant women are very recent developments. Fitness, grace, and comfort have only recently come to be appreciated for their

roles in a healthy woman's life. Being physically active and enjoying the benefits of exercise can directly affect a woman's experience of pregnancy and her self-image. Body image during pregnancy will also be affected by each woman's perception of herself, her role as a woman, and the role of her body in her goals and aspirations.

Self-Image and Body Image

I have come to believe that one's self-image is described by a number of different levels of knowing about oneself. First, we know ourselves on a historical level. We know what and who we are based on our past learning. The historic self is a self-image created for us by our parents, our culture, our lovers, and all of our previous experiences. The impact of school and our interactions with teachers and peers contribute to our sense of history about self and self-image.

Historical self-image can create conflicts for pregnant women. If they are career women, they face changes in work, role, and responsibilities. If they are athletes, they face new challenges and possibly new limitations. If they have always wanted children, they may or may not find that pregnancy

99

lives up to their expectations. And if a woman has never expected to be a mother, she will also anticipate a shift in lifestyle and social role.

Second, we know ourselves on a phenomenological level. That is, we know ourselves as we are being ourselves and as we are experiencing our lives in the present. The interactions that currently describe our lives and the behaviors that have meaning to us on a daily basis contribute to our phenomenological self-awareness.

During pregnancy, the daily experience of the expanding body creates new sensations, limitations, and opportunities for self-definition. New and different social interactions occur that present shifting definitions of competence, performance, and social role.

Third, we know ourselves because we have a body image. Body image is an element of self-image; it is a level of self-knowledge that has three components. The first one is the self that we know and recognize from the exterior; that is, each of us has an image of our own appearance. It may be accurate or vastly off target, but it is our impression of our physical selves. During pregnancy the exterior body image undergoes considerable adjustment. Body boundaries enlarge and become diffuse, and this can cause dismay and amusement, delight and confusion.

The next component of body image is the self that we know of on an interior level, a level of self-knowledge that is considerably less well-defined because most of us simply do not understand anatomy and physiology, nor do we know or think about what is happening inside of our bodies. This level of awareness is awakened during pregnancy. Suddenly, organic functioning and female physiology become interesting topics. Placement of internal organs, once taken for granted, and the preservation of the fetus, become important. Figure 9.1 illustrates some of the dynamic changes that occur within a woman's body to stimulate this new interest in the interior self.

Finally, there is an ideal body image: The ideal is our future self, our dream of self, and perhaps the unattainable self. The ideal female body image is portrayed through the media, and many women understand that this presentation of femininity is hopelessly unfair. However, it remains the driving force behind the motivation to join health clubs, try new diet plans, and be a part of the entire beauty and cosmetic industry.

It is easy to understand why self-image and body image issues arise during pregnancy. The once-familiar body images, both interior and exterior, are rapidly affected by new images. And for some,

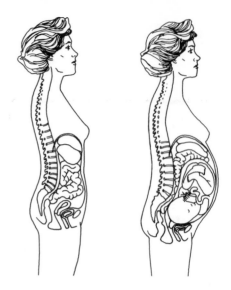

Figure 9.1. As pregnancy progresses, interest in internal self-image is awakened by the dynamic changes that occur within a woman's body.

images of the ideal self create frustrating encounters with the pregnant self. For the group leader, it is always important to try to imagine or to remember what it feels like to be pregnant. Remember to offer support and show your appreciation of every woman. I always tell pregnant women that they are beautiful.

How Body Changes Affect Self-Image

It has been observed that, as pregnancy progresses, our lovers lose their desire, our mothers reveal details of childbirth that are appalling, our employers frown, and even our best friends offer sympathy. If that isn't enough, our bodies begin to betray us. Thighs grow softer, paler, and wider. Brassieres grow painfully tight and panty hose practically choke us. And in an effort to maintain a semblance of what is most admired in our world (i.e., slimness), we exercise. Carefully prescribed routines of maternity exercises become a source of hopeful salvation. Yes, most pregnant women exercise with the secret prayer that after 9 months as an elephant, they will return to their pre-pregnant state: slim, trim, and beautiful once again.

Beautiful? We admire track stars and ballerinas for their trimness and beauty. Their bodies are firm, their movements agile and graceful. Whereas, as pregnancy progresses, simple chores become more difficult and we grow sluggish, breathless, tired, and irritable. Do we consider ourselves beautiful? Are the words *sexy* or *mysterious* part of our cultural definition of a pregnant woman? Probably not.

The fact is, in many other cultures the transformation of the female form during pregnancy has been considered quite magnificent. In the ancient caves of Pech-Merle in France, pregnant figures were depicted as having a divine quality, describing the rapture of the union between the physical and spiritual worlds. Cultures that worshiped the goddesses (Ishtar, Aphrodite, Isis, Astarte, and Ashtoreth) enjoyed and integrated the collective creativity and fertility of women into functional components of rituals and celebrations. Festivals of fertility, planting, and harvesting reflected the feminine symbols of reproductive energy. There were no illegitimate children in those cultures, for each child was born unto its mother and the line of descent was matrilineal.

In our modern, industrial community, we have not had the time or the inclination to celebrate our fertile heritage. The seasonless, endless routines of office and industry do not lend themselves to the full appreciation of what is rightfully female. Sadly, the symbols of our basic biological femaleness have been altered to fit the attitudes and aspirations of a media culture that has created an unattainably perfect, symmetrical female ideal.

Today's woman is well aware that her fingernails should be long, her heels high, her breasts firm, her hips slim, and her belly flat. The pregnant woman, who once dreamed of attaining this anatomical perfection, finds, as if by some magical stroke of misdirected yearning, that her biological functioning has become her greatest obstacle to perfection.

Body image, self-image, and self-esteem are linked to mental images and visual cues that we create for ourselves. For the pregnant woman, self-worth and self-esteem are linked to values that, overnight, become outdated and inappropriate. For some women, the passage of time and welcoming signs of life are valued experiences that help them accept their changing profiles. These women are especially lucky. For others, there is a clash of images and ideals as they face what we can call a crisis of body-ego.

Body-Ego: A Woman's Issue

Our body is our first reality. It is the essence of our being. Before we could talk, run, or choose to eat spinach but not peas, we lived in and explored our bodies without regard for social standards or limitations. We explored our genitals and our toes, for each was a pleasure point and ours was a journey in search of pleasure. We learned quickly to avoid pain, and we were easily seduced by a gentle caress.

There is evidence that as infants in our mothers' arms, our sense of self and our knowledge of being alive and of being loved came to us through our skin. Our sense of touch and tactile awareness gave us comfort and security. It warned of exposure and vulnerability. Cradled against our mother's warmth, we learned the predictable care-giving touch that gave us our sense of worth and taught us that we would be handled gently, cleaned, fed, and kept warm.

Unlike our other senses, which reveal themselves in fairly specific organs, the sense of touch is felt in almost every part of the body. Inside and out, top to bottom, there are sensory neurons that respond to the environment. They send messages of pleasure and pain. We learn quickly what is irritating and what is rewarding about our world.

In developmental terms, a sense of trust or mistrust, worth or worthlessness evolves from these very early tactile experiences. The nature of the infant's tactile gratification enables him or her to acquire a sense of physical and somatic boundaries so that further understanding of the physical and cognitive worlds can be achieved. The ability to understand time, space, shape, and boundaries builds on this foundation of initial, infantile bodily perceptions.

Studies have shown that infants left in cribs and neglected for long periods of time tend to develop self-stimulating and/or self-abusing behaviors. They may bang their heads or chew on their hands to gain necessary sensory and tactile stimulation. These children have not received the gentle and loving handling that promotes the largely positive body-ego perceptions of the healthy child.

Tactile stimulation takes on a variety of potentially pleasurable forms in adult life, including massage, bathing, eating, and sexual stimulation. Skin-to-skin contact or solitary sensual satisfaction is essential for the maintenance of positive body-ego. It is logical to assume that the more positive and pleasurable the rewards of the stimulation, the greater the desire for recurring experience and validation.

Pregnancy can create a highly unusual set of tactile possibilities, as well as a myriad of unpredictable responses. As the physical body of the pregnant woman changes, so do her pleasure points and tolerance levels. A touch that was previously erotic may become painful. A position for lovemaking that caused great arousal may become impossibly uncomfortable. Hormonal responses to pregnancy include congestion of the vulva and increased sensitivity of the genitalia. Orgasm previously achieved through gentle stimulation may require entirely different and more specific stimulation (or vice versa). In fact, the inability to achieve orgasm when lovemaking positions are modified leads some women to withdraw from the sexual experience during pregnancy. The body-ego suffers greatly if the love pair cannot find ways to reaffirm the woman's desirable, sensual, bodily beauty during pregnancy.

The body-ego demands that we maintain a homeostasis of satisfied appetite and comfortable elimination. During pregnancy, our internal cues readjust repeatedly, and appetite as well as nutritional needs are subject to surprising shifts. A sudden craving or a burst of nausea can disrupt an entire day. We may find ourselves famished at mealtimes, only to suffer with heartburn throughout the evening. We can't get enough chocolate, and suddenly shrimp with cottage cheese and catsup sounds like a gourmet treat. Previously predictable eating patterns and bowel habits are no longer the rule. The body-ego requires that we be able to anticipate, influence, and appease appetite, but some women find themselves anxious and out of control because of inconsistent and inconvenient internal cues.

Weight plays an important role in the body-ego crisis. Regardless of how logical it sounds for a pregnant woman to gain weight, our thin-conscious society has created a culture of scale watchers. This scale watching was not originally a female condition. Thirty years ago, physicians believed that they could control high blood pressure in pregnancy (formally referred to as toxemia of pregnancy), which has as one symptom rapid weight gain, by imposing strict limitations on weight gain during pregnancy. Women were weighed at each office visit and chastised if they added an extra pound. Those who gained little or nothing at all were praised for their good behavior. A woman friend reminisced that after the birth of her three children in the late 1940s and early 1950s, she looked like an "emaciated sacrecrow." She added, "I barely had enough strength to go home after my 10-day stay in the hospital. It's a good thing I didn't have to nurse!"

Body Image Problems Affect Many Women

Leslie G. McBride (1985), assistant professor of health education at Portland State University in Portland, Oregon, identified the sociocultural factors that have contributed to the current emphasis on thinness and viewed the negative impact of these factors on female self-image and body image in the context of how lowered self-esteem can lead behaviorally to chronic dieting, compulsive exercise, and depression.

This research project surveyed young women's responses to nine figure drawings. Specifically, they were asked to identify their ideal figure, their current figure, and the figure they thought the member of the opposite sex would identify as most attractive. The women consistently marked their current figure as heavier than their ideal, which in turn was heavier than the most attractive female figure. In other words, women placed unrealistic pressure on themselves to be thin. In further studies, women were shown silhouettes of female figures ranging from 20% underweight to 20% overweight. Over half of the women identified their ideal figure as the one that represented a woman who was 10% underweight, where 29% identified the 20% underweight silhouette as representing their ideal self. Physicians use 20% below average weight in diagnosis of anorexia nervosa!

An individual is at critical risk for developing negative images and opinions about body and self during adolescence. Professionals working with women who have eating disorders and others with severely distorted body images report that adolescent onset of this type of disorder represents the young person's attempt to gain control over the physical changes taking place within her body. Those of you working with pregnant teens need to be particularly aware of and sensitive to the body image concerns of adolescents and of their needs for control.

Strategies for preventing overwhelming problems of body image include stress management skill training, body image and self-esteem building, nutrition education, and weight management skills.

Emotions in Motion: The Body and Its Ego

Deep inside the pregnant woman there is a great mystery, a growing awareness of sensation and a stirring within. At first, it seems as if there may be a butterfly inside, or a tiny bubble that pops repeatedly as it bounces off some inner organ. Later, the kicking and tumult become a track-and-field event. As the fetus grows ever stronger in utero, the inner world of the body becomes a far greater reality than ever before. To many women this is a joyous experience that enriches their self-perceptions to the point of euphoria. For others, it feels as if they are possessed by a hidden and frightening force. Certainly, emotional and intellectual differences contribute to the quality of the experience of pregnancy. Previous pregnancies, expectations about pregnancy, and prenatal education contribute significantly to the experience. Yet, to some women, the pushing and pulling, and the aches and spasms of muscles under great stress are the distress signals of a body-ego in trouble.

Wide swings of emotions, called emotional lability, can be as disconcerting as any of the physical changes of pregnancy. Some women sail through pregnancy, feeling healthy, positive, and secure. Others face critical emotional challenges. Those women for whom the need for self-control and a sense of personal or professional dignity depend on clear thinking and steady handling of responsibilities may find their emotional responses to maternity surprising. Fearful moments, alarming dreams, or anxious concern for their physical survival of childbirth can combine to intensify any feelings of lost esteem. The fluctuation of emotions and perspective can leave a woman feeling vulnerable and anxious.

Assessing Body Image Issues in the Group

Group discussions about self-image and body image during pregnancy usually take on a life force of their own. Once offered the opportunity to share their feelings, women are able to discuss their concerns and perceptions quite readily. A list of factors affecting body image during pregnancy was drawn up in a workshop session I lead at a conference in Washington, DC. Several women in the group had read and were discussing *Making Love During Pregnancy* by Elizabeth Bing and Libbey Coleman (1977), *Sex During Pregnancy and After Childbirth* by Sylvia Close (1984), and *A New Approach to a Woman's Experience of Sex* by Sheila Kitzinger (1983).

We were able to divide the factors into three different categories. The first category was control, and it was defined as the individual woman's ability to influence the functioning of her body. Control factors affected each woman's awareness of her influence over internal events as well as weight gain, other physical changes, fatigue, and fear. Factors that related to sexuality and control included the physical changes of the breasts and vagina, discomfort in familiar lovemaking positions, Braxton Hicks contractions, embarrassment

about being so cumbersome, and fear that intercourse will hurt the baby. Most of the women agreed that support from and sexual acceptance by their lovers/spouses were crucial for self-esteem.

The second area identified by the women was comfort. Comfort was defined as how the body feels and how those feelings affect body image. Comfort issues affecting body image during pregnancy included feeling exhausted and frustrated about nausea, morning sickness, and the new aches and pains of pregnancy. Factors that helped the pregnant women to cope with comfort concerns included the primary support person's willingness to ease some discomforts (with massage, etc.), learning about the reasons for discomfort, and feeling the baby move.

The women wanted to define the last group of factors as visual self-image, which we decided really meant body image. The women agreed that their own expectations were the major factors affecting body image: expectations about how the body would or would not change and about past, present, and future body images. Several women identified mixed emotions about how pregnancy affected self-image, as well as competitiveness over who looked bigger, who looked better, or who was fatter. Though some women were most concerned about what they looked like while they were pregnant, others were most worried about what they would look like during childbirth. Activities that were helpful included focusing on images of mothering the newborn and talking to women who had had positive birth experiences. Avoiding horror stories about birth defects and other women's difficult births also helped relieve anxieties.

Social support became a dominant theme as we discussed how to cope with these issues of comfort, control, and body image. The support of friends and family and the approval of one's partner were very important. An understanding employer or teacher contributed to comfort in the workplace by allowing movement or adjustments in the workplace furnishings, ''flex time,'' or time off. A best friend or a friend who had recently given birth played an important supportive and educational role in most women's lives.

These revealing discussions formed the basis of a ''Body Image Assessment'' form that I developed and used with my students for over 2 years. Women were interviewed upon registering for the class. They indicated that their reasons for coming to prenatal exercises classes were to stay in shape; to learn more about the pregnancy, labor, and birth; and to meet other women like themselves.

They were also asked to fill out a self-image questionnaire (Appendix 9.1) and a body map, which we will discuss shortly. The questionnaire was designed especially for use with pregnant women, and its purpose is to explore and evaluate feelings about body image, knowledge of the body, and support systems. You may use it with your classes. It can provide you with a wealth of information about the health of the women in your groups. Remember that assurance of confidentiality will allow your students to be comfortable about sharing their perceptions and feelings with you.

Body Mapping

Body mapping is a great technique for illustrating feelings about particular areas of the body. It can be adapted to groups of any size, age, or skill level. I have often provided huge, 6-foot-long pieces of brown paper and magic markers to workshop participants or simply printed up a sample map like the one included here (see Figure 9.2).

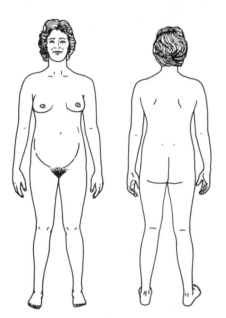

Figure 9.2. Have students circle favorite body parts, x least favorite, draw arrows where they hurt, color the parts that changed with pregnancy, and star places they like massaged.

We all have a body map, which changes considerably during pregnancy. The body, once an acceptable, dependable companion, becomes unfamiliar and unpredictable. Body landscapes undergo major changes, some delightful, some not so pleasing, and the body can become a mystery. A woman's perception of her body and the fetus within her

makes body mapping an expressive and enjoyable activity. It helps women get in touch with their feelings about their bodies and it helps them share how they are feeling with others who care about them.

Another body image assessment activity is the Body Image During Pregnancy form (Appendix 9.2). It is intended to be a fun activity rather than a serious diagnostic tool. Use it to open the group to discussion.

Also, in Appendix 9.3 you will find an Initial Physical Report form. Use Part 1 to help women identify physical problems that can be addressed through exercise and education about pregnancy. Part 2 can be used to stimulate discussion about lifestyle that can affect fetal health. The information is very useful in forming the basis of discussion planning. This form is personal and the information on it should be kept confidential.

Dance Therapy

Pregnancy is a normal part of the adult life cycle. It needn't be considered a crisis. The physical changes and adaptations of the body can be viewed as normal and healthy if women are encouraged to see themselves as healthy, strong, and beautiful.

I feel quite strongly that body image plays a significant part in how each woman accepts and then moves through her pregnancy. By addressing body image, we may be able to enhance a woman's acceptance and enjoyment of self and pregnancy. Opportunities for self-expression and creative movement experiences from the field of dance therapy may help you to understand and plan for body image work in your classes.

Movement as therapy is a field of study and practice with roots in psychiatric healing. Dance therapy's clinical applications now appear in many therapeutic environments including deaf education, head trauma treatment, institutions for the mentally ill, programs for women with eating disorders, and other specialities in the areas of exceptional education. Although the psychoeducational and psychoanalytic goals of dance/movement therapy differ from those of the prenatal exercise class, the techniques and processes that explore rhythm and breathing, time, effort, and shape are similar.

Dance therapy is a fascinating field. Bernstein, who has written a great deal on the subject (1975, 1986), has argued the relevance of dance-movement therapies, effectively reminding practitioners that individuals react and organize their movement patterns differently. With this in mind, let's look at some of the elements of dance therapy that make body image work an important activity.

Rhythm and Breathing

Rhythm is part of every movement we make. The simple act of tightening the urethra to prevent urination and then releasing it is a rhythmic process. Sucking and breathing are rhythmic processes, and one of the fascinating connections between physical fitness activities, dance therapy, and childbirth education is that they all have an intense concern and interest in these oral rhythms.

As adults we rarely consider the changes in our breathing rhythms. Well-integrated individuals are able to shift gears according to the task at hand, whether it is climbing stairs, swimming, or having a bowel movement. Less well-integrated individuals include breath-holders, who need to be reminded to breathe during exercise, and smokers, who have the tendency to hyperventilate under stress.

As pregnancy progresses many women have difficulty breathing. They experience shortness of breath, a smothering feeling, or heartburn, which all interfere with comfortable respiratory efficiency. Anatomically, the expansion of the rib cage and the abdomen should actually facilitate the comfort of breathing. The size of the fetus and the upward pressure on the diaphragm, however, may leave little room for compensatory breathing.

Breathing is an important tool in natural childbirth. As we will discuss in more detail later, the cleansing, releasing breath becomes a signal for the onset of each labor contraction. It may signal the woman to initiate her relaxation response or signal those in the room to otherwise assist her during the contraction. The breath can become part of a pregnant woman's response repertoire. To enhance the response repertoire for labor, I use the following visualization, pausing about 10 seconds between each phrase:

Breathe deeply and exhale fully. Enjoy the feeling of your breath. Visualize oxygen flowing into your bloodstream and flowing through their muscles. The oxygen flows through the placenta and down the umbilical cord. Imagine how the baby enjoys this oxygen. Now, imagine that with every breath you take, you are becoming more and more relaxed. When you are in labor, use your breath this way. Everytime you inhale and exhale, your body softens. Your face softens and your vaginal opening softens. Every time you inhale and exhale, your cervix opens more and your baby slides a little closer toward being born.

Time

A second important element in the language of dance therapy is time. Time and the effective use of timing involve the individual's automatic reactions for coping with the demands of the environment. Speeding up one's actions, slowing them down, moving with urgency, and prolonging an action are demonstrations of the use of time.

Time also involves willingness to follow through and to adapt to an action. (During labor, a woman can't leave just because the contractions hurt—she has to stay and see it through until the end!)

During pregnancy and labor, time and timing become distorted. The breathing techniques of childbirth are excellent examples of the use of time. The ability to use different levels of breathing and to coordinate the necessary relaxation response or pushing behavior require the coordination of a woman's sense of timing. A woman's perception of herself as strong and capable affects her ability to respond to her contractions and coordinate the timing of her efforts.

Activities that explore the use of time and the importance of timing can enhance a woman's perception of herself as being capable of adapting to the demands of time. You can work on this in your class by purposefully slowing down dance steps and experimenting with performing at different speeds. This will clarify body movement, potential, and self-image among your students.

Effort

Effort, in the language of dance therapy, is defined as the way a person copes with her body, expends energy, and responds to the environment. Effort describes a great deal about a woman's attitudes toward life. It is the rhythm and flow, the pace and speed of her life.

Effort is the ability to release tension, to start and stop, and to control movement. Effort is the individual's ability to channel movement; to respond to gravity; to use strength or lightness, grace or force; and to persist or draw back.

Effort is the consummate element in sexual intercourse, and, in fact, the effort of intercourse and of the rhythm of sexuality are profoundly affected by pregnancy. Childbirth is the ultimate effort!

In a prenatal exercise class, a woman's initial sluggish movements and reluctance to make the effort to move the body into position are soon replaced by her pleasurable response to the rhythm of the music, her enhanced respiratory response to activity, and her kinesthetic response to the stimulation of muscles. Teaching women how to control effort through physical and mental exercises should be one of the goals of your prenatal exercise class.

Activities that promote the release of tension are of particular value to pregnant women. You might suggest that the students imagine that they are lifting a heavy object that suddenly becomes light so that they can throw it away. In addition, use movements that stress the downward release of tension, such as wall-sits and deep supported squats.

Shape

The last term we have borrowed from dance therapy is shape. Although shape can refer to the differences between the pregnant and the nonpregnant form, in this context it refers to making the body into shapes. Shaping is the ability of an individual to understand and move appropriately according to body boundaries. During pregnancy, the body must shape itself differently; for example, it must do so to get into the car, to sleep at night, and to move from standing to sitting and from chair to floor. Women report distress, confusion, and amusement at these new and confounding shapes.

The shape of birth is also different and new. Women cannot expect to be able to shape their bodies during childbirth if they don't practice these positions beforehand. Nor can they actively participate in birth if they are required to lay down and put their feet up in stirrups. Women must be allowed to shape their bodies in response to contractions and gravity. Practice in shaping the body for birth is essential if women are to regain a sense of control over birth.

It is easy to integrate these concepts into a prenatal exercise program. I have used them for many of our movement and discussion activities. For example, I frequently ask women to draw pictures of what they think labor will look like. This enhances discussion and practice of birth positions as well as understanding how the body shapes itself for birth.

Healing

By exploring how the effort of movement changes during pregnancy and how the body feels while it is moving, we discover how breathing and rhythm can enhance the experience of movement. Through activities and discussions that encourage women to feel good about themselves, we are able to present pregnancy as a maturational journey from which they will emerge stronger, wiser, and more beautiful. Of course, sometimes we do silly things like take group photos or play belly-measurement guessing games.

There is a special group of women for whom you will have to adapt your body image activities. This group includes women who reject feeling, or are simply unable to feel, emotionally attached to the fetus: specifically, women who are not pleased to be pregnant. Try to present visualizations and activities that promote maternal/fetal attachment, which in turn may lead to more positive experience of pregnancy. Use activities that require women to give one another support; such mirroring and exploring of support positions for delivery can be helpful. Have the class rock or roll on the floor and curl into the fetal position; this helps remove some of the barriers to positive maternal/fetal visualization and attachment.

Careful and sensitive teaching is required when dealing with the differing needs of those women who will choose to parent their babies and those who will relinquish them for adoption. Personal health reports, dream sharing, and visualization techniques are useful for working with these women.

Summary

This approach to body image work focuses on the whole woman and is organized to have an impact on the woman's thinking about herself and her body. Focusing on body image helps put things into perspective. Teaching women how to cope with pregnancy and how to learn about who they are and how they feel about giving birth are major efforts towards healing self-image and body image.

The concepts of balance and healing are central to understanding how the prenatal exercise class has a positive impact on self-image. The purpose of the prenatal exercise class is to improve the functional level of the body, thereby improving feelings of self-worth, self-esteem, and self-image. The highly skilled instructor will talk about the whole woman: her changing body and her baby. This reminds the mother how special she is and how taking good care of herself means she is doing the same for her unborn child. The class is a healing environment. It stresses the balance and integration of body and mind, and of medical care and personal wisdom. Healing is directly tied to understanding the interactive systems of medicine and education. Finally, in the prenatal class women learn to accept the uncertainty of pregnancy and birth—that unexpected events are part of the open and changing system of giving life.

By inviting women to participate in an unfolding and loving environment, you are helping them to appreciate and experience each person's value and uniqueness. You can stir each person's imagination and help all the participants to perceive the unexplainable changes and mysteries of pregnancy as organic and healthy. You can even teach women how to view vulnerability as a healing process that leads, eventually, to strength. When body image and self-image during pregnancy are seen as part of a flowing continuum of life, rather than as a threatening force beyond their control, most women will find they can enjoy cooperating with their bodies with a joyous appreciation of pregnancy's inherent inconveniences.

We have already discussed a number of tools you can use to help women learn to enjoy their bodies and their pregnancies. In the next chapter we look closely at exercises and activities that promote the integration of mind and body in preparation for birth.

Self-Image Questionnaire

Please check the phrases that describe you or your feelings:

Being pregnant makes me feel fat. _____

I think I have gained too much weight. _____

Being pregnant makes me feel sexy. _____

I feel sick a lot. _____

I am tired a lot. _____

I feel angry. _____

My boss (or teachers) are very understanding. _____

I cry a lot. _____

I need more privacy. _____

This pregnancy was planned. _____

I am anxious about childbirth. _____

I have a good understanding of childbirth. _____

I feel beautiful. _____

The baby's dad is very understanding. _____

My family is very happy about the baby. _____

I have a best friend. _____

Sometimes I feel very lonely. _____

I like being pregnant. _____

I don't like being pregnant. _____

I get plenty of exercise. _____

I like the way my body is changing. _____

I wish I had a better understanding of female

physiology. _____

Please fill in the blanks:

Being pregnant is _____

The best part of being pregnant is _____

The worst part of being pregnant is _____

I wish _____

My body _____

Making love _____

Body Image During Pregnancy

Rank your feelings about the following items according to this scale:
1—Have strong positive feelings
2—Have moderate positive feelings
3—Have no feelings one way or the other
4—Have moderately negative feelings
5—Have strong negative feelings

_____ Hair _____ Facial complexion _____ Appetite _____ Hands _____ Change in waistline

_____ Maternity clothes _____ Stamina _____ Bowel habits _____ Muscular strength

_____ Energy level _____ Back _____ Stretch marks _____ Age _____ Neck _____ Gums

_____ Profile _____ Weight gain _____ Bellybutton _____ Tolerance for pain _____ Ankles

_____ Arms _____ Breasts _____ Belly _____ Eyes _____ Digestion _____ Hips

_____ Bottom _____ Resistance to illness _____ Thighs _____ Calves _____ Sex drive

_____ Muscle tone _____ Feet _____ Sleep _____ Posture _____ Ability to achieve orgasm

_____ Health _____ New aches and pains _____ Loss of menstrual cycle

Score yourself:

Total:

39–60, Excellent body image. Wow! You feel pretty wonderful about yourself and must be in excellent health. Pregnancy is probably a good time for you.

60–80, Superior body image. Good for you! You too have a remarkably positive attitude about yourself.

80–120, Somewhat ambivalent. Why? Ambivalence is a characteristic response of women who are asked to discuss how they really feel about their bodies. One woman said she was probably like everybody else: "I feel good about everything above the shoulders and below the knees."

120–160, Pregnancy and difficulty with body image go hand in hand. It may be time to start exercising regularly! You may be experiencing a physical crisis or a change in body image and self-image as a result of your pregnancy, past health problems, or stress. Let's talk!

Above 160, You sound like you need special help. Exercise should help but maybe it's time to talk to someone about how you are feeling.

Initial Physical Report

Welcome to our Prenatal Exercise Class! All the information you provide here is confidential. Please answer the questions so that we can plan your exercise and health education program together.

Your name _____

How are you feeling? _____

#1 problem, if any _____

Part 1

Please check any of the following items that apply to you:

Headaches _____   Nosebleeds _____   Changes in gums _____

Pain _____ (Where?) _____

Stiffness _____ (Where?) _____

Numbness _____ (Where?) _____

High blood pressure _____   Racing heart beats _____   Chest pain _____

Shortness of breath _____   Swollen feet _____   Swollen hands _____   Varicose veins _____

Heartburn _____   Indigestion _____   Nausea or vomiting _____   Hemorrhoids _____

Constipation _____   Diarrhea _____   Bladder infections _____

Excessive need to urinate _____   Very little need to urinate _____   Excessive thirst _____

Leaking urine _____   Vaginal discharge _____

Part 2

Important lifestyle questions for you to consider when you are pregnant:

Do you own a cat? _____

   Dirty cat litter can cause infections in pregnant women which lead to birth defects. When you are pregnant, let someone else take care of the kitty litter.

Do you smoke cigarettes? _____

   Certain tobacco products can cause problems for unborn babies. Even working in a smoke-filled room may cause problems. Try to give up smoking. There are currently many types of smoking cessation programs. Contact the American Lung Association for more information.

Do you drink alcoholic beverages? _____

   There is no known safe level of alcohol consumption during pregnancy. If you drink, now's the time to get help and give it up. Contact your local chapter of Alcoholics Anonymous.

Are you using any drugs like marijuana, cocaine, crack, speed, or heroin? _____

   Any of these can cause serious problems for you and your baby. Please work to ensure that your baby is healthy by giving up drugs. Contact your local chapter of Alcoholics Anonymous or Narcotics Anonymous.

Are you a vegetarian? _____

There are many ways to ensure that you eat an adequate amount of protein. For more information about this subject I suggest reading *Nourishing a Happy Affair: Nutrition Alternatives for Individual and Family Needs* by Leslie Cohen (1983), *The Vegetarian Handbook: Eating Right for Total Health* by Gary Null (1987), or *Food for Health: A Nutrition Encyclopedia* by A. Ensminger, M.E. Ensminger, J. Konlaid, and J.R. Robson (1986).

Do you eat raw meat? _____

Uncooked meat may contain bacteria that can cause birth defects. Make sure all meat is properly cooked.

Have you been exposed to radiation through X rays or at work? _____

Try to avoid further exposure during pregnancy.

Have you been exposed to any STDs? _____

Sexually transmitted diseases, like AIDS and genital herpes, can cause serious problems for babies. Talk to your doctor.

Are you taking any medications? _____

Some medications can be harmful to unborn babies. Take no medicine, not even aspirin, unless it is prescribed by your doctor.

Are you dieting? _____

Pregnant women should not try to lose weight. A well-balanced diet is important for your baby's development.

Chapter 10

Healing Exercises to Prepare for Birth

From the following discussion of healing exercises you will get a sense of the importance of preparing the body and mind for childbirth. The exercises I use are designed specifically for pregnancy. They promote physical strength, sensory awareness, emotional growth, and comprehension of the body as it changes and prepares for birth.

The integration of body and mind, which occurs through proper channelling of the breath and movement practice, establishes the individual's connection to self. By promoting body movement and allowing each woman to explore her potential to use the body, you help each woman to learn about herself. She will learn that she is graceful and powerful and that she can influence things that she once considered beyond her ability to change. All of these things instill the kind of self-confidence that will be of great value to her during the challenge of birth. Teaching breathing techniques is an excellent way to begin this healing, strengthening process.

Teaching Breathing Techniques

Breathing is one of the most important healing techniques of the specialized prenatal class. The effort of breathing changes throughout pregnancy, and there is a biological basis for these changes. *Prana* is a Hindu word meaning breath, or life force. I encourage women to think of breathing as *prana*: nourishment and life energy.

Now, I have never met a pregnant woman who forgot to breathe. I have met many, however, for whom shortness of breath, asthma, or chronic bronchitis created erratic and blocked patterns of breathing. I have also observed women whose anxiety or fatigue caused them to hyperventilate. This pattern was allowed to progress unchecked, and they breathed so rapidly during labor that they became lightheaded and panicky.

Therefore, I emphasize the use of slow, steady breathing as a healing technique. The proper use of the cleansing breath at the beginning and end of exercises is essential. Once the use of the cleansing breath becomes a habit for your students, it will be a logical extension to use it at the onset of contractions during labor. Similarly, once the use of steady, rhythmic breathing patterns becomes a natural response to movement, they are easily incorporated into the birth experience.

A woman who experiences the pleasure of breathing finds that proper breathing during pregnancy reduces discomfort and fatigue and improves appearance. All movement exercises should have a breathing pattern. I base most of my breathing patterns on the hatha-yoga techniques of inhalation with expansion, exhalation with contraction. Begin each exercise with a releasing breath. As the body moves up and out, the lungs are filled. As the body is made smaller, air is expelled. These are examples of activities using this technique:

1. Stretch up and out like a cat: inhale and stretch up one, two, three, and now exhale and let the cat relax.
2. Imagine your body is getting bigger, like a balloon! And now, let all the air out!
3. With your arms, make a big shape around your body. Inhale and feel the expansion. Exhale as the shape curves inward.

4. Pretend you are doing the breast stroke and inhale as you create more room in your chest.

5. Do a deep swing, as if you were preparing to do a standing broad jump. Inhale as you swing up and exhale as you swing down low.

I use breathing patterns to teach women how to breathe to specific rhythms. This prepares them to learn the various breathing techniques of natural childbirth. When we are moving together, I encourage them to think about their breathing, reminding them always that the pain of labor is in the body and breathing moves the pain up and out. These are a few of the many techniques that emphasize the positive experience of breathing and relate it to the performance of movement:

- Doing steady, uninterrupted exercise movements that flow together at a steady, even pace.
- Performing yoga *asanas*.
- Making active and conscious use of releasing breath during exercises.
- Visualizing experiences that are steady and even, and then visualizing those that have a quality of freshness, lightness, and freedom.
- Teaching tidal volume (or sleep breathing) during relaxation.
- Explaining the postural response to pain, which should be total relaxation.
- Teaching the physiological pushing breath as the breath to accompany a variety of exercises. This breath is a long, slow, gentle exhalation. It is an important substitute for the breath-holding of the aggravated ''Push! Push! Push!'' of cheering-squad births.
- Dancing to Hawaiian music or using undulating belly dance techniques that create that a series of movement transitions from tension to relaxation.

Breathing as Pleasure

Breath awareness is both psychologically and physiologically helpful. The slow-chest pattern of breathing, and the gentle or physiological pushing breath, are essentially libidinal or pleasurable responses to the stimulus of childbirth contractions. Contrast these to the frightened woman's response to childbirth tension, which is to hold her breath. If you observe breath-holding during exercise, you should read it as anxiety and seek to remedy it as soon as possible.

I suggest that during birth women become involved with the pleasurable sensation of their breath as it cleanses and gives order to periods of uterine irritability and contraction. Using the breath in a gentle, peaceful manner can feel like floating and drifting without boundaries. Relaxing deeply, as we will discuss in the next chapter, while using this breath allows the cervix to open and stretch and the baby to be born.

Suggesting that women use the breath to help them release tension confounds those women who associate letting go with losing control. Some women feel they must be active and in control at all times. These are often the women who want things to be a definite way and, as a result, are unable to achieve the release of tension that can speed labor.

The traditional breath-holding ''hutt'' for pushing during delivery could be considered an aggressive style of coping with the intensity of giving birth. It evokes the image of bearing down and then the release of a bowel movement. It contrasts vividly with the gentle pushing breath, a more natural style of breathing that brings to mind the deep and open sensation of releasing a full bladder and the deep sigh that may accompany that experience. The gentler exhalation allows participation in the sensation of the birth and reminds the mother to allow her vagina to stretch as her uterus contracts.

The bodily imperatives of birth evoke a range of respiratory responses. When I explore different ways to breathe, I also have in mind the importance of the intense and angry breath of birth; the breath of frustration, of pain, of helplessness. I have spent time with women acting out, snarling, yelling, and moaning their anxieties about childbirth. We have spent time making birth noises. We have grunted, groaned, and occasionally sobbed together.

Women who use their bodies to their full potential and who experience the integration of breathing, movement, and timing are capable of experiencing childbirth as a powerful and satisfying accomplishment. Women who are conscious of their anatomy, aware of birth's physiology, and able to use their muscles properly indulge in their own abilities. For them, birth becomes the finest victory.

Breathing Patterns for Birth

Experiencing the rising intensity of labor contractions and then pushing a baby out are profoundly important experiences in many women's lives. To those who are anticipating a first birth and those who are preparing for the next, the practice of the breathing techniques can contribute great healing energy.

A woman should begin to practice the breathing patterns for labor and delivery as early in her pregnancy as possible. The choice may be to pursue a form of exercise that includes breathing techniques like yoga or karate, or simply to begin to practice the techniques of natural childbirth.

In addition to teaching breathing patterns with exercises, you should spend time during the relaxation section of a class teaching and practicing the breathing patterns taught by childbirth educators. Most women want and need to practice relaxing and using these techniques. There is no reason to reserve the teaching of these techniques until a woman is 7 months pregnant. The more a woman knows and the earlier she knows it, the less anxious she will feel and the more successful she will be at using what she knows at birth.

For our purposes I will introduce the techniques that I use for teaching about breathing during childbirth—you may know of or prefer others. There are many varieties of breathing techniques, and cultural wisdom about which ones to use at what point in labor is always changing. My philosophy is that each woman will find her own most comfortable level and speed of breathing: There are no absolutes.

The releasing breath is a deep inhalation and full exhalation performed (a) in class at the beginning of most exercises and (b) in labor and delivery at the onset of each contraction. It is a great healer and can be used as a signal to relax throughout a person's lifetime. It is also called the cleansing breath.

Slow-chest breathing is the light, gentle breath of sleep. The lips should be parted and the mouth should be very soft. The breath is neither deep nor rapid, but slow, light, and very relaxed. This technique is used in early labor when contractions are light and wavelike. It requires no special action or activity. When a contraction begins the woman should take her releasing breath and begin using this slow and easy pattern of breathing. When the contraction is over, she should take a nice, deep, releasing breath and relax.

Accelerated/decelerated breathing is the breathing pattern called into use when contractions become stronger and the mother feels that she needs to breathe more rapidly. After taking a cleansing breath, she begins the slow-chest breathing and then speeds it up, just a bit, as if she were working extra hard, perhaps climbing a hill or riding a bike. At the peak of her contraction she is breathing lightly and rapidly, and as the contraction fades her pace slows and relaxes. At the end of her contraction she takes a cleansing breath.

The pant-blow is the technique taught for coping with transition. It is the most complicated to learn, and many women resist practicing it because it feels silly. Transition is a brief period during labor when the cervix is almost completely dilated and contractions are very strong. They occur rapidly and very close together, and the peak of each contraction is extremely intense. To cope with this degree of tension, a woman may take a quick releasing breath and place her tongue up behind her two front teeth. She should breathe in and out four times as slowly as possible, blow out crisply, and return her tongue to its position behind her front teeth and begin again. Practice of this technique should be slow. In labor most women find they pick up the pace in response to the urgency of the contractions.

Feather blowing is a technique that often causes a chuckle in class. Before a woman is fully dilated she may feel the urge to bear down. It is important to protect both the fetal head and the maternal perineum at this point, so the mother should not push too hard too quickly. Feather blowing prevents her from bearing down by requiring that she lift her chin and lightly blow out, as if she were keeping a feather dancing above her nose. During actual labor, this feather blow may become an extremely vigorous activity, but in class, keep it light. It is also used when the care giver wishes to slow the emergence of the baby's head. The mother needs to know that in the middle of an urgent need to bear down her care giver may holler, "Blow! Blow! Blow!"

Exhalation pushing is used to facilitate a gentle birth. When a woman is ready to push her baby out, she should take in several releasing and cleansing breaths and then slowly exhale and bear down on her uterus with her chest and rib cage. She should practice this exhalation pushing with her body in a C curve, pelvis open, legs wide apart, and bottom completely relaxed. I do not encourage women to push or bear down while in class.

I suggest to women that when they practice this at home they should ask their partner to place a hand on the belly just above the symphysis pubis. Pushing a baby out is not like having a giant bowel movement. A woman doesn't push to the rectum, she pushes to the vagina. Having a hand to push to can be very helpful.

Traditional pushing is a breath-holding pushing technique. During the pushing stage, a mother may be asked to give a real strong push. If she has been using the gentle pushing technique she should decide whether she wants to change the pattern. If she feels that she wants to use the traditional pushing breath, she should take two good cleansing breaths and then on the third inhalation she should catch her breath in her chest, put her chin to her chest, and bear down. This is a very aggressive method for coping with the pressure of the baby's head on the perineum. The imperatives of birth, as we mentioned above, frequently invoke great intensity. It takes a great deal of effort, and the breath should not be held for more than a few seconds at a time. I do not practice this breath more than once or twice during classes. Practice should be done with mom in a C curve, that is, with her back curved, pelvis open, and knees wide apart.

Breathing deeply, fully, and freely is a wonderful sensation. The heaviness and discomfort of advancing pregnancy does not permit a woman to enjoy deep, full respiration. I have occasionally thought that voice training would be another model of teaching to explore during pregnancy. It, too, emphasizes the use of the breath.

The following material on healing exercises addresses the importance of body awareness and surrender to and integration of the senses. Just as the breath is the essential symbol of life, so movement is the symbol of change.

Healing Exercise

Regular exercise is important for all women. Exercise has been shown to prevent osteoporosis; reduce the incidence of endomitriosis, the excessive growth of tissue from the endometrial lining of the uterus; and to prevent or to help control the onset of adult diabetes.

I often talk about how exercise heals pregnant women by strengthening the body, relieving tension, improving circulation, and contributing to a feeling of well-being and balance. Exercise makes a woman feel good about herself. When a woman exercises she encounters herself, discovers how her body works, how it feels, and what she can do to make it feel better.

The medical evidence of the value and healing effects of exercise has been presented by many researchers. In the report from the Symposium on Medical Aspects of Exercise (Goldberg & Elliot, 1985), physicians reported the beneficial effects of exercise for a variety of special populations. The reports all found that the results of regular exercise were positive.

In some classes, I begin teaching by introducing a series of movements that I call healing exercises. They are neither dance nor yoga but movement phrases that allow women to explore and discover themselves and their bodies. Our contemporary culture does not usually allow us the time to know ourselves in this way. Perhaps it is our need to conform or our fear of peer review that inhibits us. In the following section are examples of movement phrases that are designed to establish balance. They are written in the form of instructions. You may read them to your classes. Feel free to modify this and other exercises to match your students' abilities; however, always keep the ACOG (1985) guidelines and other practical safety precautions in mind. Those of you who are interested in developing your own series of healing exercises might want to refer to *Complete Relaxation* (Kravette, 1979) for inspiration. The exercises I use are similar in tone and quality to his integrated approach to relaxation and body awareness.

Healing Exercise 1: Centering

This series is done gently and slowly:

Please stand up with your feet comfortably apart. Lift your chin slightly. Inhale and exhale gently and evenly. Place your thumbs on your sternum, the bone between your breasts. Pull in slightly on your belly to reduce the curve in your lower back. Your shoulders should be relaxed, even, and not rounded forward or thrust backward.

As you breathe deeply, lift your sternum. The sternum is the body's center of lightness. As you lift it, you allow more room for your lungs to expand. You also eliminate any sunken chest or round-shouldered hunch that reflects a poor body-ego.

As you breathe, lift your chin slightly and imagine that you are adding air to the spaces between the vertebrae in your spine. Imagine that your neck is strong and that your head is sitting effortlessly on top of it. Relax your jaw. Remember, never let your head roll forward.

Make sure your weight is evenly distributed on both feet. Contract your tummy muscles. Visualize your pelvis as a bowl, and tilt the bowl slightly backward.

Lift your arms out to the side and curve them gracefully, as if they were branches on a tree, making certain that your fingers are relaxed. Bend to the side. Return to center and bend to the other side, all the while breathing gently and evenly. Inhale at the center point, exhale as you bend.

In addition to having a calming effect, this exercise does two important things. First, it lifts the rib cage to allow the diaphragm more room to move up and down, which feels great and allows one to breathe more deeply. Second, it tones the muscles of the torso, which will form the basis of the waistline after childbirth!

Healing Exercise 2: Touching the Earth

Here is another set of healing movement options. Pay close attention to the imagery and the words that describe the movements.

To begin, stand comfortably erect. Inhale deeply and exhale completely. Imagine that you are anchored to the ground, that your feet are part of the earth. Place your fists on your back and massage your lower back. Return your hands to your sides. Now, allow your head and shoulders to roll forward. Slowly, allow your body to roll down, releasing your back, vertebra by vertebra. Open your legs and bend your knees until you are hanging down with your head relaxed. Your knees are released and your arms should feel soft and floppy. (Relaxing and opening the knees wide helps prevent the sensation of a crowded uterus.)

Allow yourself to go into a deep relaxed squat. Use your hands and arms for support. Let your head and neck relax. Feel the surface beneath your hands. Notice how relaxed and comfortable you feel so close to the ground. Experiment with your center of balance. How far forward do you need to place your hands to feel stable and safe?

Now begin to roll back up, inch by inch, muscle by muscle, until you are standing firmly centered and erect. Stretch your arms straight up. Reach up over your head, place your palms together, and lift your body as high and long and tall as possible. Breathe deeply. With your fingertips and palms, pull your body slowly to center again while remaining completely balanced.

Healing Exercise 3: Shifting Center

This exercise focuses on weight and the changing center of balance.

Move your feet apart and let your knees bend slightly. Make certain that your weight is com-

fortably and evenly distributed. Slowly shift your weight from the right leg to the left leg. Hold that position and breathe. Now shift your weight from the left side to the right side. Hold that position and breathe. Your shoulders are level, and your body is in a straight line. Shift back and forth.

Now bend your knees a little more as you shift your weight. Feel the muscles of your thighs and calves. Keep breathing as you shift from side to side. Return to center. Move your feet another 10 or 12 in. apart and repeat this exercise.

Straighten your legs and place one hand over the other in front of you. Inhale deeply and allow your arms to lift slightly. Release your breath and lower your arms gently. Inhale and let your arms float up over your head. Raise your elbows as high as they will go. Place your palms together and reach as high as you can. Inhale and exhale. Gently allow your arms to fall loosely to your sides.

Healing Exercise 4: Fingertip Flick

Many women do not even realize that they feel tense until they begin to flick tension away. This exercise ends in the deeply relaxed *salaam* pose.

While seated on your knees, extend your hands in front of you, palms down. Open and close your fingers and thumbs, pretending that you are flicking tension away. Open your hands wide, stretch your fingers open and closed, open and closed. Bring your hands together until they almost touch and then relax them as your palms come together. Remember to keep your face and jaw relaxed. Repeat.

Place your fingertips on your knees and now stretch your arms out in front of you. Open your knees and place your palms on the floor. Your head should be down and your knees open as wide as is comfortable for you. Breathe deeply and relax in the *salaam* pose.

Healing Exercise 5: Kegel Exercises

During our lives, we tend to judge our fitness by the strength or flabbiness of our bellies or thighs. But there is one muscle group that we never see and rarely think about. Commonly referred to as the kegel muscles, this group of muscles is actually the support system for the organs of the lower pelvis. They act together and affect a woman's ability to control the tightening and releasing of her anus, vagina, and urethra. They also act as a sling to support the added weight of the uterus during pregnancy, and during delivery they stretch to permit the passage of the baby down and out the birth canal. This hidden muscle group includes the pubococcygeus muscle, which is part of the levator ani and is described in greater detail in chapter 2.

In the past it was recommended that women work up to performing hundreds of rapid kegel contractions to tone the vagina. More recent research indicates that fewer repetitions done carefully and slowly can also reduce incontinence and are actually more beneficial.

I recommend that you take some time teaching this exercise. For many women it will be the first time in their lives that they are allowed or encouraged to focus on these muscles.

To locate your kegel muscles, lie on your left side. Make certain that you are as comfortable as possible. Imagine that you are trying to prevent yourself from urinating. Tighten the urethral muscle and gently pull forward on it. Release and repeat that gentle squeeze. Still lying on your left side, tighten and draw in and up on your vaginal muscles. Continue to tighten for several seconds and release slowly. *(Repeat this exercise several times.)* Finally, tighten the muscles around your anus. Release slowly.

This entire area, from the urethra to the rectum, is called the perineum. This exercise will help maintain muscle tone as well as increase sensitivity and control. By isolating these muscles and becoming aware of how they feel when they are tightened, you also develop an awareness of how they feel when they are relaxed. The muscles of the perineum must be relaxed if you are going to deliver your baby. Tense, tight perineal muscles can slow down labor and dilation. Clenched perineal muscles can prevent delivery.

In the past physicians believed that women who strengthened the pubococcygeus muscle through dance or other forms of exercise tightened the perineum and increased the necessity for an episiotomy. This is not the case. Well-toned muscles stretch and allow for the natural opening of the birth canal. Slack muscles are far more likely to tear during birth than those that can stretch.

I recommend that women who have difficulty with the kegel exercise spend time at home learning to isolate the muscles. They can do this by plac-

ing their hands on the perineum to feel the muscles as they contract. They may also place a warm washcloth on the perineum to relax the area before practicing the exercises.

Talking about this exercise and emphasizing the fact that it should be done over the lifetime is very helpful. I consider this exercise the essential woman's exercise. By discussing its importance to one's experience of sexuality, as well as for prevention or treatment of urinary incontinence, you permit a woman to feel and appreciate the importance of her vaginal muscles. Many women are afraid to feel their vaginal muscles except during the sex act, and part of the fear about birth is due to a lack of understanding about the role and function of the vagina during birth. Allowing a woman to understand the elasticity of the vagina and encouraging her to enjoy the undulating, rhythmic contraction and release of her vagina is an essential, sensual experience. You may want to refer to Kitzinger (1983) for further discussion of the kegel exercise.

Healing Exercise 6: The Pelvic Tilt

The pelvic tilt is an important exercise that allows women to isolate the pelvis and to experiment with how the different muscles that are attached to it act to move it. The pelvic tilt helps to relieve backache and reduce some of the pressure women feel deep in the pelvic basin. The exercise can be done while standing, leaning against a wall, sitting, lying on the back, or resting on hands and knees (see Figure 10.1). I teach it first while women are lying down and then we experiment with the other positions.

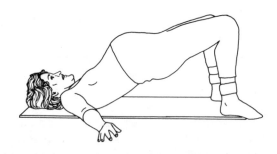

Figure 10.1. Maximum lift for pelvic tilt exercise creates a narrow triangle between the back or the pelvis and the floor. Do *not* hyperextend the pelvic tilt as shown here.

Roll onto your back, place your feet flat on the floor with your knees bent. Pull in on the tummy muscles and release. Each time you pull in, you are moving your pelvis just slightly, flattening your back into the floor. Exhale as you pull in, inhale as you relax.

The bridge exercise can accompany the pelvic tilt. Perform the exercise again and lift your coccyx and sacrum off the ground just a tiny bit. Pull in on the tummy muscles and hip flexors, tighten the buttocks, and release.

Do the pelvic tilt again, pull in on the abdominal muscles, and lift the back of the pelvis up off the ground. Create a narrow triangle with your body, your legs, and the floor. Do not arch your back. Release slowly. If the back-lying position makes you feel nauseous or dizzy, try this exercise in a different position.

Repeat the entire series.

Roll onto your side and relax.

The six exercises described above are part of a process that has to do with coming to a greater awareness of self which is a part of healing. These exercises, when put together and performed slowly, one right after the other, are a natural, noncompetitive, movement experience. The exercises flow together and have a pleasing rhythm. It is the rhythm of living and breathing.

While breathing is an automatic function about which we can become more aware, the movements we have discussed increase awareness of muscular function. There is another series of exercises that must be included in the prenatal routine to involve the mother fully in her preparation for birth. They are the exercises that teach about the postures of birth.

Preparing for the Positions of Birth

Regardless of what position a woman chooses for delivery, she will be curving and curling her body into the shape of the letter C. You will notice I said, "position a woman chooses." The positions women prefer include being propped up with pillows in a semi-reclined position; the left lateral position (lying on the left side); or squatting, sitting, or kneeling to push the baby out. You will notice that I did not include the supine, or back-lying, birth position. Any woman who is forced to recline, with her feet up in stirrups in the traditional lithotomy position, is being rendered helpless during birth. She is incapable of assuming the C curve or of using her energy and her contractions efficiently. This recumbent position is used for the convenience of medical personnel only. The only

way a woman can push in this position is to have her partner lift her into a C curve. The energy involved in doing that is wasted, and the time it takes to move a mother up and properly position her interrupts the most intense portion of the birthing contraction.

Women need to practice the positions of birth to strengthen their bodies for the effort of pushing. They need to experience the coordination of the breath and the effort it requires to assume the C position. This is how women learn about the shape and timing of birth.

Preparing for Birth in the C Position

To prepare for the open C position, women should be encouraged to stretch the hip adductors and inward rotators. They will need to become comfortable and relaxed in a very vulnerable, exposed position. Though we are fully clothed, the legs should be open wide, the perineum relaxed. The women must understand that your class is a place of great safety and that you are sensitive to their vulnerability. Begin practicing the open positions with the following exercise.

Hip Adductor Stretch

Start: Begin by hook-lying on the floor, your knees bent, feet flat on the floor, and arms relaxed at your sides.

Exercise: Place the soles of your feet together and slowly lower your knees to a wide abducted position. Do not arch your back (see Figure 10.2).

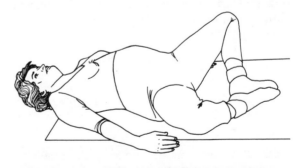

Figure 10.2. Hip adductor stretch. Place the soles of the feet together and allow knees to fall open gently. Do not arch the back.

Counting: Lower to a count of 4; hold for 4 counts; return to start to a count of 4.

Breathing: Inhale to begin, exhale as legs open, and inhale as knees close.

Variation: With buttocks against the wall, slide legs down and place soles of the feet together (see Figure 10.3).

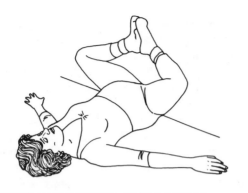

Figure 10.3. Hip adductor stretch variation done against the wall.

Preparing for Birth in a Side-Lying Position

Most women are unaware of the lateral, or side-lying, position for birth. Don't be surprised by the number of raised eyebrows as you demonstrate this position. Because many women labor while lying on their sides, practicing the position as an option to use during delivery is very important. The more options a woman perceives that she has, the freer she will feel to choose her position for birth.

The Side Curl

Start: Begin on the left side, with head resting comfortably on left arm. Legs are relaxed. Body is slightly curled forward.

Exercise: Pull the knee to the chest, grasp it on the front of the shin or hook the elbow under the knee. Do not grab the inside of the knee with the fingers. Curl the body into a C curve, look for the baby, and release (see Figure 10.4).

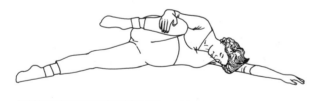

Figure 10.4. Side curl exercise for birth in the lateral position. Some women are more comfortable with bottom knee flexed. Encourage women to look for the baby.

Counting: Inhale to a count of 4; exhale, bring the knee to chest, and curl to a count of 4; and extend the leg and inhale to a count of 4.

Breathing: Inhale to begin, exhale on up-and-curl count, and inhale on release. Rest after several repetitions to avoid hyperventilating. Remind women to open the knee out and around the

uterus. This avoids crowding the uterus and encourages the open C curve.

Look for the Baby

Start: Assume same position as side curl.

Exercise: Bring the knee up towards the chest and then abduct (lift and open) the leg so that the pelvic opening is visibly widened. Support the leg on the outside of the calf. Do not pull the knee back.

Counting: Lift and look for the baby to a count of 3; release to a count of 3. Release and repeat the entire exercise.

Breathing: Same as in side curl.

The Open Book

Start: Side-lying position as in the side curl. Bend the knees and the hips and bring the knees to a 90-degree angle with the hip.

Exercise: Lift the thigh as if you were opening a book (see Figures 10.5a and b).

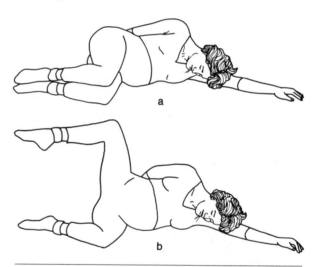

Figure 10.5(a). Starting position for the open book exercise. **(b)** The upper leg is lifted in one motion.

Counting: Lift and open to a count of 3; lower slowly to a count of 3.

Breathing: Inhale on lift, exhale on lower.

Preparing for Birth in a Squatting Position

Although the squatting position is not for everyone, it does open the pelvic outlet as wide as possible. In a relaxed, deep squat the perineal tissues are as relaxed as possible, and gravity serves to ease the baby along most effectively.

Do not practice squatting for prolonged periods to avoid overstretching the tissues of the hip and knee joints. During pregnancy, women who practice the squatting position should relax their vaginal muscles and do their kegel exercises. They should practice with their hands supporting their body in a slightly forward-tilted position. This is also a very good position for labor. If a woman wants to deliver her baby in a squatting position she will probably be supported on either side by her birth attendants. Or, she may lean back and be supported from behind. In class we experiment by suporting one another. It is very helpful to practice the breathing techniques of childbirth in the squatting position.

Skier's Squat
Start: Stand with feet comfortably apart and your back pressed firmly against the wall.

Exercise: Lower your body as if sitting in an imaginary chair. Make certain the back is pressed firmly against the wall.

Counting: Hold lowered position for a count of 10 and return to standing. Repeat twice.

Breathing: Exhale as you lower yourself and inhale as you stand.

Peasant Squat
Start: Stand with feet spread wide apart.

Exercise: Bend the knees and squat down with feet flat on the floor. As you lower your body, use your hands on the floor, wall, or ballet barre to support yourself. Totally release the perineal muscles. Look for the baby. Slowly return to standing (see Figure 10.6).

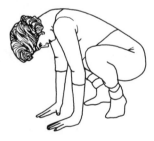

Figure 10.6. Exercise for birth in a squatting position. Remind women to relax their mouths and perineal muscles. Remember to support the body when practicing the deep squat.

Counting: Bend down to a count of 4; hold for a count of 4; and and slowly return to standing to a count of 4.

Breathing: Regular and steady.

Chair Squat
Start: Stand, use the seat of a chair for support.

Exercise: Bend into a deep, relaxed squat. While squatting, release perineal muscles.

Counting: Bend to a count of 4; hold to a count of 4; and return to standing to a count of 4.

Breathing: Exhale on the descent; while in hold position use regular steady breath; inhale on return to standing.

The Cookbook Squat
Start: Place a thick cookbook or telephone book on the floor.

Exercise: Use support. Squat down and sit with your buttocks on the edge of the book, and feet flat on the floor.

Counting: Same as in chair squat.

Breathing: Same as in chair squat, or practice physiologic or gentle pushing.

Preparing for Birth in the Semireclined Position

Some women will be most comfortable choosing a semireclined position for labor and birth. To assume this position she may use pillows or roll up the head of the hospital bed; or, if she prefers, her support person may sit behind her. Many women find it comforting to rest against someone else during delivery.

Seated C Curve
Start: Sit with torso erect, back straight, shoulders directly above hips. Rest the hands on the inside of the thigh. Legs are open, knees bent, feet flat on the floor (see Figure 10.7). Assuming this position may take practice.

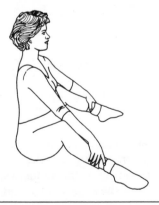

Figure 10.7. Starting position for seated C curve exercise. Back should be straight. Women should inhale deeply and exhale as they curl.

Exercise: Inhale deeply and exhale fully. During the exhalation, lower the head and curl the body forward. The pelvis should tip back slightly. Look for the baby. Keep feet flat on the floor. Inhale and lift the head and chest, straightening the torso.

Counting: Inhale to a count of 3; exhale and curl to a count of 4; inhale and return to upright position to a count of 3; hold and then repeat (see Figure 10.8).

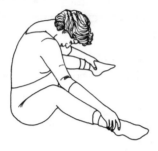

Figure 10.8. Head and neck should be relaxed; women should curl forward by tilting the pelvis back.

Breathing: Inhale when torso is erect, exhale as it curls forward.

Variation: Allow the feet to roll out and the legs to open wider as the body curls forward.

Supported C Curve

Start: Sit on the floor. Lean against a pile of pillows or the wall. Bring the knees up toward the chest, feet flat on the floor. Hold onto the outside or fronts of the knees.

Exercise: Inhale deeply; as you exhale, curl the body forward, performing a slight pelvic tilt. Allow the legs to gently drop open. Inhale and return to start.

Counting: Inhale to 3; exhale and curl to 4; inhale and return to start.

Breathing: Same as in seated C curve.

Strengthening the Abdominals for Birth

In addition to practicing the positions of birth, women should work to strengthen those muscle groups that directly contribute to the efficiency of the second stage of labor, the birth of the baby. The abdominals are important muscles in any birthing position. They, as the perineal muscles, work most effectively when they are strong and toned.

The Lithotomy Stretch

Start: Begin in back-lying position, knees bent, feet flat on the floor.

Exercise: Bring the knees up to the chest. Hold onto the outside of the calves. Open the legs as wide as possible. Lift the head and shoulders. Feel the abdominals working. This is also a good hip stretch (see Figure 10.9).

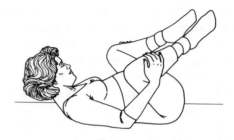

Figure 10.9. The lithotomy stretch: This is not recommended as a birthing position. As an exercise it helps to strengthen abdominal muscles and stretch hip extensors. Open knees as wide as necessary around the abdomen.

Counting: Bring knees up to a count of 2; lift the head and shoulders to a count of 4; lower the head and release the legs to a count of 3; and repeat.

Breathing: Inhale and exhale as head and shoulders lift, inhale on release.

Modified Sit-Up

Start: Assume same position as in lithotomy stretch. Keep feet flat on the floor.

Exercise: Lift head and shoulders and reach arms through the legs. Lower to the floor with a controlled motion.

Counting: Reach up to a count of 2; come down to a count of 2.

Breathing: Exhale on the reach, inhale on the lower.

Variations: Reach to the right side, reach to the left side. Lift only head and shoulders in advanced pregnancy.

Activities That Help Prepare for Labor

Although it is difficult to teach a woman what it is like to experience labor or birth, it is possible to show her what to expect through different movement activities, which you relate to many of the sensations of birth. For example, work towards learning to channel and release tension through movement as a way of preparing women to cope with the intense activity of labor. There are at least three techniques you can use to develop this skill. The first is moving with controlled exertion and tension (staccato) and then changing the effort to a loose, languid flow (legato). It is very helpful to explore the different sensations of movements that change from rigid and tense to soft and floppy. The second technique is moving in response to gravity and then using one's strength to draw back. To accomplish these exercises, I count out the pace and allow a woman to sense and then experiment with how she can initiate, sustain, and then release a movement that she controls. This kind of experience contributes to self-esteem and to the ability to focus and anticipate bodily responses.

Another aspect of preparing for birth is to focus on controlled movement—that is, being able to start and stop a movement at will. This is especially important during the moments when the infant's head is being born; at this point, the care giver will ask the woman to stop pushing. This is a difficult and confusing request! To acquaint women with this concept, use activities with a definite start and stop. For example, ask them to hold a position until you tell them to start moving again. The timing of your instructions to start and stop should be irregular so that the women have no idea how long they will hold or release a movement.

Exercises for a Woman With a Breech Baby

On occasion a woman will share with us that her baby is lying in a breech position and that her care giver has indicated that she will probably be a candidate for a cesarean section. A baby in a breech position has settled into the pelvis with its head up instead of down. A woman in this situation may ask you if there are any exercises she can do to turn the baby around.

There is no guarantee that any exercise undertaken to turn a breech presentation will be successful. However, I believe it is important for a woman to feel that she can at least try to make a difference in the outcome of her baby's birth.

The mother should pile lots of pillows on the floor to protect her neck and shoulders and to lift her hips. She should lift her hips and buttocks up as high as possible and place her legs up on the couch. She should recline in this inverted posture for 10-20 min twice a day in an effort to disengage the breech. If she feels sick or short of breath, due to pressure on the vena cava, she should discontinue this posture immediately. In addition, the woman can perform the pelvic tilt exercise and rest as often as possible with her hips elevated above her shoulders. Again, this may compromise the function of the vena cava, and the mother may not be able to maintain this position for long periods.

Please remember that this is not a childbirth education text. If you want more information about positions of the fetus in utero, or about childbirth in general, consult your local library, an obstetrician's office, or your local childbirth education association.

Summary

Exercises that are designed to integrate the body and mind are healing. Those that familiarize women with the positions for birth promote dignity and appreciation of the body. As women practice them they grow more comfortable with the images of the body during birth. Use them consistently in your classes to enhance strength, self-esteem, and self-image. We move now from integration of the physical experience to exploration of the inner world of the pregnant woman. In the next chapter we will discuss teaching relaxation skills—a significant part of preparing women for birth.

Chapter 11

Teaching Relaxation Techniques

Tension is the greatest barrier to birth without medical intervention. Tension tightens muscles, increases the perception of pain, and creates a panicky, frightened response to labor. Yet tension is a primary element in most women's lives. During pregnancy family problems, work problems, and concerns about their own health and the health of their unborn babies create tension for many women. If she has had difficult labors, a woman may be afraid of the next one. If she has never given birth, she may be filled with worry about the great unknown. What will it be like? Will she survive? How much does it really hurt? Will the baby be okay? Will the baby's father be able to help her? Will her body ever be the same again? Will she ever feel normal?

This anxiety can build for many months, and by the time most couples arrive at their prepared childbirth classes they are anxious and worried about birth. If women expect to learn about relaxation for childbirth at this point, it is almost too late. The numbers of couples in a class and the immense pressure to present the required curricular materials force many childbirth educators to offer 2-hr lectures loaded with pertinent information that fails to heal the anxieties, ease the worries, or sooth the tensions. Information comes at the expectant mother and her birth attendant in a spitfire presentation. Certainly, these classes clarify the mechanics of birth, define new terms, and describe the stages of labor. The classes also provide technical instructions about why it is good to relax during contractions. But breathing techniques and relaxation practice sessions tend to be too late, too short,

and too much under scrutiny. The secret fears surrounding life and death, survival and release, remain the silent undercurrent of tension.

Teaching Women to Heal Tension

Tension is a natural response to the pain and physical changes of labor. In most other instances of extraordinary physical challenge, the flood of adrenaline into the body would elicit a fight-or-flight response. In fact, many women really do say, "Okay, I quit! I'm leaving!" when they are in labor, only to realize they are about to give birth! So the goal in teaching relaxation skills is to help women, who would rather not be in pain, cope with pain and relax their bodies, which allows labor to progress and birth to occur.

Helping women to heal their tension through the acquisition of useful tools that really work during labor is one of the essential responsibilities of the healing maternal educator. There is much to be said for teaching breathing techniques. The real secret, however, is in offering relaxation techniques.

In an exercise studio, an examining room, or a classroom, healing is a process, a collaborative effort, that requires a woman to be open to sharing and receiving and the healer to be open to listening and giving. It is a delicate process. When you teach the techniques of relaxation you are moving into a realm that is private and personal. You are actually saying to women, "Let me in. Let me show you and share with you ways of healing your fear. Trust me. Trust me as a knowing, caring person.''

Teaching relaxation and visualization in class is an intimate, private affair. I always turn the lights down very low or off completely to darken the room. I play soft harp or flute music designed for meditation. The room is quiet and the mood is set. I do this to create a private space for each person in the room. Sometimes there are 2 or 3 women and sometimes there are 30. You may wonder why I believe each woman has a right to her private space. Let's look closely at the conditions imposed upon the mothers who give birth in most hospitals.

Hospital Delivery and Tension

In most modern hospitals, the birth process has become segmented and linear. Women in labor must check in and then settle themselves into a labor room. If there is no labor room available a woman may be placed in a ward or in the hall. Often she will be hooked up to a fetal monitoring machine that may be left on for half an hour or for the duration of her labor. The fetal monitor records how the baby's heart rate is affected by the mother's contractions and has become a standard labor room accessory in most hospitals. The mother may have an intravenous drip taped to her hand and be told to stay in bed. She may be examined once, twice, or several times by the same or different nurses. Her pubic hair may be shaved. She may be required to accept an enema. Her chosen medical care giver may or may not appear during this time. When the time for delivery nears, she is moved to an impersonal and uncomfortable delivery room. After the doctor delivers her baby and she is allowed a fleeting glimpse of it, she is moved to a recovery room. There, she is keenly observed or completely ignored. Her belly is palpated to determine whether her uterus is contracting properly. She may be required to use a bedpan. Throughout the whole process she is probed and propped, wheeled and watched.

Can you think of any mammal who would ordinarily choose this sort of disturbing treatment during birth? If you have a female house pet, you may have seen her build a birthing nest. It is usually in a private place, rarely in full public view. When she is ready to have her babies, she goes to her private place to begin her labor. Would you think to move her as she labored? Would you dream of examining her to determine her dilation?

Would you require that she stay still during labor, wear a fetal monitor, or lay her on her back to deliver? Would you bring in crowds of people to discuss her progress, or the weather or golf? Would you turn on the lights or make an announcement through a loud speaker?

No, of course not.

But, alas, the average hospital environment is not nearly so respectful of a woman's privacy or dignity. It is only recently that some women have been allowed to labor and give birth in the same bed in the same room. It is only recently that the baby is not automatically whisked away from the mother, but allowed to stay and to be nursed and held by the woman whose body warmed and protected it from conception.

Birth in most hospitals could be described as a series of disturbances. And the women who willingly give birth in hospitals have unwittingly signed away their rights to self-determination, privacy, and dignity during childbirth. As a result, their labors may be excessively long and difficult. They are examined and reexamined, interrupted and monitored. Too often they are told to remain in bed, chided for wanting to crouch or squat, told to be quiet and not to push when the urge is strong, and instructed to listen to what is best for the provider in charge.

I tell women in childbirth education classes that birth is a magical thing and that their bodies are magnificent, beautiful, and dignified. Shortly thereafter, I tell them that the tradition of obstetrics has been to speed the fetus through its perilous journey down the birth canal, to reduce what appeared to be the female agony of childbirth, and to prevent maternal or fetal death. To achieve these ends, medical personnel have come to view the laboring woman as an inefficient organism with a body gone haywire. Labor is considered disorganized, in need of skillful management by drugs and specialists. By concentrating on the fragments of the birth process instead of the wholeness and rightness of the body in labor, giving birth in a medical institution has been reduced to a mechanical function.

Birth is no longer magical or mystical, personal or private. Although it is not generally admitted, anyone who happens to be on the floor may just take a quick peek if they so choose. And, if a woman's chosen care giver cannot be there, a total stranger may order an intervention, perform an episiotomy, deliver the baby, or perform a cesarean section. The hospital is not a haven. It is not a refuge. The hospital is a place where a woman in labor *will be* disturbed.

Therefore, I teach relaxation skills to empower and enable every woman to create a sphere of privacy and self-control in an environment that would choose to deny her the right to her privacy. A laboring woman in a hospital needs to close her mind to the distractions, the clocks, and the other women who are facing the same critical experience. She needs to create a safe, private, and comfortable nest amidst the noises, strangers, and lights.

Properly taught relaxation and visualizations for childbirth can help her to do that. Let us explore the creation of the relaxation experience.

Teaching Birth Harmony

I attended Lamaze classes when I was expecting my first child. I had no idea what contractions, or the rhythmic tightening of the uterine muscle, were. There I learned the meaning of effacement and dilation, or the thinning and gradual opening of the cervix that occur to allow the fetus to emerge from the uterus. I learned about the stages of labor: the gradual opening of the cervix, the birth of the baby, and finally the expulsion of the placenta. I also learned very quickly that the best thing to do was to keep an eye on the clock. By watching the clock, I would be able to time the length of each contraction and predict when the next one would come, and successfully deliver my baby.

Nothing could have been further from the truth. During my labor I timed each contraction, and the energy I expended watching the clock and waiting for the spasms to pass was poorly spent. The strain of experiencing the contractions and counting the seconds was tedious. My perception of each contraction was that it lasted a very long time instead of less than a minute.

The second presumed usefulness of the clock was even further from the truth. My contractions were never regular. I never knew when the next one would come. I was filled with anxiety. Did this mean that I was laboring too quickly or too slowly? Was my body failing me? Did this mean I would have to have a cesarean? The clock-watching that I thought would make me feel secure only made me feel anxious and afraid.

My advice: Throw the clock away. Educators might want to discuss time as an element for describing the experience of labor, but the length of labor is an imposed concept of ''good time'' encased in a bodily process that is timeless. We should teach women that the process of birth in-

volves a combination of efforts based on harmony rather than time.

Harmony is the experience of several elements occurring simultaneously to produce a desired effect. Birth is the culmination of efforts and energies that are serendipitous. They have occurred together, in stages and in cooperation, to achieve the physical separation of infant and mother. Harmony is not an intellectual construct. It is an interpretation that allows for pain but believes in the health and goodness of the birth energies. It encourages a woman to be strong and cry out and grasp for others when she needs them. Harmony accepts that childbirth is not fun and denies that it should be painless. Harmony elicits from each woman the acceptance of the dignity and responsibility of birth.

Birth harmony accepts the kinetic aspects of mammalian birth and allows for the integration of the bodily elements that flow together to create it. It allows a woman to welcome the intensity of her contractions and the power of her uterus as both overwhelming and invigorating. Accepting the harmony of those kinetic impulses allows her to visualize her cervix opening, her vagina softening, her baby stretching her perineum, and her body giving way to the infant as it emerges. Birth harmony encourages the disintegration of clock time in favor of the diffuse, experiential time of labor and birth. Birth harmony invites the spiritual, the ethereal, and the otherworldliness of a time that transgresses common boundaries.

It is essential that everyone involved understand that birth is not an event limited to the body, but a part of a sequence of changes and adjustments that a woman and her family make for many months. For the mother, the birth culminates in a great physical challenge. Yet, those around her have interacted with her and her changing body and have felt the child grow within them as it has grown within her. Pregnancy is not just an individual affair. Family members, friends, and lovers are all living inside physical bodies, vibrating around the universe together. They share many feelings and many fears, and what a woman does to exalt or diminish her pregnancy or the health of her child is felt by everyone.

Childbirth and the child itself are not things that belong to one woman then, but are the magnificent transformations of energy from many sources. Each combination of energies and power is a masterpiece. To expect that time, with its pattern of hours and minutes and seconds neatly lined off around the circle, would be useful to a woman in labor is not part of nature's plan.

Time in labor is different from time in any other situation. In labor a woman's sense of time and the boundaries that keep the rest of us in regular time disappear. She becomes removed from ordinary people. She is in another world. She trembles and she moves without regard for others. She is within herself yet in need of support. She uses whatever space she has to create her nest. In her own home she nestles with loved ones. In the hospital, she struggles in a narrow bed or in a tiny cubicle to find a peaceful place as her body readies itself for the torrent of birth.

What can be done to help a woman prepare for this? How can we educate women to understand the importance of relaxation during childbirth? What can we do to help women to integrate the ancient female wisdom about birth as a healthy, holistic experience with the modern, technical environment of most hospital births? Let's address these questions with ways you, as a healer and teacher, can help.

Discussing Fear and Pain

Fear and pain accompany every birth. Fears of the unknown and of death are commonplace. Fear of letting go of the child and fear of becoming a mother are not new. Tearing or ripping apart, bleeding, failing, and producing a deformed baby are the secret fears of a million women. Some women fear that they will never be the same; others are afraid of never being loved again.

Pain in childbirth is real. It can be excruciating or dull and throbbing. It can be radiating, searing, or hot. The pain can feel like stretching or like drowning in a storm at sea. It can be specific or it can be diffuse. Medical researchers still do not know exactly what causes pain or how it comes to be felt. Theories of pain perception propose that pain is a response to negative stimuli, transmitted from the nerve ganglia through and up the spinal cord to the hypothalamus and then to the cerebral cortex. The nerve fibers themselves are large and small and react to the initial stimulus with vibrations and chemical reactions that send messages to the brain for interpretation. Once the interpretation of pain is received, a system of feedback mechanisms goes into action. Women in pain react with fairly predictable responses. Women's perceptions of pain, however, may vary considerably depending on past experience, preparation for childbirth pain, expectations, and social and cultural influences. The perception of pain is both

physical and psychological. Any two women will feel pain differently.

Larry Dossey (1982) has discussed how Western medicine copes with pain. He points out that in our tradition pain is considered negative information, and therefore it is dealt with in two ways: denial or suppression. In terms of childbirth preparation, the denial model was taught by early advocates of painless childbirth. This is a terribly mislabeled approach to preparation for childbirth because, although the idea of breathing techniques and relaxation are explained, the expectation of a painless childbirth is upheld as the ideal experience. When the pain of childbirth becomes too real and too difficult, a woman collapses. She feels as if she has failed because she has been working under a modus operandi that has prevented her from developing realistic expectations and the psychological skills for coping with her pain.

The suppression model is the medical model that considers pain to be negative and treats pain through prevention and intervention. The dominion of medicine over childbirth, I believe, is based on the fundamental belief that pain must be controlled. The technologies of pain prevention are at the command of physicians who, fearful of the birth process itself, and even more fearful of losing control, have found it wiser to interrupt and to manage rather than to allow birth to occur undisturbed.

Some effort has been made to understand the experience of childbirth pain as a reflection of values and expectations. The affective nature of pain, the meaning given to the perception of pain signals, and the cultural rewards for suffering in childbirth are important to our understanding of traditional delivery room behaviors. However, it may be far more worthwhile to reconsider our treatment, denial, and suppression of childbirth pain in light of its definition as an integrated response of a body immersed in a transformation.

Coping With Childbirth Pain

The transformation of birth is profound. The pain of birth is transient. Proper training in the skills of relaxation and visualization can allow a woman to release the pain, survive it, and cope with it; and when it is gone, there is euphoria. After childbirth, women commonly report a sense of transcendence and a sense of unity with all women. Achterberg (1985) wrote that this commonly felt sense of unity may be the result of the release of hormones during the extraordinarily focused demands of labor and delivery.

It is to the purpose of reaching this transcendent euphoria that we address the teaching of relaxation skills. First, women must learn how to create a private place in a hospital that is designed to discourage privacy. Second, they need to learn to meditate and concentrate on images of power, strength, confidence, and success. They need to do this to stimulate the release of endorphins and to free and make harmonic their birth energies, beyond fear, pain, and time. To do this, they must begin to learn the art of relaxation and visualization.

Considerable research exists on relaxation techniques and the related biophysical changes measured in subjects who practice them. People who practice Transcendental Meditation, which requires that the meditator practice twice a day for 20 min, frequently have lower resting pulse rates than others who do not meditate. Individuals who have high blood pressure frequently experience significant decreases in blood pressure while practicing meditation and relaxation. Those who suffer from skin irritations, ulcers, insomnia, headaches, and a wide variety of psychosomatic responses to stress can certainly benefit from learning one of the many relaxation techniques available to the consumer.

Women who understand how to allow their bodies to relax during labor usually feel more self-assured, are less irritable, and find it easier to achieve an acceptance of self and the biophysical experience of the self in labor. This does not mean that they do not experience pain or discomfort. But they attend to its meaning by relaxing their bodies completely, allowing themselves to breathe lightly, in concert with their contractions, and, by doing so, allowing their babies to be born.

Teaching Women About Relaxation

Tension, in and of itself, is not bad. We need it to achieve and to accomplish our goals. But we live with an unnecessarily high level of tension. Women in our stressful world, facing childbirth with fear and prospective parenting with anxiety, need to learn effective methods of tension reduction.

Now, you may think that women learn relaxation techniques in childbirth education classes. But most women do not get to childbirth education classes until the last 6 or 8 weeks of pregnancy. These are skills that should be introduced early in pregnancy and practiced and refined for months

for use at birth. It is ridiculous to wait until a woman is 32 weeks pregnant to finally introduce relaxation skills if she expects to be able to use them in labor. This is why we need to redefine prenatal health education and preparation for childbirth.

For these and other reasons, our neo-modern view of preparation for childbirth is a system that needs reopening and reexamining. All of us— teachers, nurses, nutritionists, fitness advocates, midwives, physicians, and childbirth educators— need to examine our roles as members of the team that supports women throughout their 9 months of transformation. As a team we must help women to organize the gestalt of childbirth—that is, to convey the meaning of childbirth as part of a whole system of living and growing. We need to emphasize the important human ability to integrate information continuously. The ongoing process of assimilating information and ideas enhances experience, making learning increasingly valuable. Preparing women for childbirth should not be a 6- or 8-week course done in early, middle, or late pregnancy, but a healing journey during which the dialogue must be open and the flow continuously interactional.

Educators need to be sensitive to the multiplicity of factors that effect each childbearing woman and aware of how the manner through which she, the mother, is educated, will maximize or minimize how she will manage tools and information. Age, marital status, cultural heritage and health all effect how a mother will accept and use prenatal education.

The encounter between a woman, or a woman and her birth attendant, and the maternal educator should be an intimate exchange. A healing approach would be to offer compassion, insight, and concern into the nature and meaning of the female's bodily responses to pregnancy and labor. There should be an emphasis on the satisfying, healing nature of preparation for childbirth and the accessibility of the related biological, physiological, and social information.

Relaxation in the Classroom

Learning to relax as a response to a labor contraction is not as hard as it may sound. The natural response to pain is tension, dismay, and the desire to escape. Understanding why the pain of labor occurs and knowing that it will end with the birth of a child is helpful to many women. Those who are uncertain about becoming a mother or who are uncertain about the meaning of birth resent the pain. Women who understand its physiological basis and who are ready to welcome the child may face the pain with self-reliance and acceptance.

The relaxation process is both a mental and a physical response. It involves an intellectual focus, a physical activity, and the assumption of personal responsibility. A woman who is confident of her ability to relax experiences it as part of a healing process. In the face of the unknown, consciously relaxing the muscles of the body is an active choice to experience the self during birth.

The material that follows explores some of the relaxation techniques that I use with pregnant women. Many of the techniques constitute hypnotic suggestion or autogenic training, but in no way is this the practice of hypnotism. Research into the procedures of childbirth educators indicates that a substantial amount of suggestion does occur. But I am not advocating the use of hypnotism to cope with childbirth pain. A woman may put herself into a trance-like state, but it must be she who controls it, she who elicits it, and she who decides on the images and suggestions.

Meditation and Relaxation

The word *meditation* calls to mind images of gurus and strange incantations. Your students may respond this way, but once you get started they will understand that learning to relax through the use of pregnancy meditations can be one of the most powerful, enlightening, and enjoyable experiences of a lifetime. During pregnancy, meditation can be wonderfully relaxing. During birth, relaxation and meditation can create a sense of physical comfort and privacy.

According to the more formal definitions of the word, the type of practice described here does not constitute meditation. Historically, meditation has no real objectives, except to enhance spiritual unity and oneness. In this context, meditation refers to an act of concentrating on images and ideas that lead to an acceptance and tolerance of childbirth pain.

The first relaxation I teach is referred to as conscious release. It is a concentrated "effortless effort" to eliminate the tightness and tension in the body. It is especially important for a women to learn this technique during pregnancy so that during labor she is able to identify areas of muscular tension and work calmly to release them. For instance, if she is experiencing back pain, she must

be able to identify the location of discomfort before she or her partner can work to reduce the pain. During intense contractions, if she realizes that she is grinding her teeth or clenching her buttocks, she can use the relaxation process to cope with the pain-induced tension.

The following is an example of how to lead women through the relaxation process. After experiencing the conscious release of muscular tension several times, women should be able to relax their bodies by using the releasing breath as a cue rather than going through the entire process. Read this meditation quietly. Make sure that the room is dark and the women are comfortable. It is helpful to play music (e.g., flute, harp, or synthesizer). No one should feel any pressure related to time. This relaxation lasts a full 20 min. Your responsibility is to set the mood, to read this slowly and clearly to your class, and to let them relax for the full 20 min. Pause briefly after reading each statement.

Conscious Release Meditation

Thank you for taking the time out of your busy day to relax.

Please lie down on your left side or assume a comfortable, well-supported sitting position.

The next 20 min are going to be yours and yours alone.

This relaxation period is especially designed for you. It will include the release of tension and several guided visualizations.

Let's begin your relaxation.

Close your eyes and begin your relaxation by taking several nice, deep cleansing breaths.

Inhale deeply and exhale fully. Take your time and relax as you exhale.

With each breath feel your body relaxing and any tensions you feel in your body beginning to fade away.

The deep cleansing breath is also called a releasing breath. It will be helpful during childbirth and it will signal your body to relax at the onset of each contraction.

Inhale deeply once again and then let your breath return to its own gentle rhythm.

This gentle breathing pattern is like the relaxed gentle breath of sleep. It is as soft and gentle as sleep itself.

Lightly focus your attention on your head. With each breath you take, release any tension you feel in your head.

Feel your scalp relax.

Breathe deeply and release the tension in your forehead.

Breathe evenly and release the tension about your eyes, letting any tension lines melt away.

Release any tension you feel around your ears.

Relax your jaw. Let your mouth be soft and allow your lips to open.

Your head and your face are completely relaxed.

Now focus your attention on your neck and shoulders. This is where we carry the weight of the world. Release your tension now and relax your neck, all the way down, from your head and across into your shoulders.

You may move your head until it sits comfortably on your neck.

Relax your shoulders. You may shrug your shoulders if that makes you feel more comfortable. Let go of all the tension in your shoulders and your upper back.

Move your focus to your upper arms. Allow you arms to relax completely. Relax your whole arm. Feel the tension leave your elbows and your forearms.

Let your wrists hang softly. Gently relax the fingers on your right hand. Now do the same for the fingers on your left hand.

Your fingers should be limp and completely relaxed.

Bring your focus to your upper back.

Breathe deeply and begin to relax the muscles in your back.

With each breath move your focus down through your spine and feel all the muscles across your back relaxing.

Move down through your lower back, releasing all the tension. Let your whole back relax.

Bring your focus down to your hips and buttocks. Relax your hips and buttocks and feel any tension or tiredness melting away. You may feel that you are sinking against your chair or bed as you relax and release your hips.

Move your focus around to your chest. Breathe deeply and release the muscles of your chest.

Relax your rib cage and then your tummy muscles.

Release tension across your whole belly, moving down, down, into your pelvis.

Now I want you to focus on the muscles of your vagina.

Tighten your vagina. Now relax it.

Remember to keep your whole body relaxed.

Take in a gentle breath. Tighten your vaginal muscles. As you exhale, release them.

During labor, with the onset of each contraction, you will release and relax your bottom and your vagina. Your vagina is the baby's birth canal. It will be soft and open for your baby's birth.

Breathe slowly and gently, as softly as you breathe when you are asleep.

As you breathe, move your focus down to your legs.

Release the tension in your thighs and then in your knees.

Relax your calves and ankles.

Relax your feet. One at a time, relax each of your toes on your right foot, and then each of your toes on your left foot.

Breathe deeply and release your whole body.

Scan your whole body for any tension. If there is tension anywhere, take a moment to relax and release it.

Feel the softness of all of your muscles and the gentleness of your breath.

Imagine now that you are part of the great mother earth.

Your body is a beautiful, sloping landscape of gentle hills and soft valleys, bathed in the warmth of a soft glowing sun.

Your body is a healthy part of nature.

Your body is strong and you are healthy.

You are feminine and you are beautiful.

Your energy comes from deep within you, and your wisdom is as old as the earth herself.

The sunshine warms you, and the warmth spreads from you to your baby and to all those whom you love.

Breathe deeply and release any tension. Check yourself. Make sure that your jaw is soft and your body is completely relaxed.

Inhale gently and exhale softly.

Begin to focus on your internal world: the world of your baby.

Your womb is dark and cushiony.

Your baby nestles within you, nourished by gently pulsing veins and arteries.

Imagine your baby within your womb.

Peaceful. Secure. Protected by you. Your baby is special and beautiful.

You will love and cherish one another beyond all boundaries.

Your internal world is a miracle unto itself and unto the universe.

Relax your body. Make certain no tension has crept in anywhere.

Slow your breathing and allow yourself to relax completely.

Let go of any thoughts or worries.

Find yourself at peace with yourself and your body.

Now, breathe in deeply and slowly and then breathe out slowly.

Whenever you are ready, at your own pace, let yourself come back from this deeply relaxed state. You might want to stretch slowly and gently. When you are ready, get up slowly. Try to retain this relaxed and peaceful feeling.

I hope you and your students enjoy this guide to conscious release. This can be a source of strength for expectant women that can be renewed throughout their prenatal experience.

Teaching Breathing for Labor and Birth

The releasing breath that we practice each week in prenatal exercise classes is part of the relaxation process. By using the releasing breath as a cue, a woman learns to release the tension in her body just by breathing in and out. In addition, as she breathes, she assures a continued flow of oxygen to her bloodstream, her muscles, and her baby.

Breathing itself can be a form of meditation. The breathing techniques of childbirth preparation can become the focus of the relaxation practice. I introduce one level of breathing each week so that after 5 weeks with me women are completely familiar with the breathing techniques for labor.

The entire series can be practiced as a labor simulation. Women must be reminded to relax completely during practice contractions and to release all accumulated tension completely in between contractions.

These are the breathing techniques many women learn in Lamaze and prepared childbirth classes. Remind the women in your class that learning them in an exercise class is not a substitute for the prepared childbirth class. This format may be especially useful to the childbirth educator who is searching for ways to incorporate practice of the breathing techniques into her program.

When members of the class are comfortably reclining or leaning back against a wall, preferably supported by lots of pillows, you can begin a relaxation exercise and allow them to get completely relaxed by talking them through a somewhat shortened version of the conscious release process described above. (Another example will appear in the next chapter.) Then begin your breathing meditation. Pause after reading each statement.

Level 1: A Guide to the Breath of Early Labor

The earliest stage of labor is called entertainment. During this stage the cervix begins to dilate. Contractions are usually mild and cramp-like. Though many women feel that they need no breathing techniques early in labor, as contractions begin to grow stronger, slow-chest breathing can be very helpful.

Releasing Breath

Take a releasing breath. Inhale deeply and exhale fully. Focus on your breathing. Become aware of the speed of your respirations and the depth to which you are comfortable inhaling. Feel the warmth of your breath and the pleasure of your gentle, rhythmic breathing.

During this relaxation we are going to practice the breathing techniques for early labor.

Take a deep, cleansing breath and relax.

Feel your body sinking into the mat. Allow your muscles to relax and your tension to disappear.

Imagine that it is early in the morning.

You have had a long, deep, and comfortable night's sleep.

You awaken to the gentle tightening of your abdomen and you realize that you are having a contraction.

It is mild and yet insistent. You feel your belly tighten and then relax. Be aware that your natural response may be to tighten the muscles of your bottom and your vagina as the tension builds.

Consciously make an effort to relax all of your muscles.

When a contraction starts, release every muscle of your body. Soften your vagina. Relax your buttocks. Release your jaw.

Waste no energy.

Another contraction is about to begin. This time, as it starts, you will take a releasing breath and settle into a gentle, even breath. It will go slowly, lightly, and steadily throughout the contraction.

The contraction is beginning.

Take a releasing breath and just breathe.

Relax your body.

Relax your face and your back.

Relax your tummy and your bottom.

Relax your feet.

Allow your uterus to do its work. (*Pause for 15-20 seconds here.*)

The contraction is peaking now and you remain completely relaxed.

Your breath is slow, comfortable, and easy.

The contraction is over. Take a releasing breath and imagine that you are drifting off to sleep.

(The total length of this simulated contraction is about 1 min.) Repeat this activity three times. Allow 2-3 min between each contraction practice.

Level 2: A Guide to the Breath of Active Labor

The next week you may introduce Level 2: accelerated/decelerated breathing. Use the following relaxation format to guide the women in practicing the breath of active labor. Begin with the conscious release process, and have the women practice the Level 1 breathing. Then move right into Level 2.

Accelerated/Decelerated Breathing

Your contractions have gotten stronger. You have rested in bed and dozed between them and now they seem longer and stronger. With the next contraction, you will practice the accelerated/decelerated breathing pattern. It is not complicated. It is not hard. You merely increase the pace of your breath to meet the intensity of your contraction. You will not feel tense. You will not have to move. Your breath is light.

Your body guides you perfectly.

The contraction is beginning.

Take a releasing breath and relax your body completely.

The contraction is beginning to build. Breathe slowly and evenly.

As the intensity of the contraction builds, pick up the pace of your breath.

Breathe more quickly, as if you were working harder, as if you were climbing a hill or riding a bike.

Your breath is still soft.

As the contraction passes, slow the pace down. Return to the gentle, even breath of sleep.

When the contraction is over, take a releasing breath and relax.

This simulated contraction lasts about 1 min. Practice the contraction two to three times, allowing 2-3 min between each complete exercise. You may want to interject that by this time women who are planning to deliver in the hospital may be having contractions in the car or elevator on the way to the labor room!

Level 3: A Guide to the Breath of Transition

The pant-blow breath of Level 3 is for use during the most intense period of labor. Referred to as transition, this period falls at the end of the first stage of labor when the cervix opens to full dilation. Women usually feel tense and anxious as the torrent of energy and activity fills their bodies and the pain of the impending birth can be excruciating. Practice the pant-blow technique very slowly. Inform women that during its actual application, the pant-blow breath will naturally assume a more rapid pace. During relaxation practice, lead up to the pant-blow technique by practicing Levels 1 and 2 at least twice. This helps to set the stage for this level of breathing. Remember to pause briefly after reading each statement.

Pant-Blow Breathing

Your labor has progressed for several hours. Your contractions have gone from mild to intense. Sometimes you have wanted to walk around. Other times you have leaned heavily against your partner and birth attendants, and their support has helped you through your stronger contractions.

Your labor is even stronger now, and you know this means that your baby will soon be born. As the next contraction begins, you will practice pant-blow breathing. Use this technique at the end of labor when the contractions are very long and very strong.

When the next contraction begins, take a quick releasing breath, relax your body, and place your tongue up behind your two front teeth. Gently breathe in and out four times. After four breaths, blow the air out and begin again. I will count the first two patterns for you and afterwards you will count them for yourself.

Your contraction is beginning. Take a releasing breath and place your tongue up behind your two front teeth.

Breathe 1, 2, 3, 4, and blow out.

Repeat 1, 2, 3, 4, and blow out. (*Go slowly. Practice this for at least 45 seconds. During labor, contractions may last up to 90 seconds and may start again immediately. Women must be prepared for this.*)

The contraction is over, take a releasing breath and completely relax your body. If you feel tension anywhere, release it.

Relax completely.

The next contraction is beginning. Take a releasing breath, relax your body, and place your tongue up behind your two front teeth. (*Repeat the entire contraction.*)

After practicing the breathing techniques, allow women to relax completely. Consider using a visualization (chapter 12) to enhance their relaxation. Remember that it is very important to tie the skills of relaxation and breathing together.

Level 4: A Guide to the Breath That Controls the Speed of Birth

The feather blow is used during the second stage of labor to prevent a woman from pushing too soon or too hard. This is to prevent injury to the emerging head of the fetus or the incompletely dilated cervical tissue. The feather blow can also be practiced during relaxation. After practicing Levels 1, 2, and 3 of breathing, lead the women in the following exercise:

Feather Breathing

Imagine that you have progressed through your labor. You feel pressure across your back and through your bottom and you want to take a deep breath and push, but your care giver has asked you to wait. Your cervix is not fully opened.

With the next contraction, you will have to lift your chin. Do not tuck it down to your chest, but lift it up, away from your neck. Blow out lightly as if you were keeping a feather dancing just above your lips (or as if you were blowing out a candle).

The contraction is beginning. Lift your chin, do not curl down, but lift and blow. Pretend you are blowing out a candle.

Good. Take a releasing breath and relax.

Teaching About Pushing and Relaxing

The pushing stage of labor can be very brief (5-10 min) or it can last for several hours. Some women need to move around during the pushing stage. They need to find the best position in which to give birth and they should be free to do so. Gravity helps a baby move and shift and turn through the pelvic opening. When I introduce positions for childbirth, I emphasize the importance of experimenting with different delivery positions until women find the one that is most comfortable. During relaxation practice I encourage women to try the side-lying position, the all-fours position, and the semirecumbent position. Those who wish to practice squatting are encouraged to do so but not without support.

The mechanics of pushing are not that complicated. Some contractions are quite mild and others create an urgent need to bear down. The intensity of a mother's pushing should be equal to the intensity of her contraction. During a long contraction a woman may bear down at intervals, each lasting 5 to 8 seconds. Between each push a woman should take a cleansing breath. She should never push if the urge to do so passes. A milder contraction may not be long enough to include any more than one or two pushes. Women shouldn't worry about missing the chance to push. The pushing contractions will continue until the baby is born.

Before you use the following activity, make sure that everyone has relaxed completely. This exercise involves both pushing and relaxing techniques. Remember to pause after reading each statement.

Pushing and Relaxing Techniques

Now we will practice the breathing techniques for birth. I do not want you really to push out or down, but you should practice how it feels to breathe and bear down just slightly.

It is especially important to relax your bottom and consciously open your vagina.

The hardest thing is to coordinate pushing, which is a lot of work, and relaxing. Sometimes it feels awkward and uncoordinated. It takes everyone a few contractions to get the hang of it.

Remember that if you lie there and do nothing at all, your baby will be born anyway because your uterus does a great deal of the work on its own. You are breathing and bearing down only to help. It is a natural process.

When you feel the urge to bear down, you are nearing the celebration of birth.

When your contraction begins, take two releasing breaths. On the third inhalation, catch your breath in your throat and chest and then slowly, gently release it with a sigh or a groan.

Make it long and make it your own.

Your contraction is beginning. Breathe in deeply and exhale fully. The urge to push is strong. Breathe in and out, and then breathe in and catch your breath. Put your chin down and curl your body forward. Exhale and sign deeply as if you are groaning the contraction away.

Good. Let's do it again.

Inhale deeply again and, as you exhale, keep your chin tucked down, relax your bottom, open your birth canal, and let your baby out. Remember to look for your baby.

Now, because this is practice and not the real thing, I want you to take a deep cleansing breath and relax completely.

You might want to finish with a visualization or repeat the conscious release process to assure that the women are completely relaxed. Practicing the pushing technique can be very stimulating and very tiring. Women may have questions about the mechanics of pushing or about positions. Leave lots of time for discussion.

Summary

The actual practice of these skills makes it possible for women to perform them competently during labor and birth. Please remind your students that these are practice sessions that do not substitute for the prepared childbirth class.

The monologues presented here demonstrate the importance of teaching relaxation techniques along with breathing techniques. The tone and the regularity of your teaching will contribute to the effectiveness of learning. Perhaps the most important skill for you to learn is how to relax and control your voice. In fact, you may need to practice speaking slowly and clearly. Time yourself and determine whether you are rushing women through their relaxation. People tend to think that time spent not speaking is dead time; in fact, this quiet time is deeply restful and important to those who are learning to relax. The moments between your words are as vital as the words themselves.

Having worked to achieve a physically relaxed state, women will be ready to move on to additional techniques that contribute to the healing of childbearing. The next chapter explores alternative techniques for relaxation including creative visualization, mantras, and massage.

Chapter 12

Reducing Tension Throughout Pregnancy and Labor

Coping with stress is a daily event. We are constantly bombarded by information, aggravation, and frustration. During pregnancy, anticipation of labor and delivery and the upcoming shift into the parenting role creates additional stress and apprehension. There is a wonderful variety of body skills you can develop and share with women to increase their comfort and ability to manage the stress of their lives.

The fitness instructor who is familiar with the imagery of childbirth and the physiology of labor is at an advantage when teaching relaxation and visualization skills. Though it is not absolutely necessary to understand the physiology of labor to be successful at teaching relaxation, insight into the dimensions of labor and its emotional components are crucial to a successful prenatal class. I recommend that you read *Textbook for Childbirth Educators* (Hassid, 1984).

When you practice the relaxation techniques in class, remember to play soft, evenly paced music. Choose music for meditation, music for harps and flutes, or particularly restful pieces that are at least 20 min long. The proper music sets the mood for relaxation and is very soothing.

You may want to explore visualizations that provide sensory information about hospital routines as well as the description of the dilation and expulsion process. Help women to visualize the hospital in which they will deliver while they are completely relaxed. Explore feelings about entering the hospital and going into the birthing room. Help them to visualize walking down the hall and experiencing a strong contraction or remaining completely calm during an internal exam.

Positive Mental Rehearsal

Women's belief systems enter directly into their experience of female rites of passage. Longitudinal studies on adolescents show that attitudes towards menarche directly correlate with gynecological distress patterns during adult life. Research reported by Paxton (1981) suggests that accurate information, presented before the event, could have made the transition and its consequences less painful. Early attitudes and experiences that connect negative aspects to female physiology predispose women to the experience of painful menstruation, impaired well-being during pregnancy, and negative psychological responses to gynecologic operations (p. 50).

Negative images can contribute to the pain or unhappiness of childbirth. Fear and tension consistently lead women to panic and feel pain. The message you can communicate is that if positive images can be created to replace the fear, women can gain a new perspective on childbirth. The mental rehearsal of labor, as well as repeated practice of breathing and relaxation techniques, may directly contribute to the prepared woman's ability to respond to the experience of labor and to cope with the physical and emotional challenge of birth.

Creative Visualization

Creative visualization is the most exciting form of prenatal and postpartum relaxation. There are thousands of images and experiences to visualize, and each woman has an equally large number from which to draw.

Visualization is the ability to create a mental picture. In the how-to books for achieving success, people are encouraged to visualize their lives as treasure chests and then to imagine that they are opening the treasure chests of success. Not a bad idea actually, but visualizations for pregnancy and birth focus on other ideas. For instance, visualizing the baby as it lies comfortably curled up in the womb, or visualizing the baby's face, hair color, or sex can contribute to a joyous sense of well-being. Women should all learn to enjoy the mind's ability to imagine, create, and visualize.

During preparation for birth and the birth itself, a woman can visualize the baby as it moves down the birth canal. She may be able to visualize the opening cervix and the wide, stretchy, smooth skin of her vagina. Although birth has been viewed as a perilous journey, a mother should visualize it as a joyous achievement and a gentle passage. Imagine the baby's head as it descends and eventually emerges. Sense how the body is opening, widening, and making room for the baby. Imagine the baby sensing the joyous anticipation of its mother and father as it is being born. There are no limits to visualization. Anything you want to create, you can create.

A woman may want to visualize healing hands moving over her body. She may release her pain, fear, or tension up to those hands. She may visualize herself being completely surrounded by a protective glow of white light. No harm will come to her or to her baby while the light protects her. She may visualize herself painting, dancing, or participating in any activity she likes. She should visualize the success of her birth and the joy of receiving her newborn into her arms.

Remember that the differences in some of the relaxation techniques we will discuss may be important to you as a teacher or to the women in your group. For example, a demonstration of acupuncture, the ancient art of inserting needles along specific meridians in the body for relief of pain, may not go over quite as well as a demonstration of acupressure, which is the art of fingertip pressure on the body to ease discomforts. So, choose your alternatives carefully. If you are not comfortable demonstrating a technique, contact other professionals in your community and seek their advice. Help to balance out the delivery of services and systems by inviting others who are knowledgeable about prenatal physiology to come into your class and share their knowledge.

Teaching Pregnancy Meditations

The following are meditations you may choose to use for your classes. Some are shorter than others, and each invokes a series of images that are experientially pertinent to pregnancy.

Take your time when you are leading relaxation meditations. Begin each with a full body release. Women should grow increasingly competent at relaxing their bodies, but do not rush them. Allow at least 10 min for a full body relaxation and another 5-10 min for any visualization or imagery practice. Pace yourself and use your voice as an instrument of healing. Get a drink of water and take the time to clear your throat before you begin. At the completion of your relaxation practice, always remind women to get up slowly. Encourage them to stretch and move carefully. No one should ever jump up suddenly, which not only diminishes the peacefulness of the relaxation, but may lead to orthostatic hypotension (chapter 2). Explain to your students that the relaxation time is extremely important, and that they should avoid having urgent or pressing responsibilities immediately after class.

Every woman experiences the challenges and changes of pregnancy in a unique way. The following meditations were written to meet the needs of many different kinds of women. You may find that all or none suit the women in your group. Feel free to write your own or ask class members to share others they prefer.

Early Pregnancy Meditation

The first meditation includes a short body relaxation and then explores the inner world of a woman's reproductive system. You should allow at least 20 min for this meditation. Pause briefly after each step.

Relax by taking several deep cleansing breaths.

Inhale again and slowly exhale, feeling the tension melt away from your body. Inhale deeply once again and then establish your own gentle, rhythmic breathing.

This breath is called the tidal volume, and it is the same gentle breath of sleep; it is as soft and gentle as sleep itself.

Move down through your body and consciously release the tension you may have in your face and neck.

Loosen your jaw.

Relax your shoulders and upper arms.

Make sure that your wrists and fingers are soft and relaxed.

Release your chest. Breathe gently and release your upper back.

Feel the tension disappear as you release the tension in your lower back.

Move around and relax your belly.

Now release your hips and your bottom.

Relax your vagina.

Breathe gently in and out and release any tension in your thighs, knees, and calves.

Relax your ankles and toes.

Check your whole body.

Relax and breathe.

Take several releasing breaths, and, as you do, feel any remaining tension leaving your body.

Take another releasing breath and now, for the first time in your life, try to visualize your ovaries. They are soft, egg-shaped organs that nestle inside you.

Each month, one of your ovaries has produced a ripened egg. It has traveled through the funnel of one of your fallopian tubes and down the branch of tube that leads to your uterus.

Each egg has 23 chromosomes. Each sperm has 23 chromosomes. Together, these 46 chromosomes are the genetic code of humanity. The code is miraculously intact. From it, a healthy baby grows.

Now that you are pregnant, that egg has become an embryo and it has nestled inside your womb, a tiny spot of life in the warmth and darkness.

Visualize your womb, dark and cushiony. Your lover's sperm has fertilized your ovum, and in this warm darkness the two cells have joined to create one tiny spirit. This tiny jelly-like cell is safely embedded inside your uterus and there inside you, it shall grow.

Think about the idea that a woman with child is the perfect example of energy in unison.

Feel the softness of your muscles and the gentleness of your breath.

When you are ready to get up, breathe deeply and exhale slowly.

Do not arise quickly.

Feeling Love Meditation

This meditation should take at least 15 min. Lead a total body relaxation before beginning the visualization. Again, pause after each step.

Take a releasing breath and relax your body.

Close your eyes and spend a few moments focusing on the quiet darkness.

Now, with your eyes closed, visualize the face of someone you love. It may be a friend or a lover, a child or an adult.

Imagine that you can hold that person's face gently in your hands.

Explore how you feel as you gaze into the eyes of your special loved one.

Exchange places and imagine that your face is being held by that person. Feel the warmth. Feel the love. Feel how good it is to be held and comforted by that person.

Imagine a conversation you might have. (*Allow several minutes to pass before moving on.*)

Embrace that person. Hold that special person close to your body and rock together.

We rock to create peacefulness.

Imagine your bodies blending together, merging into one strong spirit.

And now, slowly say good bye to your loved one.

Gather your energy and your dreams, and return to the wakeful state.

If you have time, repeat this exercise and have the women visualize the faces of others whom they love.

Great Mother Earth Meditation

This meditation should take at least 10 min. Lead a total body relaxation before beginning the visualization. (A longer version of this meditation appears in chapter 11.)

Take a releasing breath and settle yourself into a comfortable position. Feel free to shift about if you need to.

Imagine that you are part of the great mother earth. Your body is a sloping landscape of gentle hills and soft folds of earth.

Your body is a stable healthy part of nature, with a spirit that soars high above the land.

You are very strong.

You are very powerful.

You are very beautiful.

And you are very wise.

Your energy comes from deep within you, and your wisdom is as old as the planet herself.

The sunshine warms you and the star shine comforts you in the darkness.

Close your eyes and relax.

Loosen and relax any tension remaining in your body.

Visualize the sky full of color, at dawn or at dusk.

Breathe deeply and inhale the fresh clean air.

Sense the comfort of your child nestled deep within the warmth of your body.

Rest peacefully throughout the night.

Inner Sanctum Meditation

This meditation should take at least 15 min. Do a total body relaxation before beginning the visualization.

Inhale deeply and relax. Begin to focus on your internal world, the world of your baby.

See the interior world of safety, of nourishing pulsing veins and arteries.

See the purity of your womb, its sturdy security.

Imagine your baby as she or he floats inside you. Her or his energy is peaceful. She or he is a total person.

You and the baby shall be friends forever, beyond all boundaries.

Visualize your placenta, shiny and rich with veins and capillaries. It is sparkling and lively.

Imagine the umbilicus, a loving cord that acts as a river, bringing nourishment to your baby. Its internal tributaries carry away what is not used and not needed.

Your interior world is a miracle unto itself.

Pregnancy is the normal yet ecstatic progress of your body towards its maturational fulfillment. Even the uterine process of involution, which is the shrinking of the uterus after childbirth, is a part of its inborn but untested capacity.

The process of lactation, of producing milk, is the natural biological maturity of the breast. Be they large or small, round or pendulous, the breasts have the capacity to produce milk and nourish a child.

Breathe gently and deeply and relax.

Journey Meditation

This meditation should take at least 20 min. Include a total body relaxation before you begin the visualization.

Relax yourself and breathe deeply and evenly until you can feel your tension floating up and away.

We are going on a journey together.

Imagine that you are at the edge of a wide green meadow.

The sky is a soft shade of blue. A few white clouds float above you. The sun is shining and the air is the perfect temperature.

As you walk across the meadow, you notice how soft the grass is and how sweet the air smells.

A butterfly flits by and you realize how beautiful and delicate its wings are.

As you cross the meadow you notice the trees on the other side. They are tall and slender. Their roots firmly anchored into the earth, they sway gently, their upper branches delicately reaching to the sky.

You have come to an old stone staircase. Walk down it slowly. At the bottom you come to your favorite resting place.

The sand beneath your feet is soft and warm.

The pond is calm. The water is smooth and glitters with the warm light of the afternoon sunshine.

Weeping willows line the edge of the pond. Birds call softly.

Relax here. Allow yourself to feel totally comfortable. Totally safe.

And when you are ready, you will end your reverie. Turn and go back up the steps.

Go slowly, breathe deeply.

Return across the meadow. As you walk, notice the figure of someone you know coming toward you.

As the person grows closer, you realize who it is. It could be your parent, your child, your lover, or a friend. Embrace that person.

If you would like, visualize another person to join you, and together you may finish your journey.

Close the meditation with a releasing breath. Keep your body relaxed for as long as possible.

Postpartum Meditations

After delivery, mothers find that parenting a newborn is one of life's most wonderful and most stressful experiences. The sheer energy that feeding and caring for a new baby requires can create a sense of overwhelming fatigue. The physical work of mothering can create muscle strain and easily tire already slackened muscles. Understanding how to relax her body allows a mother to heal some of her own discomforts during a time when she is really focused on caring for her infant.

Creative visualization for parenting can be just as colorful and varied as those for pregnancy. A woman may visualize soothing a fretful infant or celebrating her baby's first birthday or holiday. A mother may be able to visualize herself leading her child through a difficult journey, healing a sickness, or comforting a sorrow. She may want to focus on the joy she shares with the baby's father, the strength of her bonding, and the importance of the new circle of family life.

Using the Childbirth Mantra

Mantra is a Hindu word meaning a sound, word, or phrase that is either given to or chosen by a person. It is repeated quietly during meditation, or during any other activity that requires relaxed concentration. Some people are turned off by the idea of repeating words or names to themselves because they think it is meaningless and silly. Childbirth mantras are neither meaningless nor silly. They allow for a specific focus, and they are particularly useful when the turmoil of labor challenges even the most relaxed woman. If you are interested in helping women to develop their own childbirth mantras you might discuss the option of repeating simple words or phrases that are especially relevant to the laboring mother. The mother can use her mantra as both a focus and a form of instruction to her body. She may repeat her mantra to herself or out loud. During contractions, when it is most difficult to relax, her mantra may be extraordinarily helpful. She may choose words and phrases like open, down, relax, this is for the baby, be born, be soft, I love you, begin, rest, and be peaceful.

As you may imagine, there are thousands of mantras. Some women invoke the name of God, others call upon saints or goddesses to help them. Whatever the mantra is, it should bring a woman peace and send positive vibrations through her body. She may meditate on any set of words. The wisest thing for her to do is to focus on a word or phrase that helps her to relax. Tell her not to be disturbed if she cannot think of the right mantra right away. Let her experiment. She should try to use all of them, invent more of them, and free-associate until she can come up with just the right words.

During the birth of my second child, I used the mantra "relax and open" over and over again. Between pushing contractions, I concentrated on the phrase that I now use every day: "You are the light of the universe and the light of the universe shines through you."

If, during pregnancy or labor, a woman chooses to use a word like *open* or *release* she may in fact be able to visualize the opening of her cervix, the releasing of her perineum, the opening of her birth canal, and the descent of the baby. During postpartum, a new mother may chose to meditate on the words *healing* and *strength* and visualize her body recovering from birth, healing, and growing stronger. Women who are aware of their own anatomical structure are able to visualize specific organs or muscles and may find themselves able to ease aches and pains, strains, and soreness.

If you or the women in your class have never relaxed through meditation, you may all need to be reassured that the capacity for thorough relaxation exists in all of us. It requires only time and willingness, a bit of practice, and a sense of safety.

Meditation is a lifetime skill. We all need to learn ways of reducing the tension of our lives. The months of pregnancy and the years of parenting can be surprisingly stressful, and having the ability to relax, meditate, or use visualization is a gift. Use it!

Active Meditations

Active means doing. Active meditations are those that cause you to be doing something. Some mothers find that active meditations during pregnancy help them to relax and to find comfort. Others, especially those who are comfortable about labor and delivery, are able to perform active meditations while in labor. An active meditation during labor could be anything special that a woman and her birth attendants do. It could be taking a hot bath, or creating a candle lighting ritual. Women who labor at home may find that cooking the evening meal is a centering meditation. Practicing yoga or the techniques of massage can be active meditations. Some women choose to hold a special stone, crystal, egg, or gem during labor. Dance may be part of an active meditation. Swaying gently to music and releasing tension through movement is an excellent active meditation. Some women actually sing during active meditations. Here is a poem, ''You Are My Sister,'' written by an ancient Sufi dancer (Inglehart, 1983). It was used by a woman friend of mine as an active birth song meditation.

> You are my sister
> You are my mother
> You are my lover
> You are my friend.
> You are the Center
> And the Beginning,
> You go far beyond the End.
> I love you
> You help me see
> See in you
> See in me
> For I am in you
> And you are in me. (p. 56)

You can imagine how surprised the nurses were when this beautiful woman started to sing during her labor. But she was able to hum or sing throughout most of her contractions. It relaxed her and allowed her to focus on the joy of the coming birth.

Another active meditation is self-massage, often called effleurage by Lamaze teachers. Self-massage is the gentle stroking or touching of any part of your body while you relax. Traditionally, it is taught as a light, circling motion of the hands over the uterus, the womb. You may use this light stroke on any part of your body. I heartily encourage women to share this particular form of massage with their birth partners.

A particularly beautiful active meditation has been performed by Native American women for many generations (Inglehart, 1983). Before a woman is to give birth, another woman brushes her hair over and over again. A second woman gently massages corn meal on the bottoms of her feet to symbolize the hard work she will be doing. She has planted the seeds and now she will harvest the fruit of her great efforts. She will need to be cared for during her labor so that she may be caring and nourishing to her infant. Remind the women in your class that it is wise for them to be kind to themselves and allow others to be kind to them.

Healing Tension Through Massage

In our earlier discussions of the anatomy and physiology of pregnancy, our purpose was to understand how pregnancy creates changes within the mother in relationship to exercise. Massage is another physical experience that is also affected by the progress of gestation.

The female torso undergoes a gradual widening throughout pregnancy. The breasts enlarge as milk ducts multiply, and venous circulation increases. The effects of hormones soften the cartilage that supports the joints, allowing slight flexibility in the pelvis, thus subtly widening the hips. The abdomen widens as the fetus grows. The uterus expands and the lower floating ribs flare out. And, of course, the mother gains weight and fat is deposited across her hips and buttocks.

All of these changes contribute to both the magnificence and the strain and fatigue of pregnancy. In early pregnancy, the fatigue may be felt more along the cervical vertebrae, and across the upper back, neck, and shoulders. As pregnancy progresses, the strain is felt in the lower back as the weight of the uterus pulls the top of the wedge-shaped sacrum forward. The increased flexibility of the sacroiliac joint, which permits this movement, contributes to the lower backache many women experience.

A massage is probably the kindest gift you can give to a pregnant woman. Whether it comes from a professional masseuse, a lover, or a friend, a massage releases tension, soothes weary muscles, and allows the mother to feel as if someone else were sharing her burden. Massage is also an opportunity for estranged lovers to reestablish contact. When intercourse is contraindicated by maternal condition, massage can be a sensual, nonorgasmic loving exchange. Massage also encourages circulation, which is good for the mother and the baby. The skin glows after a massage, and the stiffness that some women experience because of edema may be eased by a good massage. An entire class period just on massage is time well spent. You may want to have a special event and invite the women and their partners to join you and a professional masseuse for a massage workshop.

Healing is an active and interactive exchange. Healing is something one does for oneself, with others, for others. A caring friend or lover may offer great healing energy to the pregnant woman, and she may respond with deep relaxation and relief. Although this text is designed for instructors, I hope that they will recommend it to pregnant women so that they can discover these healing alternatives.

Introducing Massage

The potential masseuse should consider the mother's body as a beautiful, changing, natural landscape. It is a joyous adventure to explore its valleys, sloping sides, and changing contours. Inkeles (1983) reminds us that when you "please the mother, . . . you benefit her child" (p. 98). Imagine that the massage is sending warmth into the mother's muscles and that her blood is full of oxygen. The oxygen is nourishing her whole body and the baby, and as the mother breathes, she is breathing for the baby too. Imagine that the massage is stimulating the mother's circulation and that her blood is clean and rich and strong, moving through her body, clearing away toxins, and bringing energy to all of her organs.

Encourage the use of the varieties of self-massage in your prenatal classes. These can be effective as a tension-releasers during labor. Effleurage, foot massage, and even the practice of Shiatsu, which is acupressure massage, are appropriate for pregnancy and can be practiced alone or with the help of a healing friend.

Guidelines for Massaging Pregnant Women

Becoming a competent masseur or masseuse takes considerable training. There are licensing procedures in many states that carefully monitor the practice of massage. Therefore, it is not appropriate to claim that you are teaching massage if in fact you are not legally permitted to do so. You may, however, provide information about massage that can be very helpful, and you can encourage women to seek out licensed practitioners who understand the physical discomforts of pregnancy. Chiropractors also provide services for pregnant women. The following list of suggestions may help you to teach your group about massage. You may want to create a handout for women to share with their partners. For more details, consult Inkeles (1983).

- When you give a massage, use your whole hand, allowing your fingers and palms to touch the woman's skin sensitively.
- Keep your strokes smooth and rhythmic. Vary them, but change the style, speed, or rhythm carefully.
- Listen and watch for nonverbal cues. Smiles and deep sighs are good signs. Squirming tells you something very different! Stop if she says "ouch" and avoid repeating the painful mistake.
- Use plenty of pillows. She should be well supported, with all joints flexed and relaxed. Beyond midpregnancy she should not lie on her back for more than a few minutes. Encourage her to recline and turn slightly to the left to avoid compression of the vena cava.
- Don't push too hard, go too fast, act bored, or watch the clock!
- Do not massage directly over varicose veins. Use very light fingertips over varicosities and always stroke towards the heart.
- Massage the places that hurt. Ask her what she needs and where she would like to be massaged. Remember, in the beginning, no one is an expert at massage. Learn and enjoy the massage together.

Foot Massage

A foot massage may be precisely what a woman wants. During pregnancy the feet are often tired at the end of every day. During labor and delivery, a woman who enjoys a foot massage may find it immensely relaxing. These are the items and procedures you might follow for a pleasant foot massage.

Fill a basin with warm water. Allow the mother to soak her feet in the warm water. Towel dry the feet. Make certain that you dry between each toe. Apply warm baby oil or body oil. Massage the feet deeply and thoroughly. Apply gentle, consistent pressure. Massage corns, calluses, and bunions. Dry the feet. Pat them gently. If you do it right, she'll tell you it's divine.

Head Massage

You may want to instruct the women on how to do a head massage on themselves! Pregnant women frequently get sinus headaches for which they hesitate to take any medication. They are also prone to the same tension headaches everyone else gets. To administer a self-head massage, follow these steps:

1. Lie down and take several releasing breaths.
2. Place the hands on the forehead and gently begin to massage the forehead, out to the temples, across the cheekbones, down the sides of the nose, across the upper jaw, over the chin, and back to the hinge joint of the lower jaw.
3. Return to the forehead and proceed once more to massage outward, over the ear and down around the base of the skull. Allow the massage to cover the entire skull.
4. Repeat the entire massage. Each woman should be able to relax and use her hands, not her neck, to lift her head, turn it gently to the left and right, and place it back down.

After a head massage a woman should rest quietly before getting up. Proper and sensitive head massage can alleviate a headache or stop one from becoming too intense. Now that's what I call self-healing!

Perineal Massage

The perineum is the portion of the body that must stretch during childbirth and that has traditionally been the site of the episiotomy. Tight, tense muscles and a fearful mother can impede the birth of the baby. Relaxed muscles and a mother who is not afraid of opening her body completely to the emerging child contribute to the ease of the baby's passage.

A woman can massage the perineum by herself or with a partner. It should not be an ordeal. I usually demonstrate perineal massage on myself, in my sweatpants or leotard, leaning back against pillows or a wall. The purpose of my demonstration is to clarify the importance of being comfortable with one's body and especially with one's more intimate parts. When I place my hands on

my own perineum, women see that it is okay to touch and to learn through touch how their bodies feel and respond to relaxation. I always point out the bony perimeter of the pelvic outlet, demonstrating on my own body that the space is wide enough to permit the passage of an infant's head.

Releasing perineal tension requires that women unclench their gluteus muscles (the buttocks) and relax their faces, especially their mouths. At home they may experiment with their ability to relax by placing a warm washcloth against the perineum or by massaging that area gently with oil. A woman may choose to use her thumbs, her fingertips, or her whole hand. At home she or her partner may place outward or downward pressure on the vaginal opening so she can practice keeping the perineal muscles relaxed even when unfamiliar sensations are occurring. The purpose of perineal massage should not be to prevent episiotomy. Rather, it is to gain sensory awareness of tension and the individual's ability to release it.

Classroom Activity: The Group Massage

Sometimes I invite a masseuse to come into the class and demonstrate massage for pregnancy and labor. This is always a wonderfully successful event and everyone just loves it. If time or scheduling does not permit this, use the following activity. Remember to provide soft music and turn the lights down or off.

Divide the class into groups of six. One woman should lie down on her left side on her exercise mat or blanket. Use all available pillows and blankets to make her as comfortable as possible. The others should station themselves around her with one at her head and the others at her arms and legs. Members trade places after each massage. You will be amazed at the intense caring and sharing that will occur.

Each person should receive a massage. Each person should be made to feel completely relaxed, supported, and cared for with a full 5 min of undivided attention from her peers.

Experiment. As each woman receives her massage, the group can be very quiet or the person massaging the woman's head can talk to her about breathing and releasing to the touch of the massage. If possible, they should pretend that she is in labor, and the massage should respond to the rhythm of her contractions. The group may choose to explore images that are soothing. Some groups have focused on images of soaring birds and parting clouds whereas others have focused on water or on images presented in our meditations. Those who are massaging the arms, legs, or torso can experiment with different strokes. They should be careful to support the limb if they move it in any way.

When the group has completed its massage, encourage discussion about the experience. Has each group created its own ritual? Has a pattern emerged? Have women discovered any healing images or words? What did they experience? (Allow plenty of time for discussion.)

Pleasing tactile experiences integrate the body and mind, support positive body image, and encourage strengthened body boundaries. Massage is an essential tool for healing. It is also an act of love and caring.

Learning About Shiatsu

Another very interesting form of massage is called Shiatsu. It is a fascinating form of Asian massage that is rapidly gaining popularity in our culture. Perhaps the reason for the increasing interest is the awakened understanding that every culture has its own healing traditions and that each, in its own way, is valuable.

Shiatsu is the Japanese version of acupressure. According to Waturu Ohashi (1976), founder of the Shiatsu Education Center of America in New York, Shiatsu massage is part of a healing philosophy that believes that the body systems are a reflection of the energy forces of the world. Those forces are called yin, the passive, feminine force, and yang, the masculine, more aggressive force. The energy forces are connected within the body by meridian lines that connect with and govern the functioning of the organs. The proper pressure applied at specific points on the body releases and expresses the bodily energy forces.

The proper practice of Shiatsu massage takes considerable time to learn. One perfects the practice of Shiatsu by developing the sensitivity of the fingers to the body and its musculature. It is interesting to point out that the Eastern system of health and disease focuses not on isolating the sickness, but on healing the integrated elements of the body. It seeks primarily to right the imbalance of the energy forces within the human system. During pregnancy, when the organic systems undergo significant changes, a sensitive masseuse may be able to ease many of the musculoskeletal discomforts as well as those that are related to changes in the functioning of the internal organs.

A special abdominal massage, *ampuku*, is considered important during pregnancy because, according to Eastern tradition, the essence of the human spirit and the source of human energy is the *hara*, or the abdominal region. Massage of the *hara* should be beneficial to both mother and child. According to Shiatsu traditions the pain of labor contractions can be eased by applying pressure-point massage to specific locations along the sacrum and the ankle and foot, which stimulates the spleen, liver, and kidney.

In Eastern massage, the ear is one of the most important and sensitive areas of the body. If you look carefully at the structure of the ear, it is shaped very much like a curled human fetus, which may be what led ancient practitioners to consider it to be a miniature of the entire human system. A woman may find that the gentle massage or pressure-point treatment of the ear during pregnancy or labor is particularly relaxing.

With training, the Shiatsu practitioner may be able to locate and apply pressure to bodily meridians during childbirth that release pain, increase or regulate contractions, speed dilation, or reduce backache. The usefulness of this form of massage deserves careful study.

After childbirth it is recommended that the midpoint of the sternum be massaged for greater milk production. A point midway between the seventh vertebra and the edge of the shoulder should be massaged to ease breast-feeding backache.

Acupressure is receiving increasing attention as a natural healing technique. It appears to be useful for relieving a wide range of discomforts, and it may be a particularly valuable technique for self-healing in women. If you are interested in learning more about acupressure, see Bauer (1987), which describes and illustrates specific treatments for use throughout a woman's reproductive life.

Shiatsu or acupressure therapies should be administered carefully, and those who are interested should pursue study or receive treatment with individuals who are well trained and able to integrate the delicate needs of the woman and her unborn baby.

Rolfing

Rolfing, or structural integration, is a form of body work developed by Dr. Ida Rolf. Rolf theorized that because the human body is under constant gravitational stress, many disorders are really the result of physical imbalances, improper postural alignment, and weakness in the supportive muscles and ligaments of the body.

Rolfing consists of deep tissue manipulation. The rolfer's goal is to realign the bodily organs and tissues to create a system that is enhanced by its vertical posture, rather than slumped and curved or weakened.

Dr. Rolf's theory advises that women be rolfed before they conceive. The process of postural realignment for women is designed to reestablish balance in the key areas of the torso: through the shoulders and rib cage for improved respiration, through the torso and abdomen for increased muscular efficiency during pregnancy and labor, and in the pelvic basin for strengthening the muscles that support the organs of the pelvis.

Although it is not advisable to go through rolfing during pregnancy, St. Just (1984) suggests that the real benefit of rolfing may be felt during postpartum. After a woman has a child she should begin working to reestablish postural alignment, balance, and comfort. Special attention and careful body therapy during postpartum may help to heal the slackened abdominal muscles, stabilize the pelvis, and correct any displacement of the sacrum. Rolfing can be an intense, emotional, and painful process. It should not be undertaken lightly.

As we move away from skills of the body we need to focus on intellectual and cognitive events that can help reduce prenatal anxiety. The birth plan and labor rehearsal are activities that come directly from childbirth education. They are typically used in prepared childbirth classes to help couples think and plan for their births, to reduce anxieties about what will or will not happen, and to prepare for what to do when the big day arrives. I frequently use these activities in the exercise class to stimulate discussions or to encourage visualization and organization of the upcoming event.

Making a Birth Plan to Reduce Tension

There are other hands-on activities besides massage and relaxation that help reduce tension. These include clarifying images and designing a typology, or an organized presentation, of the events surrounding labor and delivery. Offering women the opportunity to create a birth plan is a revealing experience for many women who have no idea of what the procedures for birth might involve. For those who have chosen care givers who are hand-patters, the birth plan is a real awakening! Yes, there are things to think about besides the pain! Yes, there are reasons to know what to expect! And no, the care giver can't take care of everything. The mother must be responsible for herself!

Discussing a birth plan in your class is a great way to stimulate the mental rehearsal of birth. Carolyn Hecht (1982), a childbirth educator, uses a form titled "Prepared Childbirth Options" (1982, pp. 35-38). It is a flexible, useful tool for discussing options and desires for the management of childbearing. It intellectualizes the process and breaks it down into concrete, manageable pieces. The skilled prenatal educator should be able to help a mother visualize and understand the processes outlined in the compartmentalized birth plan.

The creation of a birth plan is now a standard feature in many childbirth education programs and perhaps is one of their strongest tools. Although the birth plan was once considered revolutionary, many care givers now offer to sit down with a woman and her partner to develop a birth plan and thereby discuss some of the options available to them in the hospital. Of course, some care givers still object to the procedure, feeling that it is inappropriate or that it sets up too many expectations.

However, the birth plan is not a list of demands; it is a list of choices, factors to be considered, and options to be avoided if possible. It is a statement of opinion, not of prediction. A woman and her chosen birth attendants and care givers should discuss the birth plan thoroughly. Each should be respectful of the others' opinions, but in the end, the pregnant woman must be comfortable with her plan. If she is not, then the plan has only added to, and not reduced, her tension. The woman should review her choice of a care giver if that person appears inflexible, offended by the concept of a birth plan, indifferent, or arrogant.

Many months before her due date arrives, a mother may begin to think about the kind of birth she imagines she will have. Obviously, no birth is totally planned, and efforts to create the perfect birth experience will probably end in disappointment. The more a woman feels that she can influence her birth experience, however, the calmer and more competent she will feel as she prepares for the birth of her child.

There are going to be items on this list that you as an instructor may not have considered or even heard of until this time. Identify those items and discuss them thoroughly with your service team. Make certain that you understand all explanations. You may have some women in your group who have a lot of questions about these options and others who have already decided for or against some of those same things. You must be well informed to enter into a discussion about birth plans.

I encourage women to make copies of their birth plans. If they have questions I cannot answer I encourage them to write them down and to ask their care givers, while I make a note to ask my own advisors the same question. Then, the next time we meet we can compare answers. I also suggest that women ask to have their birth plans placed in their folders so that when they get to the hospital it is there for the medical attendants to refer to; or, better yet, they can bring a copy with them to the hospital and tape it to the wall.

Women who are opting to have home births or who have the opportunity to give birth in a newer, family-centered maternity hospital may find that some of these requests do not apply. However, most women will find themselves in situations where routines tend to supersede individual choice, and it requires strength and determination to retain control over the birth. You will find a copy of the birth plan in this chapter's appendix (Appendix 12.1). I urge you to read over this plan before continuing.

You can imagine the gasps of surprise and the wide-eyed response that this sample birth plan receives from a room full of pregnant women! New ideas! New solutions! New possibilities! Opportunities for self-determination! For influence! Suddenly it seems possible to experience birth without feeling fear and being overwhelmed by unfamiliar places, strange medical routines, and the vulnerability that images of childbirth can conjure. Suddenly birth can be faced with calm, competent, adult decisions based on careful and thorough consideration of the issues. None of these ideas, suggestions, or wishes is extraordinary, out of the question, unsafe, or impossible.

Planning a Labor Rehearsal to Reduce Anxiety

A second activity for relieving some of the anxiety about childbirth is to have a labor rehearsal or a mock labor. This allows a woman, or a woman and her partner, to role-play her labor and birth. It helps them prepare for the sequence of events as they may happen. Of course, the actual event will be different, but having practiced their responses to certain predictable events, the woman and her partner are more confident in their ability to deal with those that are unpredictable. This technique

is used in many prepared childbirth programs and is an excellent teaching tool. As with all other techniques, use it only if you are well prepared to answer questions and present unbiased and accurate information.

You have awakened at 2 a.m. with mild menstrual-like cramps. What should you do?
Go back to sleep.

Now it is 5:30 a.m. and your membranes have ruptured. What do you look for?
The color of the fluid should be clear or milky, not green, yellow, or brown. It should be odorless and possibly tinged with blood.

How might your contractions change after your water has broken?
The cushion between the baby and the cervix is gone so the contractions may be stronger.

Your contractions are fairly mild, yet you need to use a breathing technique. Which one should you use and how do you do it?
Use slow-chest breathing and simply relax your body at the onset of each contraction.

How will you know when to go to the hospital? What will you bring? Where will you park?
Check with your care giver about when to go to the hospital. Have two bags packed: one with things for labor and the other with clothes and supplies for your stay on the maternity floor. Bring clothes for the baby to come home in! You have already driven to the hospital and figured out where to park, and you know how to get in.

It is 8 a.m. You are driving to the hospital and a contraction begins. It is much stronger. Coach, what should you do?
Keep your eyes on the road and your hands on the wheel at all times. Tell mom to relax and breathe gently.

After being admitted to your birthing room you find that your back really hurts. Can you and your coach think of three or four different things to do to relieve discomfort?
The pelvic tilt on your hands and knees, a back rub, a warm shower, or a hot pack on your back.

What different positions can you assume during your labor?
Standing, leaning, sitting, crouching, squatting, lying on your side, or cuddling with your coach. Don't forget to go to the bathroom during labor!

A nurse has come in to examine you during a contraction. You are 3 cm dilated! Good for you! Now the resident doctor and an intern have come in to examine you. How do you want to handle this?

You have many choices. If your water has broken you should not be examined. Another exam is probably unnecessary anyway. Be polite but refuse.

What can you do about dry mouth?

Suck on a lollypop, ice chips, a popsicle, or candy.

Cold feet?

Put on socks; get a foot massage.

Tension?

Relax and breathe, meditate and visualize, share your feelings and allow others to soothe you, try a warm washcloth or massage.

It is 11:30 a.m. Your nurse has examined you and you have progressed only about 1 cm. She indicates that unless your labor picks up your doctor may suggest Pitocin, which is a synthetic drug used to stimulate contractions. What can you and your coach do to help your labor to progress?

Close the door. Start kissing and hugging. Use nipple stimulation. Relax. Try massage.

If Pitocin is prescribed, what will happen to the quality of your labor?

It will get longer and stronger very quickly. Coach should be prepared to work harder.

Contractions are coming faster now. You may need to focus inward. What level of breathing might you choose to use now?

If you cannot stay with slow chest breathing you may want to use accelerated-decelerated breathing. (Usually this shift occurs without forethought.)

You realize that you are breathing too quickly and getting dizzy. Your fingers are tingling. What is happening and what can you do?

You are probably hyperventilating, which means you are breathing too fast and not taking in enough fresh oxygen. Slow yourself down. Breathe into your hands or into a brown paper bag.

It is 1:15 p.m. Your contractions are coming one on top of the other. What is happening?

You are nearing birth. Your contractions are beginning to push the baby out and your cervix must still finish its dilation. The contractions are quite long. You may want to use the pant-blow breathing technique. Relax as much as possible. You should not be left alone. Coach or birth attendant should stay close by to help you pace your breathing.

You feel the urge to push but you have not been examined yet. What should you do?

Feather blow.

Your care giver has examined you and you are fully dilated! You are allowed to push. Practice the two kinds of pushing techniques.

Gentle physiological pushing and breath-holding pushing.

Do not push in class! Now change positions and practice these two techniques in other optional positions for childbirth.

Squatting, on hands and knees, side-lying, leaning on pillows, sitting on a chair.

Congratulations, your baby is born!

Mom, you are asked to bear down again. Why?

To deliver the placenta.

Obviously, the labor rehearsal does not cover all the possibilities that could occur during a birth, nor has it attempted to do so. The purpose of the rehearsal is to relieve tension. Any activity that makes the birthing process more manageable is valuable to the expectant woman.

Summary

Teaching women how to relax is no easy task. It requires time and patience. You cannot hurry a woman through a relaxation meditation, and you should never rush or disturb her while she is relaxed.

Our cultural style expects things to come easily, to be fixed quickly, and to be manufactured with perfection. The art of relaxation is, however, a discipline that must be learned. Most women who understand how their bodies feel when they are relaxed are able to detect tension during labor and release it effectively. Obviously, some will choose to use drugs for the same purpose. Our goal is not to insist that women go through childbirth drug-free, but to help them feel competent enough to try to use the tools of relaxation. If they are able to relax completely during contractions, use the breath as they need to, focus on an image, request a massage, or use a mantra, they have learned a magnificent lesson in self-awareness.

As we learn to relax and use relaxation techniques throughout our lifetimes, we perform an act that emphasizes health. Relaxation is as important as exercise in promoting a healthy outlook and a sense of well-being. Disease and disability in our culture may be related as much to psychosomatic factors as it is to physical or biological causes. The consistent application and appreciation of relaxation techniques promotes the physical, mental, and social well-being of an individual. The integration of body, mind, and spirit is essential for true physical well-being.

Learning to relax is a priceless skill. A day spent actively engaging in life's challenges, working, exercising, eating, and socializing, is a day spent being whole. Relaxation is a vital component to the health and wholeness of existence. Teaching about relaxation may take a great deal of thinking, planning, and integrating. Bits and pieces of information may have to be explained, like pieces of a puzzle that, when it is done, clearly details the once abstract image in a surprising and pleasing form.

Another important issue for you to discuss in your classes is the relationship between tension and the negative cultural behaviors of smoking, substance abuse, and obesity. When dealing with pregnant women, you must present all the pertinent information that is known about the effects of these behaviors on the fetus and on themselves and their self-image. For example, in a discussion of alcohol abuse, I describe the physical abnormalities observed in the infants of alcoholics. Fetal alcohol syndrome is characterized by infants with heads of small circumference, narrowed eye lids, small noses, and some malformation of the upper lip. Severely affected infants are affected both physically and mentally. Although an occasional drink may be harmless, there is no known safe level of alcohol consumption during pregnancy. I highly recommend that a pregnant woman with a drinking problem see a counselor who specializes in women's issues and alcoholism.

I use visualizations for healing all abusive behaviors. For example, for dealing with smoking cessation, I use the following visualization. Read it very slowly.

Visualization

Visualize yourself walking through a beautiful meadow. The grass is soft beneath your feet. The air is the perfect temperature and you are breathing the sweet clean air. You breathe deeply and fully. The air is sweet, the scent of the flowers and the warmth of the earth surrounds you and fills you with clean, healthy energy. The baby within you senses this joyous purity. It is comforted by your peace.

Imagine that you have come to a stream. It is running happily, gurgling over the rocks and into pools of crystal clear water. Reach into your pocket and pull out your last cigarette. Hold it in your hand. It feels cold and dead against your skin. Break it into tiny pieces. Tear it into a thousand shreds and let it fall from your fingertips. Let the water carry away the tobacco and the shredded filter.

Breathe deeply. Your mouth may water a little. Your palm may feel cold. But the cigarette is gone.

Your baby nestles peacefully within you. Your baby grows; its brain grows, its body becomes strong, and its organs are nourished by your healthy body.

Whenever you want to reach for a cigarette, breathe deeply and fully. Remember the sweetness of your breath and the warmth of the oxygen that nourishes your child. Set yourself free. Be free of the poisonous smoke forever.

The material in the next chapter attempts to address the needs of women in special populations. There are many women for whom exercise and physical activities have not been made available. Prenatal exercise instructors must make a conscious effort to include women with special needs.

The Birth Plan

I, _____, understand that the Birth Plan is a list of flexible options and that no birth can be totally planned. Circle numbers next to statements you will discuss with your care-giver.

1. I would like a prep/partial prep/mini prep/no prep at all. (*A prep is the complete or partial shaving of pubic hair.*)
2. I would/would not like an enema. (*Giving enemas used to be routine to prevent the accidental delivery of feces. Enemas used to be considered essential for the maintenance of a totally sterile field for delivery, but this is no longer the case.*)
3. My partner may/may not be present for the prep or enema.
4. I may refuse all internal exams by any person other than my chosen care giver except in case of an emergency.
5. I will/will not wear a fetal monitor for brief/extended periods of time.
6. I will have all optional medications explained to me and I will fully understand their possible effects on me and my baby.
7. I will be fully informed as to the necessity of any intervention or examination.
8. I will/will not accept a glucose IV. (*An intravenous drip does not necessarily keep a woman hydrated or provide enough energy-generating glucose to make it worthwhile. Women should go into labor well hydrated and be permitted to drink or eat lightly if they choose. Prohibitions against eating and drinking arose during the time when many women gave birth completely anesthetized because physicians feared they would aspirate the contents of the stomach if they vomited into the anesthesiologist's gas mask. Some care givers feel they want to keep a vein open in case of an emergency, but a prophylactic IV is not necessary.*)
9. I will be permitted to ambulate during labor (*walk around, sit, take a shower*).
10. I may have fluids during labor.
11. I may have a light meal during labor (*very light!*).
12. I will have the lights on/off and the door closed whenever I choose during my labor.
13. I will give birth in the position of my choice.
14. I would like to use a birthing chair if one is available.
15. I would prefer to deliver my baby in a birthing room. (*A birthing room is a room designed to allow a woman to labor and give birth without having to move to a different room.*)
16. I will not be moved to a delivery room unless it is an emergency. (*A delivery room is a place for surgery.*)
17. I will nurse my baby as soon as it is born.
18. During my vaginal birth, my partner will support me in whatever position I choose for birth.
19. I would prefer perineal massage or warm compresses in an effort to avoid an episiotomy.
20. I would like my coach to apply the compresses or massage.
21. I would like my other children present for the birth. (*Having children attend the birth is very controversial. If it is important to you, you will need to spend some time locating a birthing center and a cooperative care giver. Children should also be educated about the birth process. Standard sibling classes do not prepare children to attend a birth.*)
22. I would like a second or third support person.
23. I will bring a battery-operated camera, tape recorder, or video equipment.
24. I would like to use the tub or shower during labor.
25. I will choose to use gentle pushing or traditional pushing as either is appropriate.
26. I agree to cooperate with my care giver's instructions but retain the freedom to also make decisions regarding the birth of my baby.
27. My partner may help deliver the baby after the head and shoulders are born.
28. My partner would like to cut the umbilical cord.
29. I would like to touch the baby as it is being born.

30. I want to wait until the umbilicus stops pulsing before it is cut.
31. My baby will be treated gently and with respect.
32. My partner/I will clean and bathe the baby after birth.
33. We would like to use the Leboyer bath for our baby. (*A Leboyer bath is the practice of submerging the newborn into a warm bath to simulate the weightless, watery environment of the womb.*)
34. I will be informed of any injections of Novocaine in the event of an episiotomy or repair of perineal tears.
35. If drugs have been used to anesthetize any area of my body, I will be informed of the sensitivity recovery time.
36. After birth neosporin or erythromycin to prevent blindness caused by undetected venereal disease will not be administered to the baby's eyes until at least 1 hr has passed.
37. I will go directly from my birthing room to the maternity floor, not to the recovery room.
38. If I choose, I will leave the hospital with my baby 6-12 hr after birth if we are both in stable condition.
39. The baby will not go to the nursery but will stay with me at all times.
40. Uterine massage will be administered carefully, gently, and with respect for my body.
41. I may have fluids and food as soon as I want them.
42. I may use the bathroom as soon as I want to.
43. I want to shower as soon as I am ready to do so.
44. I want a heating pad or ice bag for afterbirth contractions. (*Many women use relaxation breathing techniques to cope with the pain of these contractions.*)
45. I will not be examined by any residents or physicians who are strangers to me.

In Case of Cesarean Delivery

1. In the event of a Cesarean birth, I would like my partner to remain with me at all times. (*Partners should attend childbirth preparation classes, and one class should include a discussion and film about cesareans.*)
2. I would like to remain alert for surgery. (*Be fully informed about choices and effects of anesthesia.*)
3. I would like a bikini incision. (*A horizontal rather than a vertical incision.*)
4. I want to touch my baby as soon as possible after birth. (*Women used to be prevented from touching their babies for fear of contaminating them and the sterile field.*)
5. If a cesarean is needed, I do not want my arms strapped down.
6. My partner will be able to hold the baby after birth.
7. After surgery, the catheter will be removed as soon as possible.
8. I will be treated kindly by hospital staff as I heal.
9. My partner may remain with me and visit at any time during my recovery.

Chapter 13

Prenatal Exercise for Women With Special Needs

One of the most important exercises of my life was working with a committee of women preparing for a conference on women with disabilities. Our topic was medical discrimination. We met each week for many months to explore the range of medical, social, and emotional factors related to being a disabled woman in search of health care services.

The week before the conference, Mary Isom, a peer counselor/case manager at Alternatives for Reaching Independence through Services and Engineering (ARISE), the Center for Independent Living in Syracuse, New York, summed up our experience together as one of the most empowering she had ever had. By talking together, we had found the words she had never been able to express concerning her frustration and despair about the discrimination against disabled women and their subsequent ill-treatment.

Millions of disabled women are mothers. Their disabilities are physical, intellectual, or emotional. As care givers and professionals, we must recognize that the needs and interests of these women are not unlike those of all women. Our wisdom, experiences, and knowledge apply to disabled women as well. As teachers, we need to reach out to this special population and become sensitive to their needs.

The material in this chapter requires you to consider your skills, your prejudices, and your willingness to extend yourself to women whose lives may be seriously affected by disease or disability. The chapter does not address all the kinds of disabilities that affect childbearing women; however, it does attempt to raise our collective consciousness regarding all women with special needs. In your professional role, you may encounter women whose physical or emotional problems are extraordinary. If you need additional help in adapting materials and techniques, consult with other professionals who are caring for the particular woman in question.

The special concerns of rural women and teenagers are included at the end of this chapter. Not all teenagers or rural women have special needs, but as distinct groups they are not always served adequately by standard care-giving systems. The special problems involved with teenage pregnancy are attributed to physical maturity and the likeliness of poor prenatal care. Rural women's needs are special because of their isolation. The circumstance of poverty in members of either group also contributes to their identification as women with special needs. Specific activities and program ideas are suggested for improving the fitness component of prenatal care for these groups.

Women at Risk

The information in this chapter concerns women at risk during pregnancy. A high-risk pregnancy is one in which the maternal or fetal condition poses a probable threat to the health and well-being of mother or fetus (Benson, 1983, p. 99). Women in high-risk categories are statistically more likely to suffer from certain diseases, disabilities, nutritional deprivation, wife abuse, child abuse, neglect, and neonatal or maternal mortality.

Women with cognitive or developmental disabilities, emotional handicaps, and certain physical limitations are at critical risk in the areas of sexuality and reproduction. Women with limited ability to comprehend the world are often sexual victims. Their infants become fragile and vulnerable children whose early years are most critical.

Women with physical handicaps are often assumed to be mentally handicapped and have been victims of severe stereotypes. Untold wealth of talent and ideas has been lost because of incorrect assumptions about physically disabled women's cognitive abilities. Their needs and potential contributions have been virtually ignored, along with the fact that many disabled women are intelligent individuals of enormous dignity, loved and admired by family and friends, and capable of bearing children and caring for them.

Organizations that advocate equal rights and recognition for the disabled have done considerable work in the area of disability and sexuality. It has been essential to recognize disabled women as individuals who are capable of loving and making love. Acceptance and recognition of sexuality is an essential element in the liberation of the handicapped.

Exercise and fitness programs that include women with disabilities should offer opportunities for self-expression, education about pregnancy, and movement experiences to ease pregnancy-related discomforts and to help readjust maladapted movement patterns. It is important to help all women define themselves as capable and knowledgeable about their bodies and childbirth. This can be done through the acquisition of specific skills and participation in programs that include childbirth preparation and movement activities designed to improve body image and self-image.

Women With Emotional Disabilities

Women who are psychiatric outpatients or troubled women who come as independent agents to clinics have complicated problems. Histories of abusive behavior, substance abuse, and encounters with the judicial system are not uncommon among these women. Your judgment about a woman's problems is totally irrelevant to your professional obligation to her. Unless the courts have determined that she is unfit, you must assume that she will be responsible for the care and nurturing of her child. You should treat her with respect and care for her as you would any other pregnant woman.

The needs of institutionalized women will differ from those whose therapy needs and social support are met by community centers and day treatment or outpatient programs. Life in an institution creates its own set of problems. The institutionalized woman is confined, and she lives on a schedule that may not reflect her own biorhythms. Meals may come too early; she may be famished by mid-afternoon but have no appetite at all by the evening meal. Exercise or recreational activities are usually scheduled at the convenience of the staff. If you provide services in an institution, evaluate the time and location of your sessions. Make sure that the mother has eaten within the last 2 hr and that the space available to you is private and comfortable.

You may find that your client has trouble keeping track of reality; she may comment on irrelevant things or lose track of ideas or directions for activities. A pregnant inpatient may be on medication that affects her movement or balance. Find out what medications might be affecting a patient's movements, mood, or behavior. Abrupt changes in behavior, emotional outbursts, or physical changes in the pregnant woman should be reported immediately to the supervisor, social worker, or floor nurse.

Women with special emotional needs should understand the goals of the exercise program without being overwhelmed. This means that you must introduce specific goals for exercise carefully and slowly. Fitness levels may be significantly lower in special populations. You can increase the success level of participants by using approximations of exercise form, simplified routines, and direct verbal commands.

Integrate program materials and educational agenda with other learning/living situations. Women with learning difficulties or social and behavioral problems often have difficulty with carryover—the ability to transfer knowledge and learning from one situation to another. Pay attention to the kind and quantity of information you provide. Role-play real-life situations to make classroom learning part of long-range behavioral modification.

These women may find that exercise programs make them feel anxious. Indeed, moving one's body in new and different ways is physically and emotionally challenging. However, as women begin to move more freely, strengthen their muscles, understand their changing bodies, and perhaps rediscover their own potential for movement, they take major steps toward regaining their health.

As a maternal health and fitness educator, I firmly believe that the maternal fitness program, as well as the childbirth education program, can have a great impact on women. Pregnancy is a time when women are most open to education, and the effective use of our skills is critical if we are to make an impact on the experience of pregnancy and birth.

Women With Physical Disabilities

The rights of disabled women are intimately tied to the rights of all women, for over the generations of obstetrical care, we have all lost control of our bodies. It is only recently that disabled persons were assured the right to free public education. Disabled women still have not been assured of their rights to be sexual, to bear children, and to fulfill their maternal aspirations if they so choose.

Women who do not engage in exercise due to physical limitations suffer from the psychological and physiological effects of sedentary living, which include muscular atrophy and reduced cardiovascular stamina. Research has shown that nonexercisers perceive themselves as heavier and flabbier than they really are (distorted body image) and that they tend to envision physical exercise as much more strenuous and difficult than others with similar physical capabilities who engage in regular physical activities (Nelson & Mondanaro, 1982, p. 254). The effects of a lifetime without exercise include chronic fatigue, low back pain, osteoporosis, and eventual complications related to decreased cardiovascular fitness (e.g., heart attack and stroke). All women should have the opportunity to exercise.

Women who have been discouraged from using their bodies and those who have never tried or have been unable to ride a bike, throw a ball, dance, or lift weights have missed the opportunity to experience the improved self-esteem and self-assurance and the sense of physical accomplishment that accompany exercise. In addition, our culture, with its emphasis on how the body looks, has tended to dismiss the disabled woman from exercise completely. Therefore, she may never have had the opportunity to discover how her body feels when it is used to its potential—when it feels strong and vital and alive.

Options for Women Who Are Unable to Exercise

Pregnant women with physical disabilities may feel that they cannot exercise. To them, movement may be so painful or severely limited that it seems senseless to try. Those who have serious organic problems may have been told to avoid exercise to protect the fetus. It is my belief that even small amounts of exercise are important for improving self-esteem, muscle tone, and overall health. The following exercises are not designed to build cardiovascular strength or lead to athletic training. They are activities to use with nonexercisers that can enhance physical comfort and build positive body image.

At the beginning of every exercise, lead the group in proper deep cleansing breaths. Proper breathing improves posture, lifts the rib cage, and improves respiration. The head should sit squarely on the neck, and the spine should be made as long as possible without causing strain or discomfort. Encourage the participants by telling them that even limited movements are important.

For some women even small amounts can be difficult. I suggest that you to use exercises that maintain range of movement and strengthen muscles isometrically. Tightening and releasing muscle groups, progressive relaxation, and induced-tension exercises are excellent therapeutic activities. Imaginary piano playing, wiggling each toe individually, miming situations with hands and fingers, and simple ankle flexing may be all the activity the woman can tolerate. But remember, all movement is important. If muscles are allowed to be idle they will deteriorate.

Large Motor Movements

Consider including the following large motor movements in your routines. Keep in mind that fine motor coordination may be the most difficult for persons with disabilities.

Opening Stretch
Arms should open as wide as possible to the side. Extend forward, out to the side again, and up over the head. Breathe deeply. Inhale as the arms extend out from the body; exhale as they pull closer to the midline.

Shoulder Shrugs and Circles

(See exercises for the neck, chapter 14.) These movements begin slowly and may increase in size and speed when appropriate.

Seated Forward Waist Bend

Inhale and then exhale while bending forward as far as possible. Obviously, a big belly will inhibit forward movement, but even little movements are important.

Torso Circle

While doing the forward waist bend, pretend you have a crayon on each shoulder with which you are drawing a circle. Move the torso in a circular fashion.

Hip Flexors

While seated, lift the thigh and place it gently back down. If necessary, place the palm or fingertips on or under the thigh bone while lifting.

Hip Flexor With Knee Extension

Do the hip flexor, but this time extend the leg from the knee.

Kegels—The Essential Woman's Exercise

(See chapter 10.) At any point you may add heel lifts, toe wiggles, or foot circles. They may be done separately or in combination with the hip flexors. (All of these exercises are also great for office workers and those who are tied to a desk.)

The Woman With Epilepsy

Epilepsy is a relatively common neurological disorder (Black, Herman, & Shope, 1982). It is estimated that 10 out of every 1,000 individuals suffer from some form of epilepsy. Seizures, the convulsive events that occur in epilepsy, are triggered by an interference in the electrical impulses in the brain. The seizures can be mild and barely noticeable or quite severe. Seizure control with anticonvulsive drugs is usually quite successful. During pregnancy, a woman may find that she is more prone to seizures. As pregnancy progresses, normal metabolic changes occur that may require an increase in prescribed medication. Special care to protect the fetus from the effects of seizures or inappropriate medication is important.

Research has shown that exercise may raise the seizure threshold. Exercise itself offers so many benefits, including socializing and body strengthening, that it may be especially important for a woman with a seizure disorder.

A woman with epilepsy may know when she is going to have a seizure because she is aware of the emotional or physical experiences that trigger her seizure pattern. Unfortunately, many people who have seizures hesitate to inform others about their condition. Thus the occurrence of a seizure is usually an unexpected event. Even if you are not aware of women in your class or facility who suffer from seizure disorders, you should be able to perform the appropriate first aid in the event of a seizure:

1. Stay calm.
2. If the woman is standing or sitting, ease her to the floor and lay her on her side to keep her air passages open and prevent aspiration.
3. Place a towel or pillow beneath her head to prevent injury.
4. Do not attempt to insert anything into the woman's mouth.
5. When the seizure is over, keep her still, cover her if she appears chilled, and allow her to rest. Call her physician for further instructions.

A woman having a seizure may twitch, gag, shake, appear to stare, or blank out. She may drool or shout, lose control of her bladder, become rigid, or hyperextend her body. It is not an easy experience for either the woman with epilepsy or those who witness her seizure. However, your care, understanding, and protection of her is vitally important.

Women Carrying More Than One Baby

Twins occur in about 1 out of every 100 pregnancies. Discovering that she is carrying twins can be an exciting experience for a woman, but it may take her extra time and energy to adjust her expectations to the coming of two babies instead of just one.

A multiple pregnancy is considered a high-risk pregnancy. The mother and fetuses require special care to ensure that they do well throughout the pregnancy and during birth. Twins are often born several weeks early, and, though they are often smaller than singlets, their combined term weight is frequently more than that of just one baby.

Until a woman knows that she is carrying twins, she will probably continue her normal exercise routines, adjusting to weight gain and fatigue like other mothers. When she gains weight more rapidly than other mothers and shows signs of rapid intrauterine growth, and when the care giver detects two heart beats, she will probably have a sonogram that reveals the multiple pregnancy. Following this diagnosis, the care giver may advise a woman to reduce or eliminate exercise. This is to prevent injury to the mother and excessive stress that might lead to the early onset of labor.

Ideally, you should encourage a woman to continue a very moderate exercise plan. Walking, gentle stationary biking, and even doing mild dance exercises would be helpful both for morale and physical well-being. If signs of hypertension, edema, uterine cramping, or vaginal bleeding develop, however, instruct her to discontinue exercise and to see her care giver. Vigorous exercise—running, dancing, or weight lifting—should be avoided.

The woman carrying more than one baby will feel bigger and probably gain more weight than the woman carrying only one child. Her system will work very hard to nourish both babies. She deserves extra special attention. If a woman in your class drops out because of a multiple pregnancy, invite her to come and watch, have friends call her, or invite her back to the class after her birth to share her experience.

Women Who Are Obese

Obesity is a major health problem for women in America. In the evolutionary context, the range of human metabolism has produced a large number of individuals who tend to be overweight. The anthropological explanation for this is that those females who were bigger, with more body fat (and thus more energy reserves) were more likely to survive food shortages, childbearing, and nursing.

It is difficult to find a clinical definition of obesity in pregnancy. However, a woman who enters pregnancy weighing 20% more than her ideal weight or a woman who weighs over 200 lb at term is considered obese. The fetus of either woman may be at risk. The risks of obesity in pregnant women include malnutrition, heart disease, and late-onset diabetes. In addition, obese women are statistically more frequent candidates for cesarean sections due to fetal distress than their leaner counterparts.

Unless it is medically contraindicated, there is no reason for a heavy woman to avoid exercise. In fact, the slow, gentle pace of the prenatal exercise class is precisely what the overweight woman needs. In class, she will enjoy the company of her peers while learning about exercises that improve posture, ease some of the physical discomforts of pregnancy, and lead to a happier, more comfortable postpartum recovery. In addition, she may be able to explore her feelings about her obesity, deal more effectively with body image and body boundary concerns, and, in fact, begin to work towards a healthier, perhaps slimmer, life-style after childbirth.

The question of weight gain and/or dieting during pregnancy is of vital concern to women who begin their pregnancies overweight. In some cases, good nutritional counseling and careful observation of a well-balanced prenatal diet may allow a compulsive overeater to lose weight during her pregnancy. However, most nutritionists agree that a moderately overweight woman should not actively try to lose weight during her pregnancy. Dieting may deprive the fetus of necessary nutrition, and the breakdown of fats during the weight loss process produces chemicals called ketones that may be quite harmful to fetal development. Advise overweight women to eat three meals a day and to expect to gain an average of 24-34 lb.

Exercise classes are particularly beneficial for heavy women who want to avoid delivery by cesarean section. Cesareans are frequently performed because of fetal distress, as determined by readings from the fetal monitor. Some of these distress readings may be due to the weight of the maternal uterus compressing the fetus. Exploring alternative positions for labor and birth during exercise classes, such as lying on her side, kneeling on hands and knees, sitting, or squatting, gives the mother more options to choose from for childbirth. In addition, she will learn to avoid the supine position for labor.

Routines for women who are obese should be very gentle, low-impact programs that protect the ankles and feet from injury. Heart rate should be monitored closely.

My experience has been that when I offer classes in a medical facility more overweight and non-exercising women enroll than do when I offer classes in a health club or exercise facility. Heavy women tend to be shy about their bodies, and the stigma attached to "fat" in our society has dealt an unfair blow to many women, who therefore feel too embarrassed to come into a health club. If you want to reach the women who really *need* exercise, consider a location that affords them the privacy they desire.

The Pregnant Teenager

Pregnant teenagers are a group of high-risk women. Though not disabled, their needs are very special.

Every year in the U.S., 500,000 teenagers give birth—more than in many other Western countries. Financial support has traditionally gone to preventive programs first; thus the role and potential impact of the prenatal educator on the pregnant girl and her future has been almost totally ignored.

Ingrid Cominski is a family therapist in Syracuse, New York. Her practice focuses on pregnant teenagers. In a personal conversation, Cominski said that, contrary to popular belief, many teen pregnancies are intentional. She continued by describing current realities.

Let's face it, the societal rewards for being "good little girls" just aren't out there for these kids. They get pregnant to keep their boyfriends, to get out of going to school where most of them have faced repeated failures, and to achieve some level of status while defining their social role. Many of them use pregnancy as a great escape from the body-image competition because by becoming pregnant, they create an excellent excuse for failing to meet the perfect appearance standards set by the media.

When a young girl gets pregnant, for whatever reason, she has little insight into the physical and emotional demands of pregnancy, birth, or parenting. Part of the prenatal education problem can be solved through a major effort to initiate campaigns that support fitness and childbirth education as the pregnant teenager's right. The Rochester chapter of the International Childbirth Education Association is just one example of a local effort to build the goodwill of cooperating agencies. The chapter now offers "For Women Only" programs in response to the need for an agenda that allows teens (and other women without male partners) to participate in prenatal education classes that are appropriate to their age, skill levels, and range of interests.

Unfortunately, few communities have programs that incorporate fitness as an educational component for pregnant teens. Young women need the same information as more mature women, and, if teens are considered as high risk, then the information needs to be made available to them as early as possible. Though many teens think physical education is boring, a well-paced, lively program of instruction and activity can be an important social and educational experience for them. The following are objectives of a teen prenatal exercise program:

- To familiarize teens with the realities of childbearing in a manner that is factual and neither frightening nor glamorous.

- To facilitate for teens an understanding of the physical and emotional changes of pregnancy.
- To encourage and support teens to be active and to feel good about their bodies through exercise.
- To assure teens that their bodies are strong and healthy, and that after their births, discounting any special maternal condition, they may resume full participation in sports and games and their babies, too, will benefit from infant exercise.

Rural Women

In a survey taken in 1985, rural health nurses were interviewed by mail about the problems and prospects of childbirth education in outlying areas of central New York (Holstein, 1985). Staff nurses from over 20 rural facilities reported on the numbers of pregnant women they see, the type of childbirth education provided, and the difficulties encountered by prenatal health care providers in areas where transportation is difficult and high rates of unemployment are the norm.

Estimated age range of the women served in the clinics was from 14 to 30 years. Up to 90% of the women served in the clinics in some regions were unmarried, and most of them were first-time mothers. Though reporting nurses indicated that adequate childbirth education and prenatal care was available, far less than a third of their clients reported regularly for prenatal checkups. Transportation and motivation were cited as common deterrents.

The nurses themselves provided one-on-one childbirth education, and over 50% indicated that home visits were a major and time-consuming part of their jobs. Some nurses drove up to 1,000 mi per month to reach their clients. Preparation for childbirth included instruction on breathing techniques and some anatomy. Most reported that nutrition was an area that should receive much more attention.

The visiting nurse is probably the most important link between pregnant women and the health care system. She is able to reach women who would otherwise receive little or no prenatal care. This skilled professional needs to provide a moderate amount of fitness education in the home. Pregnant women, young and old, should be encouraged to exercise. On a home visit, the visiting nurse should bring a tape recorder, several selections of popular and other music, this manual, and a handout to leave with the woman that describes some essential prenatal exercises.

If you work with rural women in a health center you are probably painfully aware of the transportation problems faced by women in remote areas. Even the most well-motivated woman may be unable to reach the clinic facilities. There are several ways to introduce fitness as an educational component on clinic days. You may be able to make use of one of the many prenatal exercise videotapes and eliminate the sitting portion of the waiting room experience by providing an ongoing videotape exercise program. Provide a staff-led exercise routine every half hour on prenatal clinic days. Send women cards in the mail and invite them to attend a class or participate at a given hour. Finally, advertise the new service. Make it sound fun, worthwhile, and important.

Summary

Always remember the particular environment from which a woman comes and the one to which she is currently adapting. Women from disadvantaged communities or women with special social problems need services that are accessible, nonthreatening, and tailored to their skills and needs.

Remember cultural differences and how they are reflected in dress or behavior. Some cultures require women to wear dresses, and exercise must be adapted to respect their traditions. Some cultures do not permit exercise or recreational activities on the Sabbath.

If you have a special group, or a special individual in a larger group, always be aware of the specific medical diagnosis and be able to adapt materials and methods to the needs of the participants. It is always a good idea to require written permission to exercise from a woman's care giver. Also, ask all women to fill out a health status form before they begin to exercise in your group. If a woman is unable to do so, be fully apprised of all health-related concerns by an attending care giver. Be conscious of all warning signals and be prepared for any emergency. Always have women check for diastasis recti.

If you work with women with special needs, you must be able to use a wide variety of activities, methods, and materials. The woman who daydreams during a lecture may really tune in to exercise. The woman who hates to exercise may be fascinated by charts, films, or relaxation techniques. Remember that there is always a way to capture someone's attention or to meet someone's special needs. If a woman cannot respond to one series of activities, find another way to reach her.

Make yourself clear. State your goals. Share the responsibility for learning and planning. Make it clear that you appreciate questions and suggestions. Mutual respect, consideration, and your willingness to go the extra mile can make a big difference in a woman's life.

As we close Part III of this book, we also come to the end of the prenatal material. Our emphasis has been on the healthy, balanced approach to maternity education and exercise. It is imperative that responsibilities for education be shared among those who are caring for the pregnant woman. You may have noticed that I used the term *care giver* throughout the book. A care giver can be a nurse, a midwife, a general practitioner, an obstetrician, an herbal healer, a masseuse, a physical therapist, a fitness teacher, or a friend. All of those who care for and about the woman and her child are care givers.

The materials we have covered thus far have laid the groundwork for a holistic approach to postnatal exercise. This approach draws from the wisdom of many fields. It places great value on scientific research and the healing traditions. In a sense, the sum of this approach is far greater than all of its parts. Part IV deals with the welcoming of the new mother and her newborn into the education and exercise milieu.

Part IV

Exercise After Childbirth

Some women join prenatal exercises classes right after discovering that they are pregnant. They continue to exercise throughout their pregnancies, have their babies, and enroll in postpartum classes. It is remarkable to behold the transformation of self, body, and behavior that each woman experiences. I have often remarked to myself and to the women in my classes that it is wonderful to be with them, watching and enjoying them as they are in the process of creating life.

In the next section of the book we will turn our attention to exercise during the early weeks of new motherhood. You will need to be sensitive to the physiologic changes of postpartum and the impact of the excitement and fatigue of caring for the newborn, all of which directly affect women's interest in and capacity for exercise.

I have included the progressive return to exercise that I recommend as well as activities for moms and babies, infant massage, and infant exercise.

I have always found that teaching the postpartum classes is an especially joyous, loving experience. If you are able to respond to the mother's need for exercise and her intense interest in her newborn, the class can become a remarkable example of the healing/teaching environment.

Chapter 14

Exercise for the Postpartum Weeks

The new mother experiences the most dramatic hormonal and physiological changes of her life during the early postpartum weeks. Before birth a woman's endocrine system, led by the pituitary gland and the placenta, produces large quantities of hormones to maintain the pregnancy and, after about 40 weeks, to initiate labor. After birth, her body swiftly changes over from supporting fetal growth to nourishing the baby through lactation. The level of hormonal activity changes radically. Women who opt not to nurse also experience a sudden hormonal readjustment as the body literally shifts gears when milk production is supressed.

Pregnancy is a cause for many confusing, predictable, unexpected, and normal feelings. In short, its impact creates many contradictory feelings about body, self, past, present, and future. After a woman gives birth, the enfolding of the new child into the family, the physical recovery from birth, and the changes of social roles create issues that the new mother must resolve. Understanding that these issues exist, and that they are stressful, normal, and fairly predictable, can ease the adjustments and contribute to realistic expectations about life with the new baby.

The physical changes of postpartum are thrilling and intense. Finally relieved of the heavy burden of the fetus, a woman may be both fascinated by and disappointed in her body. Most women are anxious to get their bodies back, and postpartum classes lend the support and encouragement they need.

The Physical Changes of Postpartum

During the first 72 hr after childbirth, the uterus quickly contracts to about the size of a grapefruit. The contractions that cause this involution are stimulated by the production of oxytocin, a naturally occurring hormone. Nursing stimulates the production of oxytocin. These contractions can be quite painful; however, most first-time mothers do not feel them and are surprised when they occur after the second birth. These afterbirth pains disappear after 2-7 days, during which the uterus continues to contract. Relaxation and gentle breathing help women to tolerate these contractions, which occur when the baby nurses. By 6 weeks the uterus has returned to its pre-pregnant size.

The lochia, or bleeding, that follows delivery is the shedding of the uterine lining and the healing of the placental site. It can last from 1-6 weeks. It usually starts out red and heavy, like a menstrual flow, and then slowly changes to a light brown before disappearing. A woman need not wait until the lochia disappears to resume exercise. If the vaginal flow becomes heavier or full of clots, however, she should consult her care giver, who may want to examine her. In the case of a hemorrhage or infection, she will be advised to abstain from exercise.

There is intense and dramatic distention of the perineal organs and tissues during labor and delivery. After birth the labia may be stretched and deep red in color. They will soon return to normal size and shape.

A common concern for women returning to exercise is urinary incontinence experienced while performing vigorous activities, jumping, laughing, or sneezing. This can be due to the loss of muscle tone of the urethra and urinary sphincter, a prolapsed uterus, or a weakened bladder as a result of successive pregnancies. Urethral exercises, or kegel and abdominal exercises, done correctly and routinely throughout pregnancy and immediately after childbirth are the best natural cure for these conditions. Occasionally surgical repair is necessary.

Cystitis, or bladder infections, are very common after childbirth. Pain during urinating, fever, and the passing of blood with urine are indicators of cystitis, which should be treated by a medical care giver. Women should increase their consumption of water to facilitate healing.

Those women who have had episiotomies will feel some degree of discomfort or itching as the incision heals. Usually the incision heals easily. Practicing proper hygiene, taking sitz baths, sitting on firm surfaces, and exposing the incision to air contribute to healing. Occasionally the incision may become sore or infected. If soreness persists a woman should see her care giver. A woman with an episiotomy may do whatever exercise she likes as long as it doesn't hurt.

Many women find that they perspire heavily during postpartum. This is called diaphoresis and is due to the heat production involved with lactation and the natural loss of body fluids accumulated during gestation.

Women who have been active dancers or joggers have reported that when they return to exercise they are more prone to abdominal cramping than before they became pregnant. This cramping may be due to the weakness of the abdominal muscles and the strain on the supportive uterine ligaments incurred during pregnancy. The cramp may also be a stitch that occurs as a result of immobility or tightening of the diaphragm. In the case of stretched supportive tissue, time and gradual strengthening are the best healers. During their return to exercise, joggers should be advised to warm up before running, add distances slowly, walk when they experience abdominal cramps or a stitch, and avoid straining.

Changes in the breasts during postpartum are quite dramatic. The engorgement of the breasts with milk can be a strange and sometimes painful experience. The breasts swell and can become hard heavy. The establishment of milk production is both fascinating and tiring. The nursing mother will continue to have an intense and physical relationship with the newborn, but this should not prevent her from exercising, as we will discuss shortly.

Some women also suffer from mastitis, or a breast infection, during postpartum. This is sometimes quite painful. Symptoms of mastitis, which differ from those of engorgement, include red and tender breasts followed by a fever and flu-like symptoms. Women can reduce the pain of mastitis by applying warm compresses to the breasts. If a woman suspects that she has a breast infection, she should refrain from exercise and contact her care giver immediately.

Many women feel wonderfully energetic after they have had their babies. Some return to exercise immediately, others wait several weeks. Medical research is just beginning to understand the rates at which the hormones of pregnancy withdraw from the maternal system. The rate of postnatal hormonal adjustment is critical for women who wish to return to vigorous exercise because, until the tendons and ligaments of the body have regained their pre-pregnant firmness, injuries to the joints may occur as a result of exercise stress. The potential for injury to the ligaments that support the joints, especially the knees, hips, and back, is significant during the period of relaxin withdrawal. Always advise these women to use restraint as they return to their prepregnancy exercise routines.

Preparing for Postpartum Exercise

A woman who is preparing to return to exercise should check with her care giver. He or she may have specific suggestions or restrictions. She should pay close attention to all body signals, most notably vaginal flow. An increase in the lochia may indicate overexertion. She should contact her care giver immediately if she experiences a sudden gush or heavy bleeding after the lochia has lightened.

Instruct the new mother to wait, that is, to give the body at least 4-6 weeks before resuming high-intensity aerobics or jogging. Initially, the body is still tender, and ballistic activities are neither comfortable nor necessary during postpartum. Swollen breasts may become painful from too much bouncing, and all of the body's supportive tissues are still softened and more pliable than usual. In general, your job is to remind her to start slowly and avoid injury.

A new mother should be particularly aware of her need for fluids, especially if she is nursing. She should drink a full glass of water before and after exercise. During postpartum, a woman engaging in vigorous exercise may grow quickly overheated; therefore, she should be careful to avoid becoming dehydrated.

Posture Affects Appearance and Attitude

After carrying a baby for 9 months and working very hard to deliver it, many women find that simply standing up straight is exhausting. These women maintain their pregnancy waddle and allow their bellies to protrude and their shoulders to round forward. They look and feel depressed. In addition, this improper alignment is terribly stressful on the body. Seska Dune, director of Motherhythms in Baltimore, Maryland, calls this posture the "postpartum frump!" The head and neck roll forward, increasing the convex curve of the upper spine. The shoulder girdle curves forward, towards the body, causing the trapezius and rhomboid muscles to elongate and the pectoralis and serratus anterior muscles to shorten (see Figure 14.1). The resulting depression of the chest crowds the diaphragm, making it difficult for it to rise and fall in complete respiration. The muscles of the abdomen, weakened throughout pregnancy, are allowed to weaken further. The contents of the abdomen, which rest against the flabby abdominal wall, cause the belly to bulge. Unfortunately,

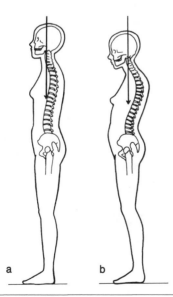

Figure 14.1. (a) Good posture includes aligning the head, neck, spine, and pelvis. (b) Poor posture, called the postpartum frump, detracts from physical and emotional well-being. Notice the forward tilt of the pelvis.

gravity works to aggravate the potbelly further. Occasionally, a woman will continue to allow the curve in the lumbar portion of the spine to create an accentuated forward tilt of the pelvis. This posture can be a major cause of postpartum backache.

Everyone looks and feels better with improved posture. You should remind the women in your classes that posture affects them in many ways.

- Proper alignment of the spine and a lifted rib cage improve respiration.
- Reduction of backache can be accomplished by aligning the pelvic basin and the spine, which lengthens and straightens the muscles of the back.
- Improved posture relieves the neck ache and dizziness that sometimes accompany a round-shouldered posture, and eliminates anterior slumping of the head and neck.
- The torso appears to lengthen, and women become aware of tucking in the abdominals to make a flabby tummy look flatter.
- Correct posture reduces the predisposition to injury caused by locked knees and poorly distributed weight.

Women in your classes should remember to stand up straight, keep their shoulders level, and center the head on the neck rather than poking it forward. They should release any hunching in the shoulders, relax the chin and neck, and allow the breath to release healing energy. If you observe new mothers waddling about, be patient, but encourage them to consciously avoid a side-to-side gait or a gait that allows the hips to dip as the weight shifts. Hips should remain level. Feet should be pointed straight ahead.

If poor posture is a result of a functional postural deformity—that is, one acquired because of obesity or years of poor postural habits, and the resulting improper alignment—an imbalance will exist between the muscular strength and the muscular strain in the body. Proper posture and consistent exercise programming can alleviate these functional postural problems.

Instructors may want to introduce postural therapy techniques such as those taught through the Alexander Technique (Barker, 1981) and the works of Moshe Feldenkrais (1977). Postural visualizations that encourage women to imagine space between each of the vertebra and lightness going up through the spine can improve posture. Exercises that improve awareness of the head and neck, as well as breathing patterns, are important tools.

Postpartum Backaches

Throughout pregnancy the muscles of the abdomen thin and stretch, while those of the lower back shorten. The small of the back, across the sacrum and sacroiliac joints, is a universal sore point. After childbirth, the stretched and weakened muscles continue to be responsible for backaches.

The Lift-and-Carry Syndrome

New mothers are the great carriers of our culture. On any given day a mother may carry her baby (in an infant carrier or car seat), a diaper bag, a play-pen, a stroller, or an infant swing. She may carry one or several items at the same time. She may load and unload the car several times a day. She may carry groceries or other young children. At the end of a day, her back is bound to hurt! If a student complains of persistent backaches, encourage her to do the following:

- She should stand close to the items she is about to lift and place her feet wide apart.
- She should lift with her feet in either a front-to-back stride position or a side-to-side position.
- The wider the base she creates with her legs and feet, the more she reduces the strain on her back.
- She should bend her knees and lift while keeping her back as straight as possible. Bending should occur at the hips and knees. Squatting to lift an infant from the floor is always better than bending at the waist.
- She should avoid twisting her torso while bending over or straightening up.
- She should make several trips rather than overloading herself, which strains the neck and back.

Although it's practically impossible, mothers should try to get adequate rest. This requires a great deal of creativity. Mothering is a lot of hard work, and pushing to the point of exhaustion only serves to predispose a woman to injury and affect her milk supply, blood sugar levels, attitude, and disposition.

Baby Feeding Backaches

Feeding a baby can be one of the most enjoyable new experiences of motherhood. It can also be one of the most tiring jobs in the world. Almost every mother knows that whether you breast-feed or bottle-feed a new baby, your body has to adjust to the new experience. Vast numbers of hours pass as a mother feeds the new baby, and finding a comfortable feeding position can be a major task.

Two of the physical problems that arise during either nursing or bottle-feeding are a stiff neck and a backache. The stiff neck comes from the strain of a poorly supported feeding position. The backache comes from hunching over into a round-shouldered position during feedings. This curving posture puts considerable strain on the back, and many women feel the fatigue as it spreads from the neck, down, between the shoulder blades, and even through the middle and lower back. It is not unusual to feel the strain around the entire rib cage. Whether she chooses to sit or recline, a mother should choose a feeding position that offers her as much comfort as it offers the infant. A favorite chair should have arms upon which the mother may rest her arm. If not, she should experiment with lots of pillows to create a comfortable nursing position. the seat should be firm enough and neither too deep nor too shallow, and the back should be high enough to allow mother to rest her head. Craning the neck to watch the baby or hunching the shoulders can lead to a weary and aching neck.

Experimenting with different ways to hold the baby, even lying down while nursing, may solve the baby feeding backache. Exercise can alleviate much of this discomfort and contribute markedly to the reduction of fatigue and contribute markedly to the reduction of fatigue and the improvement of posture. Exercises that stretch and strengthen the pectoralis minor, which is attached to the shoulder and middle ribs, are very important for the breast-feeding mother in particular. The breast is glandular tissue and fat cells. It is supported by suspensory ligaments, but the breast itself contains no muscle. Because the nursing breast is heavier than normal, toning the supportive musculature can be beneficial. Exercises should be started during pregnancy, if not before, to be most beneficial and continued throughout the nursing or bottle-feeding months.

Exercises to Strengthen the Neck and Upper Back

Headaches, poor posture, and many postpartum aches can sometimes be attributed to weak muscles in the neck and shoulder girdle. The following series of exercises is designed especially to strengthen the neck and upper back. Remember not to teach hyperextension of the neck, commonly seen in neck circles, because it can cause pain and damage to the vertebrae.

Upper Body Strengthening Exercises

I strongly recommend that women be taught exercises that strengthen the neck and the muscles that support the head while they are pregnant and before postnatal stiffness becomes troublesome. The careful use of hand-held weights can add considerable strength to the upper body.

Neck Flexion

Slowly flex the neck forward and roll the head down and then return it to center. Exhale as the head goes down. Inhale as it returns to center.

Lateral Neck Flexion

Bend the neck to the left without turning the head. Return to center and bend to the right. Exhale on flexion. Inhale on return to center.

Exhalation Neck Turn

Turn the head and look to the left. Come to center, turn, and look to the right. Exhale as you turn the head. Inhale on return to center.

Resistance Flexion

Place fingertips on forehead and gently press against the head as the neck flexes forward. Release and repeat.

Shoulder Flexion

Explore the flexibility of the shoulder girdle by curling the shoulders forward and then stretching them backward. Try moving the shoulder blades apart and then pushing them together.

Shoulder Shrugs

Without crunching the neck, attempt to lift shoulders to the ears.

Shoulder Depression

Without moving the head, push down with the shoulders.

Shoulder Circles

Forward circles should be followed by backwards circles. Move shoulders one at a time, both together, or in alternating directions.

Arm Extension

With one arm extended over the head, bend sideways and return to center; bend again and return to center. This can be done standing or sitting cross-legged on the floor. Exhale during the side bend. Inhale on return to center. Variation from yoga: clasp hands over the head, keeping elbows and ears parallel, and elbows straight.

Arm Circles

Extend arms to the side. Arm circles should be done with definite tension through the arms, down to the fingertips. Circles should go forward and backward. Progress from small to large circles.

Swim Stroke

This exercise uses arm circles that imitate the crawl stroke. It should be done to open and lift the chest, fully extend the arm, and widen the range of motion in the shoulder joint. You can also try the breaststroke.

Wall Push-Ups

Perform push-ups against a counter, couch, or wall. This exercise strengthens the neck, shoulders, and arms.

The Forearm Press

Extend arms to the side. Bend arms up at elbow. Bring palms, forearms, and elbows together in front of the body. Press together and open, press together and open.

The Scarecrow Press

Extend arms to the side. Bend arms down at elbow. Press back and push the shoulder blades together. Release and repeat.

Please note that I usually teach my students to exhale as the body is compressed and the space in the lungs grows smaller. You might want to experiment with this format and experience how differently the muscles work when inhalation accompanies compression.

Upper Body Exercise Routine

Remind mothers to breathe deeply and fully. Deep respiration and full exhalations, combined with good posture, can significantly reduce fatigue and discomfort. Choose any music that you like to accompany the following simple routine:

- Neck forward flexion: Twice.
- Neck lateral extension: Four times, twice on each side.
- Exhalation neck turns: Four times, twice to each side.
- Shoulder flexion forward and backward: Twice.
- Alternating shoulder shrugs: Four times.
- Shoulder depressions: Twice.

- Arm extensions: Bend to the side; count to 4 and hold. Come to center. Bend to the other side; count to 4 and hold.
- Arm circles: Do eight small circles forward and eight small circles backward. Repeat.
- Swim stroke: Slowly to a count of 8.
- Forearm press: Four times.
- Scarecrow press: Four times.

Finish the routine by stretching arms up overhead, gently swinging them down in front of the body, and then stretching them up overhead again. Repeat the sequence once.

Exercises to Avoid

Women should avoid some exercises during pregnancy and others during postpartum. There are even others that women should avoid for the rest of their lives! Those to avoid permanently are exercises that strain the body and do little to strengthen it.

Shoulder Stands. The excessive strain on the cervical vertebrae makes the plough or vertical bicycling a negative exercise especially when posture is an issue. Women may want to avoid it permanently if they have any neck problems.

Backward Neck Circles. These can aggravate problems with disks in the neck.

The Sitting Butterfly. This puts pressure on the inside of the knee while soles of the feet are together. This can overstretch and possibly injure the ligaments of the symphysis pubis and hip.

Back Bends. These should be limited to gymnastic performances.

Back-Lying Double Leg Lifts. Women shouldn't perform these unless they place a rolled-up towel, a pillow, or their fists beneath their buttocks.

Deep Unsupported Squats or Prolonged Squatting. Repeated deep squats can irritate the knee by stretching ligaments.

The Hurdler's Stretch. This is performed with one leg extended and the other bent at the knee and tucked backward. It should be avoided. Done improperly, it can aggravate pubic pain and overstretch the softened ligaments of the groin and the medial ligament of the knee.

The Ballet Barre Exercises. These should be carefully and gradually reintroduced with extensions performed at less than maximum to avoid injuring the ligaments of the hip. Some women find that flexing the trunk with high extended flexions of the leg lead to sciatic nerve pain.

Exercise and the Nursing Mother

Many women look forward to nursing as the opportunity to share a deeply personal, intimate relationship with the tiny baby. Some women have known since they were young that nursing would be wonderful. Others never imagined that they would want to nurse their babies.

The decision to nurse an infant is very personal. I recommend women start to nurse with the expectation that it will go well. If they find that they do not like it, they can make the transition to bottle and formula. Either choice, either way, it should be the mother's own decision. It should not be a guilt-induced decision. Pressure from a grandmother who thinks nursing is disgusting should be disregarded as quickly as pressure from a neighbor who has nursed her child for 5 years.

Combining exercise with nursing is not impossible. In fact, it's a good idea. Most women feel a tremendous desire to lose weight, get back into their old clothes, feel good about their bodies, and get over postpartum fatigue. Exercise is the perfect solution to those very common feelings.

When a nursing mother returns to exercise she may notice that her milk supply is unpredictable. On the days when she works out, her supply may be moderately or severely affected. If there is a noticeable effect, she should add several glasses of fluid to her diet to compensate for the stress and fluid loss of exercise and/or reduce the intensity of her workout. In general, however, nursing is the perfect complement to a good workout. After exercising it can be wonderfully relaxing and satisfying to lie down and nurse a baby. Women should be reminded to enjoy their babies and their bodies.

A 6-Week Postpartum Exercise Plan

The following is an example of a postpartum exercise program. Encourage and assist your students in planning their own programs well in advance of the birth of their babies. The comprehensive program that follows lasts 6 weeks.

When a woman returns to exercise after childbirth, the most important concern is muscle imbalance. She will feel fatigue in the back as the abdominals are strengthened. Therefore, she should do strengthening exercises slowly and increase repetitions gradually. During postpartum a woman should perform the following gentle exercises once a day. When she resumes her regular exercise routines she should be careful to alternate strengthening exercises with aerobic exercise to achieve a balanced level of fitness. For specific guidelines for women who exercise, consult ACOG (1986).

Days 1 and 2: Things to Do in Bed!

Resume kegel exercises: An hour after birth is a fine time to begin kegels. Contract your vaginal muscles and gently release. Repeat daily for the rest of your life! When you are ready, lie on your side and contract your urethra as well as your anus. The supporting tissues around these sphincters need the same kind of toning as the muscles that support the vagina.

Toe wiggles: Flex, point, wiggle, flex, point, and wiggle!

Ankle circles: Circle out, circle in, circle pointed, and circle flexed.

Abdominal contractions and abdominal massage: Gently pull in on the abdominal muscles and release. Gently massage the belly—it's yours, you can touch it! (You can even sleep on it now!)

Pelvic tilt: Perform as in pregnancy but now focus more on contracting the belly too. Exhale, pull in, and count 1, 2, 3, hold, and then release and inhale, 3, 2, 1.

Knee bends: While in bed, pull one leg toward you, bend it at the knee. Release and pull the other leg in toward you. This can be done in a reclined or semireclined position.

Arm extensions and shoulder circles: Stretch gently up, out in front, and out to the side. Lift and circle or shrug your shoulders. Wiggle your fingers.

Tension release: Allow yourself to do the same progressive relaxation that you learned to do for labor. This is a lifetime skill.

Relaxation breathing: Do this especially if you have had any medication during labor, although this is important for everyone. Breathe deeply and exhale fully. Allow your body to enjoy your breathing. It clears the mind and the system. If you are having afterbirth contractions, take a releasing breath, relax, and breathe gently, as if you were still in labor.

Day 3 (or When Mother Feels Ready):

Continue kegels.

Continue belly tightening and releasing.

Continue toe curls, ankle circles, and point and flex.

Continue pelvic tilt while lying down or on hands and knees.

Gentle side bends: Done standing up. Place one hand on the waist and lift the other overhead. Stretch and bend over gently to the left and then to the right. Do these with legs straight and then again with legs bent.

Neck stretch: Done standing or sitting. Inhale and then exhale, turning the head to the left. Inhale and return to center. Exhale and turn the neck and head to the right. Repeat.

Arm lifts: Done standing. There are several variations: (a) Lift the arms up high overhead, out to the side and then down to the side; (b) push your arms out in front of you, stretch them out to the side and then down; (c) clasp your arms up high over your head and stretch up; and (d) reach behind you and clasp the hands behind your back and stretch your arms. Always try to do this exercise with straight arms.

High step: Done standing in place, holding onto a chair or the wall. Lift the knee up toward the body. Repeat with other leg. (It's like marching in place.) Exhale when you bring your knee up and inhale when you return it to the floor.

Hip rolls: While lying on the floor, bring arms out to the side, knees up to the chest. Gently roll the hips to the left, allowing the outside of the left thigh to touch the floor. Try to keep the shoulders on the floor. Return to center and gently roll toward the right, allowing the right thigh to touch the floor while keeping the shoulders on the floor. Repeat.

Day 4 Through the Second Week Postpartum

Mother should be encouraged to go for a walk! She should continue to do all exercises previously suggested and may add the following:

Wall stretches: With one hand on a wall, stretch up and over the head with the other arm and touch the wall. (Do this slowly eight times.)

Wall push-ups: Facing the wall with fingers slightly turned in, do standing push-ups. (Begin with eight.) After 6 weeks, do push-ups on the floor.

Wall-sits: The skier's squat. Stand with the back against the wall. Slowly slide down the wall until the buttocks meet an imaginary chair. Flatten the back against the wall completely. Push the back against the wall. (Make sure that you continue to breathe.) Hold for several seconds and then push back up into a standing position. Repeat several times. After several weeks, work up to being able to hold the wall-sit for 15 to 30 s.

Modified cobra pose: While lying on the tummy, place palms beneath your shoulders and lift the upper torso and shoulders. Do not force the elbows to straighten. Do not exaggerate the arch in the lower back. Keep the head, neck, and spine in a straight line. Variation: Lie on tummy with arms down, at your sides, palms up. Inhale, lift the head and shoulders, and abduct arms across the back. Keeping arms straight, squeeze shoulder blades together.

Back-lying pelvic tilt with hip lift: Done in prenatal exercises. Add a hip lift to the pelvic tilt so that your body forms a triangle with the floor. Do not arch your back. Tighten your buttocks and thighs. Release slowly and, as Seska Dune in a personal communication (1986) said, "Make sure your waist touches the floor before your buttocks!" Repeat eight times.

Modified sit-ups: Start slowly. Put your hands on top of your head, or reach through your legs with your fingers. Bend your knees and keep your feet flat on the floor. Start with one sit-up and work up to more very slowly. Variations on modified sit-ups include reaching arms through the knees, reaching arms outside the knees, crossing arms over the chest, placing fingertips on shoulders, and placing palms or fingertips on top of the head. Variations for position of the legs include knees bent; feet flat on the floor; knees wide apart; knees close together; knees to chest; legs extended up overhead and crossed at the ankles; and one knee to chest, the other extended.

Two Weeks Postpartum

Continue all previous exercises and add the following:

Vigorous high steps: Much like the high step suggested for Day 3. Add an overhead stretch or swing your arms and march or work up to a gentle jog in place.

Barre work: Depending on your own strength, you can do leg lifts with a bent knee or a straight leg. I recommend doing them at the kitchen counter. Lift to the front and then to the side, keeping the supporting leg straight. Check your own posture. Pull up from the tummy and lift the sternum. Avoid maximum static and ballistic (bouncing) stretches.

Pliés and *relevés:* With feet comfortably apart and body nice and straight, bend your knees and then straighten (but do not lock) them. Tighten the bottom and lift yourself up onto your toes. Hold and then release. Repeat eight times.

Deep swings: Take a deep breath and stretch the arms up overhead. Exhale and, bending at the knees, swing the arms down as you move into a squat. Inhale and swing back up. It looks as if you are preparing for a standing broad jump. Start with four repetitions.

Sun salutation with optional push-ups: A variation of a yoga *asana*.

1. Place your palms together.
2. Stretch your arms up overhead.
3. Bend down, place palms on the floor with head down.
4. Extend one leg behind you and now extend the other leg.
5. Hold.
6. Bring one leg back toward you, then the other. Assume a squatting position.
7. Slowly return to standing. After the first few times, add several push-ups in the legs-extended position.

Gentle sit-backs: Have someone hold your feet. Place feet flat on the floor with knees bent. Clasp hands behind the head. Sit up very straight. Inhale and tilt your torso back about 5 or 6 in. Exhale and return to fully upright position. Your back and torso should remain straight. Repeat. Learn to breathe throughout the exercise. Hold yourself in the semireclined position only briefly at first. Extend the length of the hold as your abdominal strength returns. Don't be surprised if you feel very trembly at first.

Weeks 2 to 4

By the end of the second week, a woman may want to enroll in a special postpartum class, but she should always check with her doctor first. If she finds, after the first session, that she is really exhausted or if the lochia becomes much heavier, she is probably not quite ready to participate. She should reduce her level of exercise intensity for another week or two and let her body heal. The fatigue of postpartum can easily interfere with fitness aspirations.

Many women are very anxious to get back to weight-training machines. Nautilus machines are designed to reshape the body's musculature, and that is precisely what most postpartum women want to do. Traditional advice has been to wait at least 6 weeks before returning to weight lifting to allow joints to become more stable and thus avoid permanent injury. When a woman returns to the machines, advise her to work out with light weights to avoid strain and fatigue and, if necessary, to reduce them to below pregnancy training levels. Alternatively, a woman can reduce the number of repetitions.

Weeks 4 to 6

If mom has a bad case of cabin fever and there are no postpartum classes available, at this point she can try a very gentle stretch-and-tone class or a low-impact aerobics program. She should be very careful not to overdo it despite her high energy levels. For nursing mothers, especially, such activity combined with fatigue and dieting can cause an erratic milk supply.

At 4 weeks, women should still try to avoid rapid, repeated flexion of the knees and hips as well as lots of bouncing movements. Speed is a lot less important than form during this period. They should also remember to continue with kegels. The increase in activity during this period may be accompanied by leaking of urine, which occurs because bladder sphincters are still very weak. Female incontinence is quite common and though it was once considered a normal, if unpleasant, side-effect of childbearing and aging, it is not something anyone should have to put up with. Exercise (e.g., kegels) can usually reduce incontinence. Occasionally, consultation with a care giver regarding surgical repair is necessary. If necessary, women should consider wearing a minipad for exercise.

There are a number of things to remember about exercise as the weeks and months pass after childbirth. First, the ACOG (1986) recommends that standing aerobic exercise be kept to 30-min sessions. This is to protect the hips, knees, and feet and to avoid excessive stress on the cardiovascular system. Encourage women to monitor the length of aerobic exercise sessions and their own bodies' responses to strenuous exercise. Many experts believe, however, that women should not feel limited to 30-min if they can tolerate extended workouts.

The second postpartum exercise concern is for women to monitor their heart rates continually. Once a woman is past postpartum, exercise sessions should not be of such high intensity that a woman works above 75% of her maximum heart rate.

Exercise clothing and environment are the third concern. Women should work out in comfortable, appropriate exercise clothing: This includes an exercise bra, well-fitted shoes, and cotton clothing. Women should exercise in well-ventilated spaces. Aerobic dance instructors should make certain that these women especially are not dancing on a cement floor. Encourage women to try to exercise with a partner or in an area where others are working out, for their own safety.

A fourth concern is the inclusion of a warm-up and a cool-down in any exercise program. The warm-up should stretch muscles and increase the action of the heart. It never involves breathholding when stretching and avoids rapid, ballistic stretches or any stretch taken to its maximum. The cool-down period gradually returns the heart rate to normal and prevents pooling of the blood in the lower extremities.

Finally, remind your students that exercise is wisest when done in a careful, controlled manner. Flailing, uncoordinated movements, poor mechanics, poor posture, and erratic frenzied activity do little to improve appearance, health, or stamina, and may increase the risk of injury. Focus on the proper performance of exercises in postpartum classes.

Exercises for the Whole Body

These are exercises that will help new mothers with some of the residual strains of pregnancy and the new challenges of motherhood.

Exercises to Reduce Backache and Stiff Neck

These exercises should offer relief from the normal strains of the back and neck that mothers often incur when nursing or lifting their infants.

Overhead Reach
Perform alternating overhead stretches while standing. This improves respiration and stretches muscles of the back and chest.

Pelvic Tilt

Done on hands and knees. Pull in on the abdominals and exhale. Inhale and release. This is great for easing backaches.

Extended Leg Stretch

Done while sitting. Hold one leg straight out and the other bent with the heel at your groin. Reach over the extended foot, stretch, and release.

Salaam Position

Sit back on your heels, lean forward, and place your head down on the floor. Extend your arms out in front of you and relax.

Soles-Together Breather

Sit up straight and place the soles of your feet together. Inhale and then exhale as you lean forward. Your head and your neck should be completely relaxed. Inhale again and let your head lift your body back up.

Hip Rolls and Neck Stretch

Both are described under ''Day 3'' postpartum program.

Exercises to Improve Muscle Tone in the Arm

These exercises improve arm muscle tone and strength. This is important because if mothers have confidence in their arm strength, they will be less likely to injure their backs by using them to lift.

Shoulder Circles

Done forward and backward with arms relaxed and hanging down. This loosens tension and warms up the shoulder girdle for more exercise.

Arm Circles

Large and small, fast and slow. Put the energy down to your fingertips! This really tones up the upper arm.

Inverted V

On hands and knees, push up and straighten arms and legs, with elbows and ears parallel. Heels should be off the ground and feet should be close together. Feel the stretch in arms and calves. Hold and release slowly.

Push-Ups

Start doing five while standing at a wall. Put your palms on the wall, fingertips turned in slightly. Try doing them at the kitchen counter. Next, do five in the old-fashioned girls' position on the floor, resting half of your weight on your knees. Then do them with legs extended out to the back. The

stronger you are the closer together you will be able to put your feet and hands. (Everyone should be able to do 15 push-ups.)

Exercises for the Torso and Waistline

Mothers are often very eager to begin exercises that will help them regain their waistlines.

Side Bends

There are several ways to do this exercise, but no matter which you choose, do not bounce and, during postpartum, do not raise both arms up overhead at the same time. One arm should always be down, either resting on the hip or hanging down as a counterbalance to the extended arm—this is done to avoid straining the back. Stretch to each side to a count of 8, then to a count of 4, 2, and 1.

Opposite Toe Touches

While standing with feet wide apart, reach down and touch the toes or calf with the opposite hand. Do not twist the body.

Wall Stretches

Described under ''Day 4 Through the Second Week Postpartum.''

Exercises for the Abdominal Muscles

These exercises will help your students tone their tummy muscles. Many women are very eager to have flat stomachs once again and will be eager to learn how they can most easily and quickly accomplish this.

Pelvic Tilt

Pelvic Tilt With Hip Lift

Described under ''Day 4 Through the Second Week Postpartum.''

Pelvic Tilt With Knee Resistance

Lift your hips and then pretend there is a small beach ball between your knees. Squeeze it.

Supine Toe Touches

Lift the right leg and reach for the knee, shin, or toes with left hand. Lower the leg. Lift left leg and reach for shin, calf, or toes with right hand. This is also good for the arms if you use hand-held weights.

Hip Lift

Lying on your back, with your bottom as close to a wall as possible, place your feet on the wall, shoulder-width apart. Knees should be bent. Lift the hips, release slowly, and repeat.

Leg Scissors

Lying on your side, support your body by placing your hand on the floor in front of you. Do a scissors kick. This is also good for the thighs.

Bent-Knees Bicycle (Better Known as Knee Grabs)

Always exhale as you bring your knee to your chest and inhale as you release. Lift your head and shoulders for this one and do not arch the lower back to extend the other leg. Bicycle variation: With a towel or fists beneath your buttocks, bring your right knee up to your chest, and then do the same for your left knee.

Leg-Ups and Leg Crosses

Done with palms or fists supporting the lower back. Lift one leg up straight and lower it slowly. Or, lift one at a time so that both legs are up overhead together and do a V-split scissors kick. Make sure you have your fists or a rolled-up towel under your bottom to prevent lower back strain. Do not do double leg lifts.

Exercises for the Thighs

Toning and strengthening the thighs is also of concern to women. These exercises will help them do both.

Lion Pose

Use this to strengthen the inner thigh. With arms up and out to the sides and feet wide apart, turn one foot out and bend the knee.

Elbow-to-Knee Pose

While standing with feet wide apart, bend forward and work to touch elbows to opposite knees. This is a good thigh toner; however, because it is a tough one, I do not recommend it for true beginners.

Doggie Lift

On hands and knees, or resting on forearms, lift one leg out behind you, straighten it and flex and point your toe. Do not arch your back; rather, tighten your bottom. Variation: Lift the bent leg out to the side, then straighten and flex the foot.

Frog Kick

Lie on your back with the soles of your feet together and legs bent. Bring legs up, out, together, and down to starting position with the soles of the feet together.

(Do the next three exercises on your back with bottom against the wall.)

Supine Leg Opener

Do a V-stretch using the wall for support. Open and close your legs.

Supine Leg-to-Nose Stretch

With leg straight, lift it away from the wall and imagine you can bring it to your nose. Then bend it and pull it into your chest. Extend the leg back up to the wall.

Leg Overs

Cross the right leg over the left and then the left over the right.

Side-Lying Leg Lifts

You can do these with the leg straight or alternating straight and bent, and you can also vary the foot position by flexing and pointing your foot, or simply flexing it. Always bend the lower leg at the knee and hip to provide a stable exercise base.

Side-Lying Thigh Toners

Curl your legs up to create a 90-degree angle at your hips. Push the upper leg straight out in front of you and flex your foot. Pull it in and repeat. In the same position, lift your thigh as if it were the cover of a book. Keep your leg bent at the knee and lower it back down.

Wall-Sits

Described under "Day 4 Through the Second Week Postpartum."

Belly Dancing: The Secret Weapon

Aerobic exercise—dancing, walking, swimming, cycling, and jogging—and calisthenics are essential components of anyone's exercise regimen. After the initial postpartum recovery period, however, there is one style of dance exercise that will delight, entertain, and tone—belly dance.

Belly dancing is a tradition that is almost 3,500 years old. The Arabs called it *beledi*, which means native or native rhythm. Anthropologists have called it primitive; our culture thinks it is sexy. In general, belly dancing is wonderful for toning muscles, developing grace, and improving posture and stamina. Belly dancing is taught in individual or group lessons in many sites and centers. Keep it in mind when recommending routines to postpartum women. If your own facility offers a class in belly dancing, don't hesitate to recommend it to interested individuals. Direct women to a class that progresses slowly, involves more than a shimmy and avoids back bends.

Exercises for Women Recovering From Cesarean Surgery

A cesarean birth can have a profound impact on a woman's self-image and body image. In some instances, a surgical delivery creates feelings of inadequacy, powerlessness, and failure. This is not true for every woman. The consequences of major abdominal surgery for the sake of saving the woman's life or the life of her child can be significant. The physical and emotional recovery from a cesarean can be difficult, and the disappointment with the birth experience may be profound.

Women in these circumstances must learn to heal themselves and their self-image, body image, and sexuality. This takes time and patience. You can help all the women in your prenatal class by telling them what to expect physically and emotionally after a cesarean section. I have included a list of suggested exercises in this section that you can hand out to your students before they have their babies.

Exercises for Immediate Postpartum

After an abdominal delivery, a woman's body is very sore, but the sooner she starts to move the better she will feel. This is why there is so much emphasis on getting up and out of bed as soon as possible, even though the first movements are excruciating and the first walk down the hall is a painful and delicate shuffle. A woman who has had a cesarean should begin to exercise in bed as soon as she feels the surgical anesthesia wearing off. Despite the initial discomfort, she should start slowly with the following:

- Deep breathing
- Flexing and pointing her toes
- Doing ankle circles

Soon afterwards, she should begin to do the following:

- Bending her knee and sliding her leg up the bed toward her body, even if it only moves an inch, and then sliding it back down
- Doing shoulder shrugs and overarm stretches
- Performing kegel exercises
- Approximating abdominal contractions
- Lifting her head and neck off the pillow (if she has not had spinal anesthesia)
- Performing the pelvic tilt.

Post-Cesarean Exercise at Home

When a mother returns home after a cesarean and is ready to exercise, she should begin slowly. At first, just being able to go up and down the stairs is a lot of exercise. When she feels stronger, she should try the following exercises:

- Lie down on your tummy and lift your head and shoulders slowly up off the floor. Return them gently to the floor.
- Tighten up your buttocks and release them slowly. Remember to breathe deeply and slowly.
- While lying on your back, pull in on the abdominal muscles and release.
- Do the back-lying pelvic tilt.

Women recovering from cesarean births usually take 3-6 weeks, or longer, to return to regular exercise than vaginally delivered mothers. Regardless of how anxious she feels to get back into shape, a mother recovering from surgery should not exercise if her incision is not healed, if it is painful, or if there is any indication of infection. Some women have sensations of pulling or other abdominal discomfort while in certain positions for exercise. It is not unusual for women to find that they shake or experience unusual tremulousness during their initial return to exercise. Let them know that this will pass as the muscles regain tone and strength.

During the recovery from surgery, women who want to exercise should disregard former fitness standards and expectations. They should start with one repetition of an exercise or try 10 s on the rowing machine instead of 10 min. They should not do sit-ups or back-lying double-leg lifts. In addition, postoperative overexertion can force the muscles of the back to compensate for the weakness of the front of the torso, resulting in a painful backache.

An important option for a woman who has had a cesarean section is to join a cesarean support group. These are groups of women who get together weekly or monthly to discuss their feelings and concerns about their birth experiences. Some of these groups include exercise as part of the meeting. Many women feel comfortable beginning their postpartum regimen within the safety of this kind of support group. One of your responsibilities as an instructor is to inform the women in your prenatal class of all the resources available to them postpartum. Let women know about the cesarean support group and whether there is one to attend in your area.

Summary

The physical recovery from pregnancy and childbirth is a journey full of unexpected events and surprises that may not all be so delightful. The new mother is vulnerable to a variety of discomforts, and the more that you can tell her about what to expect and how to deal with the changes, the better off she will be. Above all, stress the importance of a gradual return to exercise as a way to cope with the impact of birth and the changes in body and social role that accompany it.

The next chapter describes postnatal classes and presents activities and hands-on strategies for teaching. The mother-and-baby classes are increasingly popular, and your biggest concern may be how to limit class size!

Chapter 15

The Postpartum Mother-and-Baby Class

Giving birth to a child is probably one of life's most significant personal events. When women are asked about the most important days of their lives, they frequently recall the days their children were born. On those days, lives are changed in the most intimate and important ways.

Identity

Springtime blooming
His birth and I was so naive.
A thousand books read and underlined
in search of an identity.
I remember lilacs swaying,
I was heavy with this child.
Before the torrents of sweat and heat,
then, light as the bloom before the rain
Skin to skin
Alone with him
He came.
Nativity
In search of my identity.
Mama

I enjoy teaching postpartum mother-and-baby classes and find that most women are delighted to find an exercise class that is designed especially for their needs. Exercise routines in these classes should begin slowly, and the pace should increase gradually. Weight loss and muscle toning will be most women's primary objectives. Your role is to guide their choices about exercise and to encourage them to experience their new body boundaries, explore their strengths, and develop new ones. In addition, you should try to be sensitive to the difficulties of the transition from pregnancy to parenthood as the supportive prenatal network disappears and a new ecosystem must emerge.

If you decide to offer special classes for mothers with new babies, one of your major objectives might be to help mothers to understand and develop their relationships with their newborns. Your role will be instrumental as each mother learns about living with and loving her new baby and adapting to the changes in her family's life circle.

Changes in Family Life and the Emotional Components of Postpartum

The emotional components of postpartum are considerable. After childbirth, each woman and her family experience a profound period of adjustment. A woman's physical recovery from pregnancy can be hastened or hampered by her emotional adjustment to motherhood and the social and emotional support she receives from those around her. It is important to be sensitive to the fact that each woman has carried her infant for 9 months: The pair have a basic, interactive, organic bond. The intimacy and importance of this link must be supported, nurtured, and never ignored or taken for granted.

It is very important for new mothers to understand that it is normal to feel both exhilarated and exhausted during the early weeks at home. For working women, being at home with the new baby is a new experience. A woman's competence is tested as she becomes the primary care giver of her new child. In many communities she may find herself isolated in a world of single family homes and working couples. Sometimes women elect to take extended leaves of absence from their jobs or to give up their careers completely to devote themselves to their young families. In other situations, a mother has only a brief, perhaps unpaid, maternity leave and feels anxious about returning to work so soon after childbirth. Some women are mothers at 15; others become mothers at 40. Some have one child; others have many. Each woman must adjust both physically and emotionally to motherhood.

Parenting Is Hard Work

Parenting is one of life's most rewarding jobs, but it can also be extremely frustrating. Babies can cry a lot. They are not all little angels who sleep 20 hours a day. They create mountains of laundry and have no respect for other people's appointments, needs for sleep, or desire to have dinner. Sometimes the baby's father is very understanding and helpful. Other times he may be distracted or otherwise unavailable to help. Fathers can feel shut out and helpless to soothe a nursing infant and some even resent the mother-infant attachment. Occasionally a father will feel overwhelmed by the added responsibilities of his role. If there are other siblings, they may have strong and confusing reactions to the baby. In the midst of all this, mother may feel divided and she may feel terribly tired as she tries to meet everyone's needs.

In addition to worrying about everyone else, new mothers often wonder about themselves: Am I a good mother? Am I doing this right? Am I normal? Am I more tired than other mothers? Am I too anxious? Am I too nonchalant? All mothers have their own styles just as all people have their own personalities. Some women respond to mothering with unbounded glee. Others adjust more slowly. Some women experience times of depression, which are usually the result of changing hormonal levels, fatigue, and demanding adjustments to their working, social, and familial relationships. All of this is normal, but if a mother

notices that her down days are becoming overwhelming, she should be encouraged to call her care giver, counselor, or therapist who may be able to help by listening and offering therapeutic advice and support. These women will appreciate your sensitivity to their transition from pregnancy to parenthood.

Most women are eager to get back into good shape. They really do want to feel good about themselves, their babies, and their parenting skills. Excellent nutrition, exercise, and the support of a social group (e.g., the postpartum mother-and-baby exercise class) are the key elements to developing and maintaining the physical and emotional stamina a mother needs for peak functioning and endurance.

The Cycle of Parenting Stress

In postpartum classes we are particularly interested in helping mothers to understand the process of bonding and the cycles of stress that occur during the early weeks at home. Awareness of the interdependent relationship between mothers and newborns is as ancient as mothering itself. Mothers and babies share so many experiences together that if one is peaceful, the other too may be restful; if one is tense, the other may feel the anxiety quite deeply.

The shared tension of this relationship is called the cycle of stress. It is a normal part of the mother-baby relationship. Just as love, joy and pride define parenting, sometimes stress is the major factor in the new family. The cycle may begin when the mother herself is tense or when the baby starts to cry. In the latter case, the child cries and grows tired, the fatigue creates more tension, and the mother, in turn, becomes anxious as she tries to soothe the tears. It is not uncommon for her to sob right along with the crying child. As the mother wonders what is wrong and what she can do, the cycle of stress, this wheel of energy, spins ever faster until both mother and child are a weary and miserable duo. At this point, the baby usually falls asleep, all tired out and unhappy, and the mother puts the baby down and tiptoes away, thankful for a few moments of peace and quiet so that she may recover herself.

It is to this cycle of anxiety and tension and the importance of balance and support that postpartum education should address itself. All mothers need to learn that there are ways to ease the stress of parenting and that exercise, massage, and insight into infant growth and development are important parenting skills.

Objectives for Postpartum Classes

The mother-and-baby class I teach is for mothers with very young babies. It is designed for infants up to 20 weeks old. Women are invited to come into the classes as early as 10 days postpartum. The emphasis of the class is on sharing the unique experiences of new parenthood, gradually returning to exercise, and experiencing the body in its new, nonpregnant state. We come together to celebrate and welcome the new babies.

Classes for mothers and infants include six important activity-based areas of emphasis and practice. We teach baby massage and baby exercise because both techniques stimulate infant development and strengthen the maternal-infant bond. They are also excellent intervention skills during times of parenting stress. We value education for mothers about baby behavior and infant development because reasonable expectations and insights into normal development help to create a secure and nurturing environment for the young family. By helping the new mother to reestablish a positive body image and to develop the strength and stamina she will need to continue to care for herself and her new family through postpartum exercise, we are nourishing the woman who is the mainstay for her family. In addition, these classes promote the importance of community, friendship, and support from a balanced ecosystem, which women seek intuitively. And finally, there are relaxation and comfort skills for the mother herself that, in the hubbub of family life, are quickly and easily forgotten.

Adjusting to parenthood is an important and often difficult stage. It is part of the educator's role to encourage and support the mother as she begins to meet this challenge. Parenthood is a confluent experience. Confluence is the pulling together of all the things one knows about living, loving, and giving. Confluence in adjustment to parenthood is the blending of social, emotional, and educational skills to create the experience of joyous parenting. As an instructor, you can help women achieve this by incorporating the following suggestions into your classes.

- Provide a superior class. Be informed, prepared, and professional.
- Incorporate much support information into the class.

    If a college nearby has programs on parenting, publications of interest, or workshops on child development, tell the women about them. If companies publish brochures on baby care, send for them and distribute them liberally. If there are educational films or videotapes available, set aside a class period to view them.

- Let people know what your goals are.

    You need to be able to communicate, either in writing or in person, that you are providing a unique and important service that goes beyond the basic exercise class.

When I begin a class for new mothers, I usually introduce the program by telling new mothers that one of my goals is to help them to create positive, loving relationships with their new babies. I usually discuss the importance of social support for the young family. Many women are far from close friends and family. The class is both a social group and a support system. Have the women introduce themselves and tell their babies' names. Provide a class list of telephone numbers and allow time for casual conversation.

I also point out that we will be working together on a wide range of parenting skills that become more natural with time. Nobody will be an expert right away! Many women feel uneasy about their parenting skills. The group, led by you, can offer support, compliments, and tactful advice. If a baby in the group has a problem encourage the mother to share her feelings and reactions to the problem and explore the causes and treatments you have covered in your reading.

I always emphasize that the relationship a mother has with her baby is the strongest bond she may ever share with another human being. It is filled with joy and sorrow, passion and deep concern. The range of her being is expressed within that relationship. In fact, it is a love affair that lasts a lifetime.

Weight Loss and Body Image

"Forget the baby," one woman said to me. "What about my body!?" Body image is a major concern for many women after they have had their babies. In our body-conscious society, women may find themselves preoccupied with concerns about weight, shapeliness, and clothing. As most women learn, pregnancy weight does come off. At first, the weight of the baby and placenta will disappear. And then, little by little, the additional pounds come off. Some women find that they lose weight quickly when they breast-feed because the nursing uses up a lot of calories. Other women find that they do not lose all of their pregnancy weight until they stop nursing. Every woman's body is different and each responds to the demands of child care differently. Women should not feel pressured to lose a lot of weight quickly. In the early months it is far more important for them to eat well, to maintain their own health and strength, and, if they are nursing, to ensure a rich supply of milk. We deal with body issues throughout the mother-and-baby class and discuss them specifically in Class 2.

The Postpartum Class Format

The following is a general curriculum outline for a mother-and-baby postpartum class. It is designed to be flexible based on your interests, strengths, population, and goals for the program. Strive to provide the best possible program for women and their babies. Be prepared to organize and present your thoughts, materials, and activities in an orderly and enthusiastic manner. In developing the format for my class suggestions, I decided to write out the material presented in the first class to help you get a feel for designing your classes to match your philosophy with pertinent postpartum information and exercises. I outlined the rest of the classes to provide a workable framework that I invite you to modify to match your teaching style. It is up to you whether to use a 3-, 6-, or 8-week program format.

Not every instructor will feel capable of teaching a complete mother-and-baby format like the one presented here. Don't hesitate to call upon outside help if necessary to round out the program and fulfill your objectives. By all means, adapt the information and ideas I present here to your own skills and to the mission of the agency or institution with which you are affiliated.

Class 1: Getting to Know the Newborn

As the title implies, the focus of the first class is on helping women discover what their babies are like. Specifically, I lead the class through infant observation skills and infant massage. These skills help women understand how their babies communicate their needs and how to intervene in situations that are otherwise out of their control (e.g., soothe a crying or fussy baby with massage). I also include in this class activities just for mothers—including exercises to strengthen and rejuvenate them and discussions about nutrition and relaxation to help them through the first weeks of parenting.

Infant Observation Skills

Nurses who specialize in newborn care are trained to observe and assess the physical well-being and behavior of the infants they help to deliver or care for in the nursery. Most mothers are not as well trained in infant observation skills and would benefit greatly from a quick course in normal neonatal assessment techniques.

In this class we set the stage for integrating and sharing knowledge about infant behavior and development.

TIME. Activities last 45 minutes. Schedule an hour for each class to allow time for burping, feeding, crying and changing, all of which will occur during every class. Approximately fifteen minutes will be spent on baby activities and a half an hour on exercises for moms. This will vary depending on the discussion topics.

PURPOSE. To introduce mothers to the class format. To present the philosophy of the program. To create a comfortable atmosphere for the life of the group. To help mothers to further understand and develop their relationships with their newborns.

GOALS. To discuss infant appearance and abilities at birth. To have all the mothers perform an infant massage.

OPTIONAL TOPICS FOR DISCUSSION. Introductions, infant massage, how baby experiences the world, behaviors and responses, how it feels to be a new mother, expectations about the class, special problems, exercises for mom.

REFERENCES. Heinl (1982)

TECHNIQUES. Demonstration, hands-on activities, discussions.

CLASSROOM INTRODUCTIONS. Provide name tags! Be certain to tell the group your name, then ask each mom to give her name, baby's name, date of birth, vaginal or cesarean? Nursing or bottle-feeding? General feelings, aches and pains? Main concerns?

Exercise and Instructional Format for Moms

The exercises for the first day should be very mild. You do not know how strong the mothers are, if they have been exercising regularly, or the extent to which they will feel comfortable with the exertion. Music should be for background only, not speed.

Exercises should include work on upper back, arms, and neck for relief of backache; standing torso stretches for tension relief; and pelvic tilt variations and hip rolls for relief of lower backache and abdominal muscle tone. Introduce a sit-up or sit-back. Do kegel exercises. You may follow the introduction to postpartum exercise plans presented in chapter 14.

At the end of each class, leave a few minutes for soft music and quiet relaxation. Many moms will lie down and nurse their babies. Others will close their eyes and simply enjoy the few quiet moments. Turn the lights down and just relax. I use the first class to introduce mothers to their babies' behaviors. We sit in a circle and observe the babies as I point out their reflexive behaviors. Most mothers are more than anxious to know how their babies work. During this class, I provide the women with the following information.

The neuromuscular responses of the newborn are sensitive and complicated. Because the newborn's neuromuscular system is immature, movements are uncoordinated, which historically led people to believe that the newborn was not as complex as the older child. Babies rarely move symmetrically and control over movements is drastically limited; however, they should demonstrate equal strength in both arms and both legs.

A baby demonstrating weakness in one limb or another should be carefully evaluated.

Some newborn babies can hold their heads erect for short periods of time; others cannot do this for several weeks. Both of these behaviors are completely normal.

The infant is born with a variety of reflexes that help it to survive and communicate. The moro reflex occurs when the baby is startled. The infant flexes its knees and extends its arms and fingers. The infant may demonstrate this as it is being lowered into a bath or when it is moved suddenly. This usually means that the baby should be comforted and made to feel secure once again.

Blinking, for example, is a protective mechanism, whereas the palmar grasp, an instinctive tightening of the infant's fingers around any available surface, seems to stimulate adult care-giving behaviors.

When the sole of the baby's foot is lightly stimulated it should point or curl its toes downward. The plantar grasp seems to lessen by about 8 months.

The Babinski reflex should be present at birth. This can be demonstrated by stroking one side of the sole of the baby's foot from the heel across the ball of the foot. The toes should hyperextend.

The stepping reflex is frequently the reason for a proud parent to exclaim that the baby will be an early walker. When held upright with one foot touching a hard surface, the infant will appear to be making stepping movements. This reflex disappears by 6-8 months.

The tonic neck reflex is often more dominant in the leg than in the arm and disappears between 3 and 4 months. When the baby's head is turned to one side, extremities on that side will extend while those on the other side will flex.

Many newborns placed on their abdomens will make motions that look like crawling. Stroking the back tends to stimulate a curl to one side.

Many undifferentiated infant responses take a long time to become specific. As the baby grows more attentive to its environment, it is important to remember that all babies have delayed responses to stimuli. That means that if you ring a bell or talk to your baby it may be several seconds before the baby is able to process that sound. If you turn away quickly, you may miss the response you sought!

All mothers do not bond with their infants immediately. This sometimes takes days, weeks, or years. A special love exists between mothers and their infants, but each is different and unique. Some babies are not beautiful. Each, however, is a unique and special human being and should be appreciated for its value on that basis alone.

After discussing some of the features of infant behavior that make babies so special, I encourage each new mother to use the form "Looking at My Baby" (Appendix 15.1) at home. Its purpose is to encourage mothers to get to know their infants as real people. Each baby has a personality, a style of behavior, and a special method of communicating. Mothers are most successful when they are able to tune in to their babies and respond appropriately to their needs.

Infant Massage

The success of any new family depends on communication and sensitivity. Sharing the loving touch of massage with a baby while learning to be sensitive to her own changing needs for education, exercise, and emotional support is the best way for a mother and an infant to begin their new life together. Teaching infant massage is also an excellent way to begin interacting with moms during your first session together.

Massage can be a magic family ritual and the way to cope with stress. If a baby is particularly fussy, a mother can use massage to end the tantrum. Lots of tension and anxiety builds up inside a baby that can also affect the mother. Using massage as a resource creates a feeling of success and pride for the new parent. I usually provide mothers with a handout on infant massage (Appendix 15.2). I think that encouraging them to take this information home will mean that fathers and other support persons will have the opportunity to share and learn these new skills.

Relax and Enjoy

In my first class session, I spend about 15 min on baby activities and a half hour on exercises for mom. I schedule the class for an hour so that there will be unhurried time for burping, crying, changing, and feeding. These are the natural interruptions of a postpartum class and you and your class shouldn't feel dismayed by noisy reminders of needs that must be met. While mothers exercise, the babies are placed on quilts, pads, or in infant seats around the perimeter of the room where we can all see them but where they will not be inadvertently bumped or disturbed. Occasionally we have placed them all in the center of the room while we worked out around them.

Class 2: Postpartum Body Image

The postpartum inventory (Appendix 15.3) is designed to help each woman gain a sense of her own body image and her feelings about the changes that have occurred. Throughout pregnancy, body boundaries become diffused and expansion becomes the norm. During postpartum there is a disturbance in boundaries once more. This time a woman may not be able to find the source of the disturbances as easily as she did during pregnancy. The inventory encourages women to focus on specific areas of concern, to understand and accept their own body parts, and become to more discriminating in their analysis of body image.

PURPOSE. To discuss body image concerns. To review infant massage and have each mother massage her infant. To share again the fact that babies learn to respond to the world through stimulation of all the senses.

GOALS. To orient any newcomers, reinforce competence, and improve group dynamics.

OPTIONAL TOPICS FOR DISCUSSION. Nutrition, weight loss, stress, fatigue, and other postpartum concerns.

REFERENCES. Brazelton (1969), Levy (1975), and Simpkin (1985).

HANDOUTS. Postpartum Inventory (Appendix 15.3).

TECHNIQUES. Demonstration, hands-on activities with babies, and discussion about previosly listed topics.

EXERCISES FOR MOMS. Review of Class 1 exercises; add thigh toners and introduce exercises to assess and improve posture.

Class 3: Discussing Childbirth

After several weeks together much of the initial shyness or reticence about talking openly in the group will disappear. Women will feel more comfortable about discussing their own experiences during childbirth and their feelings about postpartum and parenting. I believe it is important to encourage open discussion of the childbirth experience. Many women come through childbirth with flying colors. Their self-esteem is intact, their bodies are strong, and their childbirth memories are glowing. Other women experienced unexpected complications, because of either their babies or their bodies. Although they may hesitate to discuss their feelings, let them know that sharing doubts and disappointments is a healing experience. Your method of opening the class up for discussion will depend on your population, but always be tactful and considerate. If this discussion occurs early in the group's life, and women may be shy or afraid of sounding inarticulate. Be gentle and supportive. If, in the process of sharing their experiences, they ask questions or remark on current concerns, make note of them for further discussion.

PURPOSE.   To open discussion of the birth experience, adjustment to parenthood, plans for returning to work, and methods for coping with the newborn's siblings.

GOALS.   To support retrospective observation of childbirth and the transition into parenting. To explore child rearing and developmental philosophies and stimulate creative parenting. To perfect infant massage techniques.

OPTIONAL TOPICS FOR DISCUSSION.   Ask women to discuss things they would have done differently, their feelings about care givers, and their partners' roles in childbirth. You can also ask for suggestions for childbirth educators and introduce the topics of sex role socialization, marital sexual adjustment, social pressures, and support systems.

REFERENCES.   Close (1984), Debrovner and Shubin (1985), Brooks-Gunn and Matthews (1979), Inkeles (1983), Keeton (1985), LaRossa (1977), and Lichtendorf (1983).

HANDOUTS.   ''Impressions of Childbirth'' (Appendix 15.4).

TECHNIQUES.   Group discussion, hands-on activities, and demonstration.

EXERCISES FOR MOMS.   Introduce more exercises and varieties of those already presented in Classes 1 and 2. Begin an exercise routine with simple choreography and pleasant music. Avoid hard rock music—it wakes up the babies.

Class 4: Baby Exercise

Mothers are usually very eager to learn how to perform baby exercise. Remind those who are overenthusiastic to go slowly, and encourage those who are timid about handling their babies to provide gentle, firm support as they help them to move.

PURPOSE. To introduce baby exercises.

GOALS. To have mothers feel comfortable and confident about performing exercises with their babies.

OPTIONAL TOPICS FOR DISCUSSION. Purpose of infant exercise, how to handle the infant's body during exercise, range of movement, and equipment for exercise.

REFERENCES. Glover, Preminger, and Sanford (1978), Levy (1975), Simpkin (1985), and Singer and Revenson (1978).

HANDOUTS. ''Baby Exercises'' (Appendix 15.5), ''Childproofing Your House'' (Appendix 15.6).

TECHNIQUES. Demonstration, hands-on activities, and group discussion.

EXERCISES FOR MOMS. Review exercises from Classes 1-3 and encourage discussion about how exercise feels, what areas need more work, and what areas feel strong or weak. Increase the number of repetitions as is comfortable by this point in postpartum.

BABY EXERCISE. Learning to exercise the baby's body helps a woman to develop a warm and responsive relationship with her baby. Encourage mothers to make eye contact with their babies, to speak gently, and to encourage them throughout the exercise period. Mothers should place their babies in their laps or on a quilt or exercise pad. Introduce these exercises (Appendix 15.5) for use when the baby is about 2 weeks old. They are appropriate for most infants and can be continued until the child becomes bored and crawls away! The following are supplies you may want to have on hand for baby exercises and stimulation activities:

1. Pillows: to prop up babies and raise their visual fields.
2. Blankets or pads: to place beneath babies for warmth and protection (receiving blankets are particularly good for playing peekaboo).
3. Beach balls: excellent for placing the baby on and rolling gently back and forth to stimulate the sense of balance that helps humans maintain upright posture.
4. Soft knit or cloth balls: for tactile stimulation.
5. Cylinder cushions (either pillows or inflatable cylinders): great for stimulating arm reaching and visual and vestibular senses.
6. Scooter boards: for riding and stimulating all the senses.
7. Rattles and squeaky toys: for visual and auditory stimulation games.
8. Dolls with bright faces: for visual stimulation.
9. Mirrors: for stimulating visual attention.
10. Pen lights: for drawing attention to light (do not use a flashlight).
11. Feathers and soft scarves: for tactile stimulation.

Baby exercises are fun and easy to learn. Observing a few safety precautions will ensure that exercise time is a happy, safe, and loving experience.

- Never force a baby to exercise. If a baby really doesn't want to exercise there is usually a very good reason. Fatigue, boredom, a dirty diaper, or a hungry tummy may be the source of a baby's refusal.
- Exercise the baby gently. Never force a baby's limbs to move.
- Be sensible. Babies have the same joints and muscles that we do. Never bend any body part into an unnatural position. Exercise should never hurt.
- Always exercise the baby on a safe surface. The floor is the best choice. Remember to place a pad or quilt beneath the baby.
- Do a warm-up activity before exercising. You may want to do a full body rub or gently pat or rub each major joint. Most babies need to relax before engaging in exercises.

Once you have finished setting up the exercise space and going through the warm-up activity, lead the mothers and babies through a series of exercises that are designed to help the baby experience a full range of motion and new and rewarding body sensations and boundaries, to release tension, to enjoy positive socialization, and to experience the success of using and activating its own body.

Each exercise is appropriate for developing strength and encouraging new skills. Stress the fact that these exercises are not designed to speed up a baby's development. Also, don't expect to be able to teach all of the exercises in Appendix 15.5 in one session (it may take several!). Demonstrate the exercises on a large rag doll and then work with each mother and baby individually.

Class 5: Infant Stimulation Activities

There is a great deal of information to share with new mothers about infant exercise, development, and stimulation. By providing a bounty of information, you also share your enthusiasm. Don't worry about overburdening women with too much information.

In addition to showing mothers how to exercise with their infants, you should encourage them to explore the potential of developmental learning. Most mothers want to know about the kinds of things babies can do. Opportunities for infant stimulation activities arise daily as parent and child spend hours of time together. Introduce and demonstrate some of the infant stimulation activities (Appendix 15.7), depending on the ages of the infants in your group.

Household safety and the prevention of accidents is another topic that usually doesn't appear in a regular exercise program. However, it is a vital component of parent education. I always discuss the importance of putting the fire, police, and poison-information numbers next to each telephone in the home. And finally, because we are sharing ideas for creative play and parenting, I discuss choosing and using safe toys (see Appendix 15.8).

PURPOSE. To introduce infant stimulation activities (Appendix 15.7) and the creative use of toys and activity equipment. The group leader should bring in catalogs of educational toys and be prepared to demonstrate the creative use of cushions and pillows, scooter boards, beanbag chairs, mirrors, bells, bright-faced toys, some battery-operated toys that are visually stimulating for young children, and educational toys that you can make or acquire inexpensively.

GOALS. Each mother should experiment with the use of the special materials and props. She should observe which ones attract her baby's attention and think about what kinds of things she has at home that could become useful playthings for her baby.

HANDOUTS. "Infant Stimulation Activities" (Appendix 15.7), "Choosing Safe Toys for Your Baby" (Appendix 15.8).

EXERCISES FOR MOMS. Continue with exercise routines from earlier sessions. Increase pace and number of repetitions. I often introduce light weights in the class and talk about home exercise equipment and videos.

Class 6: Look How Much We've Grown!

I use this class to bring our experience together to a close and to reinforce the skills we have learned for attending to the needs of babies, siblings, spouses, and ourselves.

PURPOSE. To review baby exercises and further explore infant development as it occurs in the areas of cognition, coordination, and locomotor and communication skills. Invite women to share feelings and explore ideas and suggestions for future classes if this is a final class. If this is not your last class you may want to invite a guest speaker—pediatrician, nutritionist, child development expert, or nurse—to discuss a topic of the mothers' choosing.

GOALS. To further the appreciation of infant growth patterns. To determine whether mothers feel pleased with their new infant massage and exercise skills, have plans to continue exercising themselves, and feel supported and successful.

OPTIONAL TOPICS FOR DISCUSSION. Share plans for other activities in the community, extend individual good-byes to each mother in the group, and plan a reunion.

EXERCISES FOR MOMS. These should be more strenuous with an emphasis on increasing speed and the number of repetitions.

SUMMARY OF MOTOR DEVELOPMENT. All children grow and develop differently, yet, by and large, each tends to acquire the fine and gross motor skills in the same sequence. Table 15.1 (see Appendix 15.9) does not intend to define normal or abnormal development. It is designed to help you determine whether the exercises or activities you are providing are appropriate for the babies in your group. It will also help you to individualize instruction as necessary. Encourage mothers to watch for the development of the following motor skills:

Reach is first developed with near objects. Reaching for a distant object is first accomplished by rotation of the body. This requires fairly good balance.

Grasp first appears at about 16 weeks and develops for several years.

Release first emerges at about 40 weeks and progresses from full opening of the palm to more economical release of the fingers.

Information on infant growth and development is readily available. Become familiar with it and convey its importance to the women in your classes.

Fathers and Postpartum Classes

Someone once asked me if I wasn't being sexist by excluding fathers from the postpartum classes. I was really surprised. I have never excluded fathers. Nor have I ever had a father ask to attend. I have, however, always encouraged women to share the skills and techniques we learn together with the men in their lives. Fathering well is a necessary part of healthy family functioning. I think all fathers should learn to give infant massage and play easily and comfortably with their babies.

Summary

In conclusion, there are three things you should now understand from the text about being a prenatal or postpartum fitness educator. First, a good teacher takes enormous pride in her work. Teaching well requires a flexible framework, a broad and in-depth knowledge of the subject area and a commitment to excellence. I hope that this text has stimulated your interest and provided you with a firm and accurate foundation for teaching prenatal and postpartum fitness. Second, the pedagogy of maternal health education requires an activist's commitment to the importance of holistic health education. The ecosystem approach—the blending of wisdom from many cultures, science, and philosophies and consideration of the whole woman—is the pathway to better health. And third, childbearing is a basic function within the physical dominion of women only, and control of it should be returned to each of them through education and preparation for childbirth and support throughout the childbearing years. Fitness education is a logical and vital component of childbirth education. The close link between education and health makes this premise inevitable, motivating, and essential.

Women's health education should span the life cycle. Our job is to help more women lead healthier lives. We must learn to use the exercise classroom as the perfect instructional vehicle for improving women's health, for within this context women can learn that they can heal themselves and each other.

Looking at My Baby: A New Way of Thinking

How does my baby respond to light? Does it turn its head to look at it or close its eyes to avoid it?
_____

How does my baby respond to different kinds of noises? Does it attend to a rattle? to music? to my voice?
_____

What does my baby like to look at? bright toys? faces? _____
_____

How does my baby respond to the people around it? Does it look toward its siblings? frown at strangers?
_____

When my baby is startled or tense, what does it do? cry? clench its fists? _____
_____

How do I console my baby when it is tense or irritable? _____
_____

Do I consider my baby to be quiet? tense? irritable? relaxed? cuddly? How would I describe my baby's personality? _____
_____

What does my baby do when it is alone? look around? suck its hands? Are its fists clenched? Does it wiggle around in its crib yet? _____
_____

Do I understand my baby's different kinds of cries? _____
_____

Do we talk to each other? Does my baby coo to me? _____
_____

Other ideas and observations _____
_____

Infant Massage

The most wonderful part of massage is that there is no secret to it! There is no magic you must learn, and no ritual you must follow. Simply remember that your touch should be gentle because a massage communicates love, security, patience, and respect. Massage is also a beautiful way to teach your baby about body awareness, body boundaries, and the difference between tension and relaxation. It helps your baby to be comfortable in its body and to differentiate between self and the environment.

The touching and caressing of an infant's skin is a sweet experience. Massaging your baby is like singing. You croon with your touch. You send vibrations of love through your hands to the skin of the child. This kind of tactile experience can be very emotional. With your fingertips or your palms on your baby's tiny body, you both share a loving, special closeness.

When should you massage your baby? Anytime: In the morning sunshine, after a bath, before a nap; in the afternoon when the baby is fussy or before your other children come home from school; when you are changing it or when you are playing. Try it in the evening just before bedtime. You and your baby will find the best times for you. Some babies fall asleep after a massage, others are stimulated and want to play.

Where should you do the massage? Try spreading a blanket down in a warm, sunny spot in your home. Or, simply begin the massage when the baby is lying down on your bed or on the floor.

How long should a massage last? It depends on your schedule and your baby's mood. You can do a little bit of massage as part of your bedtime ritual or a full-fledged 20-min massage at midmorning. A simple back rub may soothe your baby if it is fretful.

Do you need any special equipment? If it is chilly, your baby ought to be covered or dressed in a T-shirt at least. If it is warm, a naked body is best. Some mothers prefer a diapered bottom. Others simply put a pad beneath the child and keep a spare to catch an unexpected squirt! If you'd like, use a little baby oil on your hands to reduce the friction of your rub. If you prefer to use powder, use it sparingly. Talcum powder can be very irritating to tiny throats.

How do you begin? You may begin anywhere, but for convenience let's assume that your baby is on its back and you begin the massage at its head.

Gently stroke its head, softly encircling the skull, touching the forehead, massaging the brow. Gently massage the ears and over the nose, around cheeks, mouth, and chin. Explore the baby's face. Learn its curves, its chubby places, and its smoothness. Never push hard and avoid pressure on the soft spots, or fontanelles, of the skull.

Stroke the neck and then move down to the shoulders. Let your hands curve around the shoulders, touching both the shoulder blades on the back and the collar bone in front.

Never break contact with your baby's skin from this point. If you break contact or lift both hands from its body once a massage has begun, this may signal to the baby that the massage is over. Keep one hand on it at all times.

Massage the shoulder joint, upper arm, forearm, and wrist. Never force the arm to straighten or the elbow to bend. When you come to the hand, spend a few special moments relaxing the palm and encouraging its fingers to open. Repeat on the other side.

Now focus on the torso. Traditional massage encouraged the masseuse always to rub toward the heart. This is not always important, but remember to be consistent. If you choose to do circling motions, upward or downward rubs, light tickles, or full torso strokes, remember to repeat your strokes several times. This allows the baby to detect your pattern and respond to it. After you have completed one style of movement, change to another. You and your baby will learn which patterns are most pleasurable.

Allow your hands to scoop under the baby's lower back, under the bottom and then back around to the front of the pelvis. Be certain to help the baby to relax its hips as they are often the site of great contraction and tension.

Massage the legs as you massaged the arms. Massage fully and lovingly. Be as gentle to the knees as you were to the elbows.

The feet are probably my favorite place to massage. Traditional foot reflexology teaches that every organ of the body can be stimulated and healed with foot massage. Be gentle to the ankle, never forget a toe, and cover both the arch and the top of the foot.

Turn the baby over and repeat the entire massage while it is lying on its belly. Remember that mothers and babies know each other on two levels: what they do, and how they do it.

Postpartum Inventory

My Age: _____

My Height: _____

How much I weighed when I got pregnant: _____

How much weight I gained during pregnancy: _____

How much weight I have lost since my baby was born: _____

Do I want to lose more weight? _____   How much? _____

Why? _____

    Please take a moment and close your eyes. Think about your body. When you are ready, open your eyes and answer the following questions about your body. Identify the body parts you feel have changed as a result of your pregnancy. How have those body parts changed? How do you feel about those changes? What can you do about them?

Hair _____

Vision _____

Complexion _____

Teeth and gums _____

Neck _____   Shoulders _____   Arms _____

Upper back _____

Lower back _____

Posture _____

Breasts _____

Belly _____

Waistline _____

Hips _____

Bottom _____   Genitals _____

Inner thighs _____

Outer thighs _____

Legs _____

Ankles and feet _____

Energy level _____

Appetite _____

Sleep patterns and needs _____

Menstrual cycle _____

Bowel habits _____

Headaches _____

Emotions _____

Other questions for discussion:

Do you have more aches and pains now than you did before you had your baby? _____

Does any part of your body seem to hurt more than it should? _____

Are you feeling especially worried about your weight or any particular aspect of your body and its changes?

_____

What can you do about these feelings? _____

Impressions of Childbirth

This is a page for you to write down your thoughts about your birth experience. Some women find they have very few words with which to describe their feelings. Others discover that they have a great deal to say. Many years from now your child may ask you how you felt about his or her birth. Take a few minutes to write down some of your impressions.

_____

_____

_____

_____

_____

_____

_____

_____

_____

_____

Baby Exercises

Begin with one or two repetitions only. Work up to more as baby gets stronger.

1. Hand openers

Purpose: To release tension and prepare for grasping skills.

How-to: Gently massage the baby's shoulder, arm, and hand, and encourage the baby to open its hand. The baby may be stubborn. Never force an action but always encourage cooperation.

2. Arm extenders

Purpose: For flexibility.

How-to: Gently lift the baby's arm up and over its head. There may be resistance. Work slowly and support the whole arm. Alternate one arm at a time and then both arms up.

3. Scarf exercises

Purpose: For flexibility and strength.

How-to: Gently cross the baby's arms across its body. Release and repeat with the other arm.

4. Leg-ups

Purpose: For flexibility and strength.

How-to: Support the calf of the leg and bend the leg at the knee and hip. Alternate. The exercise looks like a running step.
Variation: Move both legs up together.

5. Roll-up

Purpose: For flexibility and release of tummy tension.

How-to: Gently lift baby's bent knees to the chest and lower.

6. V sit

Purpose: For flexibility and strength.

How-to: Repeat "Roll-up" to chest and then firmly grasp ankles and open legs to a "V." Release gently and repeat.

7. Hip rolls

Purpose: For flexibility and release of tension.

How-to: With baby's legs relaxed and extended, gently place your palms under the baby's hips and roll baby to the left and right. Then with the baby's legs bent at knee, roll baby to left and right.

8. Alternating toe touches

Purpose: For strength and flexibility.

How-to: Lift baby's right leg and reach baby's arm to touch its toe. Repeat on left side.

9. Sit-ups

Purpose: For strength and balance.

How-to: With baby lying on the mat, firmly support arms and lift baby gently to sitting position. Go slowly if there is a lot of head lag but do not be afraid to do the exercise. Do not force the baby into a fully upright position. Allow the baby to come only part of the way up if it strongly resists. Gently lower the baby back down to the mat.

10. Stand-ups

Purpose: For strength and balance with a baby at least 8 weeks old.

How-to: Perform the sit-up and then lift baby with support from under its arms to a stand. Do not let the baby support its own weight. Gently lower baby back down to the mat.

11. Wheelbarrow

Purpose: For upper back and neck strength with babies at least 6 weeks old.

How-to: Place baby with chest high on a pillow, a partially inflated cylinder, or a rolled-up towel. Face the baby. Talk to it and place a bright toy in front of it. Encourage baby to lift its head.
Variation: Gently lift baby's hips and support it as you gently roll baby forward and backward on the round pillow or towel.

12. Push-up

Purpose: For arm strength and sensitivity to touch.

How-to: Support baby's legs, hips, and torso, and lift baby up off the ground. Allow its arms to hang down. Lower baby until its hands lightly touch the mat. Lower the baby to the mat and then lift it again until hands just skim the mat. Eventually the baby will reach for the mat and support increasingly more of its own weight. At first you are merely introducing the sensation.

13. Sitting arm stretches

Purpose: For balance, torso strength, visual stimulation, and head alignment.

How-to: Allow baby to relax while seated facing you against pillows. Lift baby's arms up high, then open wide and return to center.

Variation: Lift arms up high and then open slightly to the side. Allow baby's torso to lean and gently pull baby back to midline. You may repeat this series with baby seated between your legs.

14. Foot push

Purpose: For strength.

How-to: With baby lying on its back, place your palms on the soles of its feet and allow baby to push up against your hands. Turn baby over and repeat with it lying on its belly.

15. Belly reach

Purpose: For strength and flexibility.

How-to: While baby is on its belly, extend its arms out in front of it and gently lift its chest just slightly up off the mat. Repeat and then massage the baby's back.

Childproofing Your House

Obviously, a new baby won't be crawling off to cause a domestic accident. But babies grow quickly, and it is never too soon to childproof your house.

Get down on the baby's level and remove everything that can be ingested or broken or can cause other things to fall. Also look for poisonous substances or things that are capable of causing an electrical short or shock or a fire. Plug all electrical outlets. Get baby locks for all accessible cupboards. Put all cleaning materials out of reach. Put gates in front of all stairwells, doorways, and open windows. Pull all houseplants up and out of reach. Curtain cords, shade pulls, and stereo wires should be out of reach. Laundry room doors should be kept closed. Old refrigerators should be removed. Never leave a baby in an infant seat on a table or counter. Protect your child's life. Babyproof your house!

Infant Stimulation Activities

Here are some activities you and your infant will enjoy. Your baby may not be ready for all of the ideas suggested here, so exercise good judgment when playing and make playtime an enjoyable part of your life together.

"My baby has begun to feel things with its fingers."

1. Provide lots of opportunities to touch. Offer toys, food, scarves, hard objects, rubbery objects, tickly feathers, and scratchy sweaters.
2. Make a touching board with different fabrics. Try velvet, something furry, aluminum foil, and a piece of carpet.
3. Take the child's hand and guide the touching experience. Talk about it.
4. Touch the child with different fabrics. Stimulate cheeks, tummy, back, and toes!
5. Dress the baby in a variety of textures and fabrics. Touch its hand to each.
6. Take your baby's hand and touch it to various parts of your face, hair, clothing, and skin.
7. Loosely wrap a piece of yarn around the baby's hand so the baby may play with it and not lose it.
8. Hold the baby's hands together and play "patty cake" or clap to the rhythm of a song.
9. Tie a piece of yarn to a bell or rattle and encourage the baby to pull on it.
10. Massage the baby's palms and fingers.
11. Allow the baby to splash in the bath water.
12. Place a variety of objects directly in the baby's hands.
13. Encourage the baby to bring its hands to its mouth. Later put a small bit of honey or some other good tasting food on the baby's fingers and let it lick them off. (This does not encourage thumbsucking).

"My baby loves to look at things now."

1. Play peekaboo with your hands, a tissue, a washcloth, or a towel.
2. Look right at the baby when you talk to it and smile, blink your eyes, stick out your tongue, and wrinkle your nose.
3. Place toys around the playpen or crib; hang a mobile or balloons above the crib.
4. Hold a squeaky toy in front of the baby. Move it across the baby's field of vision. Encourage it to follow the toy up, down, and around in a circle.
5. Carry the baby and identify objects in your environment: trees, bricks, the refrigerator, and so forth.
6. Hold a toy up so the baby can see it. Shake another so it can respond to it, too. Encourage the baby to look at the two different toys and to reach for them if it can. Reward the tiniest gestures by placing the toy in the baby's hand.
7. Place a toy on the table in front of the baby. Allow the toy to fall off the table. Look at it together. Pick it up and repeat the activity.
8. Put a rattle in the baby's hand and shake it. If it drops the rattle, pick it up and repeat.
9. Show the baby its image in the mirror.
10. Let the baby watch a fish tank.
11. When the baby is lying on its back, place a toy on its tummy.
12. Hold an object 6 in, 12 in, and then 36 in from the baby's face. Which does it focus on? Which can it follow if you move them around?
13. Show the baby pictures of bright faces; look at books together. Look out the window.

"My baby seems to know if I am not in the room."

1. Play peekaboo with a towel or a receiving blanket so that you seem to disappear briefly.
2. If you leave the room, continue to talk to the baby.
3. Gently hide the baby behind a scarf and ask "Where's the baby?" Pull it off and laugh.
4. Place the baby in an infant seat or high chair facing away from you. Talk to it and then return to its field of vision. Say "Hi!" each time you reappear.
5. Play peekaboo with the baby in the mirror.
6. Take the baby with you from room to room, but when you have to leave it for a moment, tell it you'll be right back.

"My baby is really paying attention to its toys."

1. Hide a toy beneath a pillow or towel. Watch the baby's delight when it reappears.

2. Offer a new toy just within or beyond the baby's reach. Encourage the baby to move toward it.
3. Hang bright balloons around the house and call the baby's attention to them. Blow on them and watch them move.
4. Place a toy in each of your baby's hands and watch how it observes their differences.
5. Hold a bell and put a small cloth over your hand. Ring the bell and help your baby find it.
6. Roll a toy under a piece of furniture. Encourage the baby to feel for it and find it. If the baby is too little, do it yourself and talk about what you are doing.

"My baby is really listening to things."

1. Talk to your baby when you are out of its field of vision and encourage it to turn its head toward your voice.
2. Shake a toy or rattle to one side of the baby's head and encourage it to turn toward the sound.
3. Play music and sing or dance with the baby.
4. Hang bells within baby's reach and encourage it to turn toward the sound.
5. Pat the mattress by baby's head and encourage it to turn toward the sound.
6. Hold the baby close and whisper to it.
7. Talk to the baby in the car.
8. Identify sounds in the environment.
9. Identify people's voices.
10. Let the child bang on pots and pans, drums and boxes. Allow it to play a piano. Locate electronic toys that make a noise in response to a light touch.
11. When the baby is lying down, stand above it and then speak to it as you walk around it.

"My baby is paying attention to me when I talk."

1. Whisper softly to the baby when it is fussy.
2. Describe what you are doing even if the baby cannot understand your words.
3. Have the baby close to the table when the rest of the family is eating.
4. Speak the baby's name when you want its attention, whenever you are talking to it or moving about.
5. Praise baby for responding to auditory or visual stimulation.
6. Comfort the baby if it responds fearfully or with distress to angry voices or loud noises.
7. Provide a variety of language options when you are interacting. For example, "Up?" "Do you want up?" "Does Erin want up?" Or, "Eat?" "Do you want to eat?" "Is it time for you to eat?"
8. Choose music that you like and that seems to please the baby. Play it often so baby may enjoy it.
9. Imitate all the noises, gurgles, coos, grunts, and squeals that your baby makes.
10. When cooing back to the baby, add other sounds like "aaahhh," "eeehhh," or "ooohhh."
11. Tickle, massage, or roll the baby to encourage it to vocalize.
12. Record the baby's babbling and play the tape back to it.
13. Respond to your baby's expressions of anger, frustration, or fatigue with reasonable verbalizations that indicate that you understand it.
14. Let the baby feel your face when you speak.
15. Make conversations with the baby when you change its diapers.
16. Get a book of nursery rhymes and bone up on a few!
17. Learn finger plays and little songs that the baby can enjoy.

"My baby is really starting to move around."

1. When your baby grabs your finger, let it hang on and gently move your hand back and forth, up and down.
2. When baby kicks, let it push against your palms.
3. Change the baby's position frequently and create several different environments for it.
4. Allow and encourage it to spend time lying on its tummy or back, or sitting up in a seat, propped up on pillows, in a swing, or on the floor.
5. If the baby's head seems to sag, help it to straighten it up. If the baby seems tired, change its position.
6. While the baby is on its belly, place a toy a few inches in front of its face and encourage it to lift its head and look at it.
7. When your baby grabs your hand or finger, gently pull it so it rolls over.
8. Place the baby at the bottom of the crib so it can push against the footboard.
9. Place a small cushion or rolled-up towel under the baby's chest. This frees its arms to play. Talk to it in this position and encourage it to lift its head.

10. When the child sits on the floor, get down and imitate its movement. Continue to imitate movements at every developmental stage. Silent parallel play is supportive and comforting.
11. While holding the baby, move it back and forth, closer to and then further away from your face.
12. When the baby is able to support itself on its forearms, gently push its shoulder and encourage it to roll over and/or keep its balance.
13. While supporting the baby under its arms, let it bounce while you sing. Let the baby dance but do not encourage it to support its own weight.
14. While the baby is on its back, show it a toy and encourage it to reach for it.
15. While the baby is seated, show it several toys. Move them, talk about them, and encourage the baby to look for them if they disappear. If the baby attempts to reach for them give them to the baby.
16. Sit the baby between your legs and encourage it to support itself.
17. Both seated on the floor, roll a ball between your legs and your baby's legs.
18. While the baby's head is well supported, rub your forehead against the baby's.
19. Put the baby on a big blanket and pull it around the room.
20. Place the baby in the middle of a blanket and create a hammock. With another person's help, gently swing it from side to side.

Choosing Safe Toys for Your Baby

Toys for babies and young children should be fun, interesting, and safe. They should not have sharp edges, wires, or small, removable parts. Toys that need to be plugged in or that require batteries are not appropriate for tiny babies.

- Look for unbreakable, well-constructed toys.
- Labels should state clearly "Non-Toxic and Flame-Resistant/Flame-Retardant." All fabric toys should be washable. Check label for composition of stuffing.
- Avoid toys with many small parts that could be swallowed.
- If a toy is battery-operated, check batteries frequently for leakage.

- Cloth or vinyl books are best for the little one. Heavy cardboard books come after teething.
- "Nerf ball" toys are fun and can't cause any damage to your home, but make sure your baby is not eating them.
- Try pulling the eyes and ears off stuffed toys. If they come off they are dangerous.
- Toys should be challenging, not frustrating. You won't help your baby's intellectual growth by buying it highly sophisticated toys.
- Toys can be made at home using good judgment and safe materials. Avoid pins, tape, or glue that a small child might ingest.

Fine and Gross Motor Sequences

Position	Weeks 1-12	Weeks 13-16	Weeks 17-24
Supine	Head turns to one side. Tonic neck reflex seen. Fists are clenched. Legs resist extension.	Can hold head at midline. Limbs positioned symmetrically. Hands engage near face or chest. Tonic neck reflex fading.	Lifts head. Lifts legs.
Prone	Body flexes. May lift head briefly.	Props up on forearms. Unstable, may verge on rolling over.	May roll over. Turns head to regard sound or objects.
Ventral suspension	Head droops.	Head aligned with trunk. Legs extend.	Demonstrates alignment strength.
Sitting	Head droops.	Minimal head lag, prefers head at midline. Back rounds forward.	Lifts head. May be stable for brief periods. Enjoys high chair.
Standing	Reflexive straightening of legs. Stepping reflex. Unable to support own weight.	Makes effort to straighten torso.	Enjoys upright position. Uses arms when supported.
Reach	Diffuse	Arm activity increases.	Bilateral or sideways approach.
Grasp	None	Retains objects placed in hand.	Reflexive. Voluntary plantar grasp emerging.
Release	None	None	None

Visual Development

Weeks 1-6	7-10	11-12	13-16	17-24
Feels tactile stimulation but cannot look up or down. Can see objects in visual field.	Regards extended hand. Awareness of shape and color. Range 90°.	Eyes follow objects. Begins to associate certain objects with sounds. Range 180°.	Looks at hands. Begins to regard objects and move whole body in response to pleasing visual stimulation.	Eyes and hands coordinate. Shows interest in variety of objects.

References

Achterberg, J. (1985). *Imagery in healing: Shamanism and modern medicine*. Boston: New Science Library.

American College of Obstetricians and Gynecologists. (1985). *Exercise during pregnancy and the postnatal period*. Washington, DC: Author.

American College of Obstetricians and Gynecologists. (1986). *Safety guidelines for women who exercise*. Washington, DC: Author.

American College of Sports Medicine. (1978). Position statement on the recommended quantity and quality of exercise for developing and maintaining fitness in healthy adults. *Medicine and Science in Sports*, **10**, vii-x.

Artal, R., & Romen, Y. (1986). Fetal responses to maternal exercise. In R. Artal & R. Wiswell (Eds.), *Exercise in pregnancy* (195-204). Baltimore: Williams and Wilkins.

Artal, R., & Wiswell, R. (Eds.). (1986). *Exercise in pregnancy*. Baltimore: Williams and Wilkins.

Barker, S. (1981). *The Alexander technique*. New York: Bantam Books.

Bauer, C. (1987). *Acupressure for women*. Freedom, CA: The Crossing Press.

Benson, R. (1983). *Handbook of obstetrics and gynecology*. Los Altos, CA: Lange Medical Publications.

Berkowitz, G.S., Kelsey, J.L., Holford, T., & Berkowitz, R.L. (1983). Physical activity and the risk of spontaneous preterm delivery. *Journal of Reproductive Medicine*, **28**, 581-588.

Bernstein, P.L. (1975). *Theory and methods in dance movement therapy*. Dubuque, IA: Kendall Hunt.

Bernstein, P.L. (1986). *Theoretical approaches to dance movement therapy* (Vols. 1-2). Dubuque, IA: Kendall Hunt.

Bing, E., & Coleman, L. (1977). *Making love during pregnancy*. New York: Bantam Books.

Black, R., Herman, B.P., & Shope, J.T. (1982). *Nursing management of epilepsy*. Aspen, CO: Aspen.

Bolen, J.S. (1984). *Goddesses in every woman*. New York: Harper Colophon.

Borg, G. (1973). Perceived exertion: A note on history and methods. *Medicine and Science in Sports*, **5**, 90-93.

Boston Women's Health Book Collective. (1971). *Our bodies ourselves*. New York: Simon and Schuster.

Brazelton, T.B. (1969). *Infants and mothers: Differences in development*. New York: Dell.

Brooks-Gunn, J., & Matthews, W.S. (1979). *He and she: How children develop their sex-role identity*. Englewood Cliffs, NJ: Prentice-Hall.

Close, S. (1984). *Sex during pregnancy and after childbirth*. Wellingbrough, North Hamptonshire, England: Thorsons.

Cohen, L. (1983). *Nourishing a happy affair: Nutrition alternatives for individual and family needs*. Burdett, NY: Larson.

Collings, C., Curet, L., & Mullin, J.P. (1983). Maternal and fetal responses to a maternal aerobic exercise program. *American Journal of Obstetrics and Gynecology*, **145**, 702-707.

Cooper, M., & Cooper, K. (1972). *Aerobics for women*. New York: J.B. Lippincott.

Dale, E., Mullinax, K.M., & Bryan, D. (1982). Exercise during pregnancy: Effects on the fetus. *Canadian Journal of Applied Sport Sciences*, **7**, 98-103.

Debrovner, C., & Shubin, R. (1985). Postpartum sexual concern. *Medical Aspects of Human Sexuality*, **19**, 84.

Dossey, L. (1982). *Space, time, and medicine*. Boston: New Science Library.

Edwards, M.J., Metcalfe, J., Dunham, M., & Paul, M. (1981). Accelerated respiratory response to moderate exercise in late pregnancy. *Respiration Physiology*, **45**, 229-241.

Ensminger, A., Ensinger, M.E., Konlaid, J., & Robson, J.R. (1986). Food for health: A nutrition encyclopedia. Clovis, CA: Regus Press.

Estok, P.J. (1985). *Exercise during pregnancy: Risk or benefit?* Princeton, NJ: Continuing Professional Education Center.

Feldenkrais, M. (1977). *Awareness through movement.* New York: Harper and Row.

Ferguson, M. (1980). *The Aquarian conspiracy: Personal and social transformation in the 1980's.* Boston: Houghton Mifflin.

Flanagan, G.L. (1962). *The first nine months of life.* New York: Simon and Schuster.

Glover, E., Preminger, J., & Sanford, A. (1978). *Early lap-learning accomplishment profile.* Winston-Salem, NC: Chapel Hill Training-Outreach Project.

Goldberg, L., & Elliot, D.L. (Eds.). (1985). *Symposium on medical aspects of exercise: Vol. 69. Medical clinics of North America.* Philadelphia: Saunders College.

Goldsmith, J. (1984). *Childbirth wisdom.* New York: Congdon and Weed.

Hassid, P. (1984). *Textbook for childbirth educators.* Philadelphia: J.B. Lippincott.

Hauth, J.C., Gilstrap, L.C., & Widmer, K. (1982). Fetal heart rate reactivity before and after maternal jogging during the third trimester. *American Journal of Obstetrics and Gynecology*, **142**, 545-547.

Hecht, C. (1982). An answer to childbirth educator burn-out. *Birth*, **9**, 35-38.

Heinl, T. (1982). *The baby massage book.* Englewood Cliffs, NJ: Prentice-Hall.

Holstein, B. (1985). *The problems and prospects of childbirth education in rural central New York.* Unpublished manuscript.

Inglehart, H. (1983). *Woman spirit: A guide to women's wisdom.* San Francisco: Harper and Row.

Inkeles, G. (1983). *Massage and peaceful pregnancy.* New York: Putnam.

Jarrett, J.C., & Spellacy, W.N. (1983). Jogging during pregnancy: An improved outcome? *Obstetrics and Gynecology*, **61**, 705-709.

Keeton, K. (1985). *Woman of tomorrow.* New York: St. Martens/Marek.

Kitzinger, S. (1983). *A new approach to a woman's experience of sex.* New York: Penguin Books.

Knuttgen, H.G., & Emerson, K. (1974). Physiological response to pregnancy at rest and during exercise. *Journal of Applied Physiology*, **36**, 549-553.

Kravette, S. (1979). *Complete relaxation.* Rockport, MA: Para Research.

LaRossa, R. (1977). *Conflict and power in marriage.* Beverly Hills, CA: Sage.

Levy, J. (1975). *The baby exercise book.* New York: Random House.

Lichtendorf, S. (1983). *Eve's journey: The physical experience of being female.* New York: Berkley Books.

Liu, D. (1974). *Taoist health exercise book.* New York: Perigree Books.

Lotgering, F., Gilbert, R.D., & Longo, L. (1984). The interactions of exercise and pregnancy: A review. *American Journal of Obstetrics and Gynecology*, **149**, 560-565.

Luttgens, K., & Wells, K. (1982). *Kinesiology: Scientific basis of human motion.* Philadelphia: Saunders College.

Marsal, K., Gennser, G., & Lofgren, O. (1979). Effects on fetal breathing movements of maternal challenges. *Acta Obstetrica Scandinavica*, **58**, 335-342.

Maternity Center Association. (1985). *An instructor's guide to the growing uterus charts.* New York: Author.

McBride, L. (1985, Fall). The slender imbalance: Women and body image. *Journal of the National Association of Women Deans and Counselors*, **16**, 22.

Morton, M.J., Paul, M.S., Campos, G.R., Hart, M.V., & Metcalfe, J. (1985). Exercise dynamics in late gestation: Effects on physical training. *American Journal of Obstetrics and Gynecology*, **152**, 97-108.

Morton, M.J., Paul, M.S., & Metcalfe, J. (1985). Exercise during pregnancy. In L. Goldberg & D.L. Elliot (Eds.), *Symposium on medical aspects of pregnancy: Vol. 69. Medical Clinics of North America* (pp. 97-106). Philadelphia: Saunders College.

Nelson, M.B., & Mondanaro, J. (1982). Health promotion for drug dependent women. In B.G. Reed, G.M. Beschner, & J. Mondanaro (Eds.), *Treatment services for drug dependent women* (pp. 247-302). Rockville, MD: U.S. Department of Health and Human Services.

Null, G. (1987). *The vegetarian handbook: Eating right for total health.* New York: St. Martin.

Ohashi, W. (1976). *Do it yourself shiatsu.* New York: E.P. Dutton.

Olds, S.B., London, M.L., & Ladewig, P. (1984). *Maternal-newborn nursing: A family centered approach.* Menlo Park, CA: Addison-Wesley.

Oxorn, H. (1985). *Oxorn-Foote human labor and birth*. New York: Appleton-Lange.

Paxton, M.J.W. (1981). *The female body in control*. Englewood Cliffs, NJ: Prentice-Hall.

Pernoll, M.L., Metcalfe, J., Schlenker, T.L., Welch, J.E., & Matsumoto, J.A. (1975). Oxygen consumption at rest and during exercise in pregnancy. *Respiratory Physiology, 25*, 285-293.

Pijpers, L., Wladimiroff, J.W., & McGhie, J. (1984). Effect of short term maternal exercise on maternal and fetal cardiovascular dynamics. *British Journal of Obstetrics and Gynecology, 91*, 1081-1086.

Platt, L.D., Artal, R., Semel, J., Sipos, L., & Kammula, R. (1983). Exercise in pregnancy: 2. Fetal responses. *American Journal of Obstetrics and Gynecology, 147*, 487-491.

Pomerance, J.J., Gluck, L., & Lynch, V. (1974). Maternal exercise as a screening test for uteroplacental insufficiency. *Obstetrics and Gynecology, 44*, 383-387.

Pritchard, J.A., & MacDonald, P.C. (Eds.). (1980). *Williams obstetrics* (16th ed.). New York: Appleton-Lange.

Schutz, W.C. (1967). *Joy*. New York: Grove Press.

Simpkin, D. (1985). *The complete baby exercise program*. New York: New American Library.

Singer, D.G., & Revensen, T. (1978). *A Piaget primer: How a child thinks*. New York: New American Library.

Snyder, D.K., & Carruth, B.R. (1984). Current controversies: Exercise during pregnancy. *Journal of Adolescent Health Care, 5*, 34-36.

St. Just, A. (1984). Rolfing the female body. In K. Weiss (Ed.), *Women's health care: A guide to alternatives* (pp. 204-292). Englewood Cliffs, NJ: Prentice-Hall.

Thompson, J. (1977). *Healthy pregnancy the yoga way*. New York: Dolphin Books.

Glossary

Abduction: movement of a body part away from the midline of the body.

Abruptio placentae: premature separation of the placenta from the wall of the uterus that causes vaginal bleeding.

Accelerated/decelerated breathing: a technique used during labor to meet the changing intensity of contractions.

Acetabulum: the point where the head of the femur meets the pelvis.

Active myocardial disease: disease of the heart's inner wall.

Adduction: movement of a body part toward the midline of the body.

Adductor group: muscles that contribute to the adduction and flexion of the hip.

Aerobic: using oxygen.

Agonist: muscle that shortens and contracts during a movement.

American College of Obstetricians and Gynecologists: a national medical organization that promotes research and education on the health care of women.

Anaerobic: not using oxygen.

Angular motion: motion of the body around an axis; rotary motion.

Antagonist: muscle that lengthens during a movement, working opposite the agonist.

Anterior flexion: bending forward.

Apgar score: named for Virginia Apgar, a numerical system that rates the condition of the newborn at birth.

Assisted stretches: stretches done with help of a partner or a machine.

American Society for Psychoprophilaxis in Obstetrics: international organization that promotes the philosophy and teaching of Ferdinand Lamaze, founder of the Lamaze childbirth method and author of many books and articles on the subject of natural childbirth.

Babinski reflex: extension following flexion of the infant's toes when the sole of the foot is stimulated.

Balance: ability to maintain a state of equilibrium while at rest or in motion.

Ballistic: activities that involve jumping or jarring movements.

Ballistic stretches: activities that stretch the muscles through bobbing or bouncing.

Biceps brachii: muscle that causes flexion of the shoulder and supination of the forearm.

Biceps femoris: member of the hamstring group.

Birth harmony: a concept that describes balance of the physical, emotional, and environmental events that lead to a natural, undisturbed birth.

Blood pressure: the force that the flow of the blood exerts on the blood vessels.

Body awareness: component of a prenatal education program that promotes awareness of physical being and personal health.

Body fitness: component of the prenatal education program that promotes the goals of exercise including cardiovascular training, muscle toning, strength building, and so forth.

Body image: perception and awareness of self and body.

Body mapping: an activity that permits exploration of feelings and awareness of the body.

Brachialis: elbow flexor.

Braxton Hicks contractions: normal tightening of the uterine muscle during pregnancy; not labor contractions.

Breech position: in utero, a fetus whose head is not down in the pelvis; presenting part can be the buttocks or feet.

C curve: the preferred shape of the body during childbirth.

Catecholamines: chemicals produced by the body that affect temperature, smooth muscle, and cardiovascular and metabolic rates.

Cardiovascular training section: the portion of the aerobics class during which activities are designed to raise heart rate to within target range.

Carpal tunnel syndrome: soreness, numbness, or weakness in the thumbs, hands, or wrists caused by pressure on the median nerve.

Center of gravity: theoretical point where weight is distributed evenly; each part of the body has its own center of gravity.

Cervix: the lower portion of the uterus that thickens during pregnancy and must efface and dilate for birth to occur.

Circumduction: rotation or cone-shaped movement at a joint.

Coccyx: the last bones at the tip of the spinal column.

Common center of gravity: theoretical point of the entire body at which weight is distributed evenly.

Concentric contraction: development of tension and shortening of a muscle at work.

Congestive heart failure: failure of the heart to maintain adequate circulation.

Continuous training: fitness activities that are sustained for a period of time.

Contractions: rhythmic tightening of the uterine muscle to open the cervix and facilitate the birth of the baby. Labor contractions grow longer, stronger, and closer together. Braxton Hicks, or false labor, contractions do not.

Cool-down: section of the aerobics class during which movements are gradually slowed and heart rate returns to normal.

Corpus luteum: site of the expulsion of the egg from the ovary; produces hormones until placenta is functional.

Cycle of stress: a concept that describes the negative and anxiety-producing pattern created during frustrating parent-infant interactions.

Cystitis: a bladder infection.

Dance therapy: a psychotherapeutic technique that uses movement as its method of communication instead of words.

Dehydration: condition resulting from excessive loss of body fluids.

Deltoid: superior muscle of the shoulder girdle; also covers anterior and posterior portion of the shoulder joint.

Diaphragm: dome-shaped sheath separating the thoracic and abdominal cavities.

Diastasis recti: a separation at the midline of the muscular sheath covering the uterus.

Dilation: the gradual opening of the cervix during labor.

Dynamic balance: the ability to maintain balance while in motion.

Eccentric contraction: development of tension in a muscle while it lengthens.

Ecosystem: an environmental concept that describes the interactive patterns of individuals, groups, systems, and social structures. An ecosystem can be balanced or imbalanced, healthy or unhealthy.

Ectopic pregnancy: the fertilization of the egg outside of the uterus.

Effacement: the thinning of the cervix that occurs to permit the birth of the baby.

Effluerage: a gentle, circling, fingertip abdominal massage technique taught by Lamaze childbirth advocates.

Effort: a term from dance therapy that describes the energy expenditure of an individual or movement.

Endometrium: the inner layer of the uterus.

Endorphins: chemical substances produced in the brain that reduce the perception of pain through chemical binding with receptor sites.

Engorgement: the filling of the breasts with milk.

Episiotomy: an incision made at the opening of the vagina to widen the birth canal.

Erector spinae: major muscle group of the back; responsible for extension, flexion, and rotation.

Estrogen: female sex hormone responsible for secondary sex characteristics.

Exhalation pushing: a breathing technique that allows a woman to exhale as she is bearing down to help expel the baby.

Expulsion: the second stage of labor, during which the fetus is pushed down and out of the birth canal, resulting in the birth of the baby.

Extension: the unbending that increases the angle of the bones meeting at that joint.

External oblique: a broad pair of muscles on either side of the torso; works with the rectus abdominus.

Fallopian tubes: the oviducts through which the egg travels.

False labor: contractions that do not get longer, stronger, or closer together and do not result in the birth of the baby.

Feather blowing: a breathing technique that helps a woman control the speed of birth.

Fetal monitor: a machine that measures the condition of the baby in response to labor.

Flexion: the bending that decreases the angle of the two bones that meet at a joint.

Fundus: top of the uterus; the level of the fundus is an indicator of uterine growth during pregnancy.

Gestational diabetes: disease related to insulin production that first appears during pregnancy; may disappear entirely after childbirth.

Gluteus maximus: major muscle across the back of the ilium.

Gluteus medius: a muscle that works during abduction and outward rotation of the hip and as a hip stabilizer.

Gluteus minimus: a muscle that works during inward rotation of the hip and as a hip stabilizer.

Hamstrings: group of three muscles that act as hip extensors.

Healer: a concept that defines the role of the care giver, teacher, nurse, or midwife who offers health-promoting information, skills, and treatments when necessary, to enhance the health of an individual or family.

Health education: the provision of health-promoting information. In this context, maternal health education should be provided throughout childbearing years to enhance the well-being of an individual or family.

High risk pregnancy: a maternal condition that may pose a threat to the survival of mother and/or fetus.

Historic self: that part of self-image based on past events, interactions, and learning.

Hormone: a product of living cells that produces a specific effect on the activities of cells remote from its point of origin.

Hyperextension: extension of a joint beyond normal range.

Hypertension: high blood pressure. In pregnancy, high blood pressure can be dangerous to the health of mother and fetus.

Hyperventilation: increased respiratory rate resulting from carbon dioxide depletion.

Hypotension: low blood pressure. In pregnancy it may be a result of the weight of the uterus preventing the return of blood to the heart.

Ideal body image: an image of the perfect self that may be impossible to attain; can be very motivating or very frustrating.

Iliopsoas: muscle that causes flexion of the back; shortening may increase lumbar curve.

Ilium: one of the three sections of the pelvis.

Insertion: attachment of a muscle to a bone that is movable at a point furthest from the body.

Internal oblique muscles: a pair of diagonal abdominal muscles.

International Childbirth Education Association: a worldwide organization promoting family-centered birth. Provides classes for parents, publishes a journal, promotes research, and sponsors teacher training.

International Dance Exercise Association: a worldwide organization that promotes the training and certification of exercise instructors.

Interval training: a form of athletic training during which there are short bursts of intense activity.

Involution: the contraction of the uterine muscle to its pre-pregnant size after childbirth.

Ischium: one of the three sections of the pelvis.

Isokinetic: method of athletic training that puts maximum stress on a muscle. The contraction is controlled rather than resisted.

Isometric: contraction that does not lengthen a muscle but increases tension against a force that cannot be moved.

Isotonic: contraction during which the load remains the same while the muscle shortens.

Isthmus: portion of the uterus below the main body of the organ that softens and expands during pregnancy.

Kegel muscles: muscles of the perineum. The kegel exercise is the contraction and release of these muscles to enhance muscle tone and prevent incontinence.

Kinesiology: study of movement.

Kyphosis: excessive convex curve of the upper spine; round-shouldered posture.

Latissimus dorsi: muscle that moves the arm, causing adduction, extension, abduction, and inward rotation.

Levator ani: the pelvic floor muscles.

Levator scapulae: a muscle that works with the trapezius.

Ligament: fibrous muscle tissue that connects the bones to the joints.

Lightening: the time at the end of pregnancy when the baby begins to descend into the pelvis.

Linear: movement or thinking that occurs in a straight line.

Lithotomy: a position for childbirth that requires a woman to lie flat on her back with her feet up in stirrups.

Lochia: bloody vaginal discharge after childbirth.

Lordosis: excessive concave curve of the lumbral section of the spine.

Lumbrosacral joint: the point at which the fifth lumbral vertebra meets the pelvis.

Lymph system: a circulatory system that carries lymphatic fluids from the tissues to the bloodstream.

Mantra: a word or words repeated during meditation to promote relaxation.

Mastitis: breast infection.

Matrix: a system, design, or structure; synonyms: womb, uterus.

Maximal heart rate: theoretical limit to the number of times the heart can beat per minute.

Maximum working heart rate: the upper limit of the target heart rate range.

Meditation: an activity that promotes relaxation and the release of tension by clearing the mind and body of unnecessary distractions.

Menarche: the onset of menstruation.

Minimum working heart rate: lower end at which one can work and still experience cardiovascular training.

Miscarriage: expulsion of the fetus before viability; usually early in pregnancy but occasionally later; synonym: spontaneous abortion.

Moro reflex: a defensive reflex in the neonate that is demonstrated when the baby is startled.

Multigravida: a woman who has had more than two children.

Myometrium: the thick muscular layer of the uterus.

Obterator foramen: two pelvic openings through which blood vessels, nerves, and muscles pass.

Origin: attachment of a muscle to the bone at a point closest to the body.

Os innomita: the pelvis.

Ovaries: the small, almond-shaped organs that produce eggs in the female.

Overload: term used to describe strengthening process during which performance rate or intensity is steadily increased.

Pant-blow: a rhythmic breathing technique frequently used during the most intense labor contractions.

Pectineus: a hip flexor.

Pectoralis major: anterior muscle of the shoulder girdle that causes flexion, extension, abduction, and adduction of the arm.

Pectoralis minor: smaller anterior muscle of the shoulder girdle.

Pelvic floor muscles: muscles that encircle the pelvic outlet and extend from the sacrum and coccyx to the ischium and symphysis pubis.

Perimetrium: the outer covering of the uterus.

Perineal body: central point of the perineum between the vagina and the anus.

Perineum: area from the vagina to the anus.

Phenomenological self: the encounter and perception of self in daily life.

Placenta previa: the formation of a placenta in the lower portion of the uterus, possibly covering the cervix and preventing birth from occurring normally.

Postpartum: the 6-week period after childbirth.

Prana: life force, energy, oxygen.

Progesterone: a hormone produced to maintain pregnancy.

Proprioception: sensory awareness mechanism that provides information on movement and position of the body.

Pubis: one of the three sections of the pelvis.

Puerperal: the immediate postpartum period.

Pulmonary: having to do with the lungs.

Quadratus lumborum: extensor and flexor muscle of the back.

Rami: the bony bars that form the two large openings at the front of the pelvis.

Range of motion: movement allowed by a joint.

Rectus abdominus: major muscular sheath of the abdomen.

Rectus femoris: muscle that works to cause flexion of the hip, forward tilt of the pelvis, and extension of the knee; the only member of the quadriceps group that acts on the hip.

Relaxin: a hormone produced during pregnancy that softens all of the body's ligaments.

Releasing breath: a deep inhalation and a full exhalation that signals the body to release tension.

Resting heart rate: the rate at which the heart beats when an individual first awakens in the morning or after resting.

Rhomboids: posterior muscles of the shoulder girdle.

Rolfing: a system of deep tissue massage; structural integration therapy.

Rotation: process of turning on an axis.

Sacrococcygeal joint: point at which the coccyx is attached to the sacrum.

Sacroiliac joint: point at which the sacrum and ilium meet.

Sacrospinalis: see Erector spinae.

Sacrum: triangular wedge-shaped bone that forms the back of the pelvis and the base of the spinal column.

Sartorius: a muscle that works during hip flexion and outward rotation.

Scoliosis: lateral curvature of the spine.

Seizure threshold: the point at which the balance of stimulation and brain activity cause a seizure.

Self-stretching: stretches that the individual controls, without the use of assistance or equipment.

Semimembranosus: member of the hamstring group of muscles.

Semitendinosus: member of the hamstring group of muscles.

Sensei: the master or teacher of karate.

Shaping: a term from dance therapy that describes the individual's ability to move the body in response to the environment.

Slow-chest breathing: a light, gentle breath frequently used during the early stages of labor.

Sparring: practice fighting in the martial arts; not recommended after the first trimester of pregnancy.

Splenius: posterior muscle of the neck.

Sprinting: running relatively short distances at maximum speed; an anaerobic activity that is not recommended during pregnancy.

Stages of labor: childbirth is divided into three stages: The first stage is the opening of the cervix; the second stage is the birth of the baby; and the third stage is the expulsion of the placenta.

Static balance: the ability to maintain one's balance in a relatively stationary position.

Static contraction: muscular contraction during which no movement takes place.

Static stretching: stretches that involve the lengthening of a muscle without bouncing or bobbing.

Sternocleidomastoid: anterior and lateral muscle of the neck.

Stress reduction: activities that promote relaxation and the elimination of anxiety through specific relaxation techniques as well as the acquisition of knowledge and understanding about anxiety-producing issues.

Symphysis pubis: the bones of the pubic arch.

Synergistic: see Synergy.

Synergy: a concept that describes the healthy, interactive dependency and cooperation of functional systems; also used to describe cooperative functioning of muscles.

Target heart rate range: the zone between the maximum and minimum heart rate at which training will occur.

Tensor fascia latae: muscle that contributes to flexion of the thigh.

Teres major: muscle that works with the latissimus dorsi to adduct and inwardly rotate the arm.

Timing: A term from dance therapy that describes the individual's ability to coordinate effort and shape.

Tonic neck reflex: movement of the baby's limbs in response to the turning of its head.

Torso: the human trunk.

Traditional model: a model of health care and education that narrowly defines the roles and objectives of the health care provider and patient; occasionally referred to as the old paradigm or the biomedical model.

Traditional pushing: a breathing technique that requires a woman to hold her breath while she is bearing down to expel the baby.

Transverse abdominus: muscle that works with rectus and oblique muscles to hold the abdomen flat.

Trapezius: posterior muscle of the shoulder girdle.

Triceps: posterior muscle that causes extension of the arm.

Trimester: pregnancy is divided into three trimesters; each is 12 weeks, or 3 months, in length.

Toning section: the portion of an activity class that promotes muscle strengthening.

Vagina: the canal that leads from the uterus to the external orifice of the genital canal.

Valsalva's maneuver: holding one's breath during strenuous activity.

Vulva: external genitalia.

Warm-up: the section of the aerobic activity that promotes lubrication of the joints through the release of synovial fluid and increased circulation to the activated muscles.

Author Index

Subject Index

A

Abuse, 154
ACOG, iv, 13, 34–41, 66, 67, 68, 71, 74, 96, 116, 164, 171
ACSM, 47, 84
Activities to avoid in pregnancy, 57, 59
Aerobic capacity, 11, 23
Aerobic dance, 65–67
Aerobic exercise, 89
Aerobic options, 40
Aerobic prenatal class, 66–67
Aerobic training, 65
Afterbirth pains, 163
Amniotic fluid, 39, 96, 97
Anemia, 12, 39
Apgar scores, 22, 23
Appetite, 15
ARISE, 153
Attachment, 106, 177, 178
Autogenic training, 130

B

Baby exercises, 185, 196
Baby massage, 177
Baby safety, 185
Backache, 18, 94, 165
Balance
 function of body systems, 9–10
 level of fitness and, 164
 muscular, 52
 types of, 50
Barre work, 68
Belief systems, 137
Belly dancing, 173
Bicycling, 40, 84
Birth
 emergency procedures, for, 97
 fear of, 128

gestalt of, 129
harmony and, 3, 127
healthy, 128
imagery of, 137
impressions of, postpartum, 184, 195
as a perilous journey, 138
plan for, 92, 146–147, 150–151
positions for, 19, 91, 92, 119–122
shape of, 106
Bladder, 16
Bladder infection, 16, 17, 164
Bleeding during pregnancy, 61–62. *See also* Vagina
Blood pressure, defined, 12. *See also* Hypertension; Hypotension
Blood sugar, 19, 166. *See also* Diabetes
Blood volume, 12, 14
Bloody show, 61
Bonding. *See* Attachment
Body, experience of, 20
Body awareness, 4, 5, 116
 in infants, 191
Body boundaries, 47, 99–101, 106, 157
 in infants, 191
 postpartum, 183
Body comfort, 45
Body-ego, 101, 102
Body image, 97, 99–111, 145, 155, 157
Body landscape, 131
Body mapping, 103
Body-mind integration, 5, 6, 52, 73, 106–107, 113, 123, 148, 149
Body signals, 41, 164
Body systems, 9–23
Body wisdom, 9
Braxton Hicks contractions, 39, 61, 96
Breasts, 20, 21, 164
 infection of, 164
Breath-holding, 11, 38